THE MICROBIOME MASTER KEY

Also by B. Brett Finlay, PhD
with Marie-Claire Arrieta, PhD

Let Them Eat Dirt: How Microbes Can Make Your Child Healthier

THE MICROBIOME MASTER KEY

Unlock Your Health and Lifelong Vitality

B. BRETT FINLAY, PhD
AND JESSICA M. FINLAY, PhD

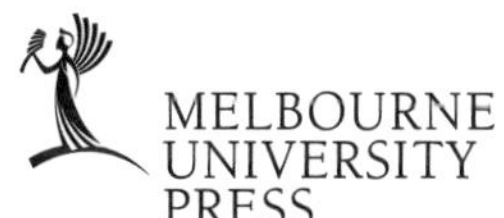

Melbourne University Publishing acknowledges the traditional owners of the unceded land on which we work, learn and live: the Wurundjeri Woiwurrung peoples of the Kulin Nation. We pay respect to elders and acknowledge the importance of Indigenous knowledge.

MELBOURNE UNIVERSITY PRESS
An imprint of Melbourne University Publishing Limited
Level 1, 715 Swanston Street, Carlton, Victoria 3053, Australia
mup-contact@unimelb.edu.au
www.mup.com.au

First published as *The Whole-Body Microbiome* by The Experiment, LLC

Cover design by Philip Campbell Design
Cover images courtesy iStock
Printed in Australia by McPherson's Printing Group

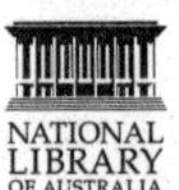

A catalogue record for this book is available from the National Library of Australia

9780522882186 (paperback)
9780522882193 (ebook)

To Jane and Matt

"Grow old along with me!
The best is yet to be . . ."

–Robert Browning

Contents

Preface

"But Dad, what do microbes do *after* the age of twelve—as in, for the rest of our lives? That's what I want to know!" During a family-vacation crack-of-dawn run along Hawaii's rugged coastline, we were distracting ourselves from the muggy heat by discussing *Let Them Eat Dirt*. The book, which Brett coauthored with Marie-Claire Arrieta, had just come out and presented a somewhat radical idea: that conceiving and raising children in a highly sanitized world is not as good as it sounds. Jessica, his daughter and fellow scientist, was fascinated by her dad's research and findings, but her mind, if not her pace, was already far ahead in the human lifespan, seeking answers for how she could apply microbial science to aging populations, her chosen demographic of research. Brett was used to this question and knew she was onto something—he had heard some variation of it many times before from colleagues, friends, and public audiences whenever he talked about the book. *I've already had my kids, and I am not getting any younger. What about me?*

Brett glanced back after pushing ahead of Jessica up a steep hill. He replied, "Well, we know that gut microbes are involved in asthma, obesity, cardiovascular diseases, and many other serious health issues. But what's really cool is how microbial communities are playing a role in aging in sites distant to the gut, across the entire body. Everything from wrinkles to Alzheimer's disease and systemic inflammation have microbial links." Between labored breaths and the occasional break to take in dramatic ocean views, our mental gears began to turn in sync.

For the rest of the vacation, when not boogie boarding and hiking (can you tell yet that we're slightly high energy?), Jessica peppered her dad for more information about microbes, health, disease, and microbial perspectives on aging. At the time, Brett already had age on his mind. Peering ahead at retirement, minute reminders of getting older that had previously remained under the surface now permeated his thoughts. Waking up to stiff muscles, he pondered: *How can I make sure that I'm still running and skiing with my kids–and hopefully grandkids–in my sixties, seventies, and eighties?* Jessica was already contemplating her own aging (even more so than the average thirty-year-old), in addition to the aging of those around her. With training and research in gerontology, she was the resident "aging expert" of our family. Her friends frequently asked for advice on how to preserve their skin and hair as they pointed worriedly to wrinkles and grays; and happy hour chatter strayed more often than ever before into discussions of ideal places to retire.

We first wrote this book about six years ago when the microbiome field was exploding. Every day, the news was filled with wonderment about some effect of the microbiome on health or disease. Fecal transfers were saving lives, and everyone wanted to know more about their microbiome. Since then, much has changed. Brett marked his sixty-fifth birthday; Jessica moved to Colorado and now has three lively, dirt-loving children; we lived through the biggest global pandemic since 1918; and the microbiome field is maturing scientifically.

We now know there are many concrete steps you can take, based on solid clinical trials, to harness microbes for the improvement of your health and well-being. Hence the need for this revised edition, which is full of life-changing findings that have come out over the past six years. We completely update the science and provide many more tangible tips and takeaways for health and longevity. The great thing about your microbiome is that, unlike your genes, you can change it! We point out where the current science is, and where the hype precedes the data (which is still prolific). Given new scientific breakthroughs, we have added two brand-new chapters–one on COVID-19 (did you know the microbiome affects COVID severity and your likeliness of contracting long COVID?) and another on sleep. We even discuss microbiome considerations in space travel!

The Microbiome Master Key is the accumulation of our shared interests in healthy aging and personal motivations to develop strategies to age better. As scientists and researchers, we wanted to see what was "out there" regarding scientific knowledge on aging and the microbiome. After compiling and distilling a massive literature review of existing studies, we extrapolated potential steps based on science that we all might take now for health and longevity, and we aim to encourage the future direction of research and clinical applications. Along the way, we encountered many questions and misconceptions about microbes and aging, which we highlight throughout the book.

Despite the title of "Dr." in front of our names, neither of us are physicians, but rather PhDs who are full-time scientific researchers. We are not geriatricians or clinical gerontologists: Jessica's expertise stems from years of studying and working closely with older adults in geographic and public health research, which is a perfect complement to Brett's expert biological knowledge of the human microbiome. The tips and suggestions throughout this book are therefore based directly upon academic research; there are no rigid or prescriptive medical recommendations. Expert interviews and key references will help you make informed diet, lifestyle, and personal health decisions.

This book approaches aging as a lifelong process. No one just wakes up one day and finds themselves suddenly old. Rather, we accumulate our health, both strengths and risks, over the entire life course. In our shared quest to have more control over aging, we hope this book offers fascinating new ways to harness the microbes living in and all around us. Long live you and your microbes!

Age is inevitable. Old is optional.

1

The Fountain of Youth Is Full of . . . Microbes?

From the moment we are born, we begin to die. Aging is a universal but uniquely personal experience. It scares us, bullies us, and motivates us to live better. Because we, as a species, are living longer and longer (more than eighty years nowadays in most high-income countries), every one of us has even more time than ever before to grapple with aging and mortality.

Despite what advertisements and doctors may tell us, there is no way to simply "turn back the clock," but we still try to delay the inevitable. We all search for ways to prolong our lives and preserve our bodies–these complex machines made of muscle, bone, and a host of other tissues, our minds, our hearing and eyesight, even our looks. The mythical Fountain of Youth is a spring that allegedly restores the youth of anyone who drinks or bathes in its waters. Since the fifth century BCE, tales of such a fountain have been recounted across the world. Today is no exception–we continue the age-old quest to preserve and restore youth, but instead of seeking the hidden location of the elixir of life, our goal is to conquer it through science. Pharmacy, grocery store, and cosmetic aisles are stocked with anti-aging products, ranging from serums and creams to fight wrinkles and banish spots, to vitamins and supplements promising an elusive "youthful glow."

Scientific studies suggest myriad ways to intervene in the aging process, including antioxidants (to limit the number of free radicals, which cause age-related damage at cellular and tissue levels), calorie restriction (which extends lifespan and minimizes age-related chronic diseases in various species including rats, mice, fish, flies, worms, and yeast), hormone supplements to treat menopausal symptoms, and a host of dermatological procedures and treatments including retinoids, chemical peels, dermabrasion, ultrasound imaging, laser resurfacing, and cosmetic surgery. While many of these methods have been touted as glamorous and high-tech, one of the most exciting frontiers of current aging science involves the oldest life forms on Earth: microbes.

Contrary to the cutting-edge scientific inventions we're using to make alternative time-reversers, these bacteria have been around for more than 3.5 billion years, from a time when our planet was covered in oceans that regularly reached boiling point. Our climate has changed dramatically, but microbes are still everywhere: in the air you breathe (they actually made the original oxygen in the atmosphere), on the chair you sit in, and in the food in your fridge. In fact, there are more microbes in a gram of feces than there are people on the entire planet!

Microbes are our constant companions throughout life. Commonly known as germs, they come in many forms, including bacteria, viruses, protozoa, algae, and fungi. While we often blame them for disease (e.g., "I've got a stomach bug"), we have only recently realized they are in fact absolutely essential for a healthy life. We could not exist without them. But what do microbes have to do with aging? Everything, actually.

We have distinct microbial communities throughout our entire bodies–not just in the gut. These communities affect how our brain, teeth, skin, heart, gut, bones, immune system, and nearly every other body part functions as we progress through life. Well-being is also intimately tied to the microbes that surround us–on our cell phones, kitchen sponges, houseplants, pets, and desks. If you move to a new home or travel abroad, you are exposed to new microbial communities that can disrupt your body's existing microflora (your entire microbial collective), for better or for worse. Your zip code is one of the best predictors of health and longevity, which is underscored by billions of invisible neighbors: microbes. Knowing that there is a continuum between you and the outside world, not a brick wall that ends at your skin, can help you stay healthier over time even if your zip code, and age, changes.

You can harness the microbes in and around you to help keep your gums healthier, bones and muscles stronger, and possibly even protect your brain from Alzheimer's disease and dementia. Of the top ten causes of death in the United States and Australia, we now realize microbes can play an integral role in all but one.

THE LEADING CAUSES OF DEATH IN THE UNITED STATES AND THEIR MICROBIAL INVOLVEMENT

Asterisks (*) denote the authors' evaluation of the strength of microbial involvement. Accidents, Nephritis and Chronic liver disease are not in the leading causes of death in Australia.

Heart disease: 702,880 ***
Cancer: 608,371 **
Accidents (unintentional injuries): 227,039
COVID-19: 186,552 **
Stroke (cerebrovascular diseases): 165,393 **
Chronic lower respiratory diseases: 147,382 **
Alzheimer's disease: 120,122 ***
Diabetes: 101,209 ***
Nephritis, nephrotic syndrome, and nephrosis: 57,937 **
Chronic liver disease and cirrhosis: 54,803 **

Data for 2022 obtained from the Centers for Disease Control (2024).

In this book, we will explore and untangle these connections between disease and our bodies' microbes to broaden your understanding of their impact on aging and mortality. Moving through the body, we illustrate how the invisible world of microbes around and inside all of us is nourishing and essential to a healthy and long life. We think through improvements to lifestyle, diet, and household practices to promote the right kind of microbial exposure. For example, instead of homes and care environments that are as sterile as possible, we envision places that are comfortable living spaces for us *and* our microbial roommates. Age-friendly environments need to foster the health and well-being of all inhabitants—microbes included.

Growing Old with Your Microbes

Aging is a natural process that occurs in all biological species, though for some it happens faster than for others. Biologically, we humans hit our prime at around age twelve. In other words, if your physiology (meaning your body and its functionality) remained at that age, you would live more than one thousand years! After twelve, the chance of dying doubles every eight years.

And yet our species somehow beat these odds with increasing success. We spoke to Dr. Anne Martin-Matthews, Professor Emerita of Sociology at the University of British Columbia and former Scientific Director for the Institute of Aging established by the Canadian Institutes of Health Research. She commented on our current staggering, and unprecedented, aging population: "Over the forty years of my career studying aging, we never anticipated how the field would be shaped by the extended longevity of the population. As recently as a decade or so ago, much of our research focused on 'older people' in their seventies and the 'oldest old' in their eighties. Now we all personally know a seventy-three-year-old with a ninety-five-year-old mother, or an eighty-two-year-old woman concerned about her elderly husband and with a 105-year-old parent still alive!"

The advent of vaccinations, antibiotics, and improved sanitation beginning in the early 1900s dramatically reduced the number of childhood deaths, as well as deaths due to infectious diseases. This resulted in a major increase in longevity worldwide: Life expectancy increased from thirty-two years in 1900 to seventy-one years in 2021, with Japan's average currently coming in highest at eighty-four! Dr. Martin-Matthews noted that the number of centenarians (people older than 100) continues to increase worldwide, along with more supercentenarians (those older than 110). This is one of the most significant social transformations of the twenty-first century.

While virtually every country in the world has growing numbers of older people, chronic ailments such as obesity, type 2 diabetes, asthma, and inflammatory bowel diseases are also rapidly on the rise worldwide. Far from being limited to high-income regions of the world, chronic diseases are accelerating in developing countries. The number of people in low- and middle-income countries with diabetes, for example, will increase by more than 2.5-fold: from 84 million in 1995 to more than 228 million in 2025. The World Health Organization (WHO) estimates that the global burden of chronic disease has risen to 74 percent in 2024, up from approximately 46 percent in 2001. Almost three quarters of all deaths in 2024 are attributable to chronic diseases.

These conditions plague many individuals' health and reduce quality of later life. In terms of incidence (i.e., the number of people affected), cardiovascular disease and brain diseases such as Alzheimer's, Parkinson's, and dementia are on a dramatic upward trajectory in our society. But despite more than twenty years of intense research, Dr. Martin-Matthews reflected there is still no "silver bullet" to address Alzheimer's disease and related dementias: "Research has primarily focused on the brain and its structural changes. Yet the reality is that we have not been able to find effective prevention or treatment measures. Multiple billions of dollars of research investment later, we're coming to understand that the issue is much more complex. We clearly need to look elsewhere. Perhaps the microbiome plays a role–maybe to solve problems in the brain we need to look at the gut and other areas of the body where microbes are involved." Dr. Martin-Matthews admits she is no microbe expert–in fact, she confessed at the beginning of our interview that she is quite the opposite.

And yet, as a sociologist and social scientist she is clued-in to possible microbial interactions. Microbes affecting our brains, as well as other distinct bodily and environmental sites, are ripe for investigation given that they offer immense potential to better understand aging. Researchers with the openness of Dr. Martin-Matthews have already drawn remarkable connections between the microbiome and conditions such as obesity, type 2 diabetes, asthma, and inflammatory bowel diseases, in one way or another. They have also found links to many other normal physiological changes associated with aging, such as loss of bone and muscle mass and skin wrinkling. This research involves microbial effects well beyond the stronghold of our gut in important body sites such as the brain, heart, and bones, as well as critical human environments, including hospitals and nursing homes. By better understanding our everyday environmental microbes, we believe we may be able to strategically manipulate them so that we can live healthier and longer lives.

In Sickness and in Health: Microbes, Our Lifelong Partners

We are inhabited by more microbes in and on our body than we can imagine: There are at least as many bacterial cells in the body as human cells. They surround and cover us. There are layers of microbes between every body surface and the environment, not only between your skin and the pages of this book, but also between the air you breathe and your lung cells. Normally we all coexist peacefully, but our microbial interface is heavily influenced by changes in our environment. Every moment has the potential to radically alter the landscape of our microbiome–and thus impact health.

Microbes are especially important at the bookends of life: the first few years of childhood and the last years of adulthood. Cohabitation with microbes begins with our journey through the birth canal, when we consume mouthfuls of bacteria. We then get a regular dose of microbes from our mothers by drinking breast milk and being held skin-to-skin. This critical microbial bolus (i.e., dose) jumpstarts our immune system and impacts brain development as we set off on our lifelong relationships with microbes. As a result, by the time we reach adulthood, there are well over five hundred distinct species living at any one moment in our intestines. The microbiome is fully formed by the age of two to three.

Microbes help break down food in the digestive tract and harness energy and nutrients. They keep our immune system functioning and help protect against pathogens that we constantly come into contact with. They even help our brains develop. As we age, however, the role of microbes changes. People over the age of seventy have radically altered microbial communities from when they were younger. The composition of microbiota (microorganisms in a particular environment) also shifts, which may detrimentally affect older people. For example, as we will see later, age causes an increase in inflammatory microbes, and a decrease in helpful microbes that dampen the immune system. Collectively, this results in an increase in low-grade inflammation throughout the body causing tissue damage, a process called "inflammaging." These changes can lead to greater susceptibility to diseases and a general decline in health. Knowing that microbes are at the heart of general body decline is a great discovery for science–and for all of us–and highlights the critical need to maintain and enhance our microbes as we age.

It is estimated that longevity is 25 percent genetic and 75 percent environmental. This is a profound statement: It means that we have the ability to control the majority of elements that affect our health and lifespans. Just because your parent had cancer doesn't mean that your fate is sealed—although you may have genes that increase your likelihood of getting it. Your future is affected much more by your environmental exposures. We now realize that when we talk about the "environment" as being that which is in closest contact with our body, we include microbes.

It is natural for our microbiome to decline as we age, but this process has undergone a radical shift because we've turned our environment into a battleground for our modern crusade against "germs." Our common understanding that some bacteria and viruses make us sick and should be avoided is very true. These are the notorious germs we continually battle—pneumonia and flus, and now COVID-19. But we've taken that truth to an extreme that is causing us to suffer dire consequences, speeding up and exacerbating the annihilation of key microbes we likely need for longevity.

As far back as the nineteenth century, pioneering microbiologists focused on chasing the microorganisms that caused infectious diseases, including cholera, tuberculosis, and diarrhea. Scientists discovered that "germs" caused rabies, anthrax, and other infectious diseases, so the hunt for disease-causing microbes escalated. Then everything changed around the middle of the twentieth century. We developed antibiotics to rid ourselves of some disease causing infections. While these wonder drugs have saved millions of lives, they have also led to our modus operandi to kill microbes—all of them—rather than try to learn more about them and live in harmony, as we had for most of history. Other inventions, such as hand sanitizer, antimicrobial mouthwashes, and household antibacterial cleaning solutions became everyday products. "If clean is good, then cleaner must be better!" we shouted from every rooftop, billboard, TV commercial, and transit station. COVID-19 further heightened our anxiety about cleanliness and germs. High on our own scientific mastery over these tiny bugs, we didn't realize that we were sending ourselves toward current disease epidemics.

A glance around our society today reveals a completely different set of diseases than those of a hundred years ago, when infections were a major killer. Obesity, diabetes, inflammatory bowel disease, allergies, and asthma are but a few examples of conditions we now realize are partly collateral damage from our war on microbes. This is because antibiotics do not just kill off the "bad" microbes, they wipe out the "good" ones, too. This is why using antibiotics can cause diarrhea, an upset stomach, and even urinary tract infections. Taking these powerful drugs will kill off the agent of disease, but they will also leave our body vulnerable in other ways by eliminating the good microbes that normally help protect us. We call it the "hygiene hangover," or the head-splitting price we pay for our century-long bender of antimicrobial precautions.

Furthermore, our highly sanitized world remarkably reduces the overall number of microbes that we are exposed to. Every generation has fewer types of microbes in and on their bodies than the previous one. More and more of us spend our days inside sanitized and climate-controlled buildings. Our bodies' ability to work as they were designed to, in the presence of abundant and diverse microbes, is being compromised as a result, jeopardizing a key part of continued human evolution, let alone personal health.

We evolved over millions of years with these invisible partners, and yet within two to three generations, many of them could be on their way to extinction.

The Book of Microbes: Exploring Uncharted Territory

What to expect when you're expecting to grow old? While there is an entire industry devoted to preparing expectant parents, scant resources guide us on how to grow old. Every day, more and more young adults, professionals, Baby Boomers, and family members with aging loved ones actively seek out advice and information. We mainly turn to online resources or other sources of oft-outdated science on aging. The supply of legitimate and scientifically based resources indeed remains scarce–and is a key reason why we're writing this book. What we present here is not an exhaustively full or definitively complete picture of the specific role of microbes in aging; instead, our goal is to provide a starting point for everyone who appreciates the fact that well-being is a lifelong process and wants to improve their health as they age. We aim to provide practical actions that one can take based on sound science.

In each chapter, we explore the fascinating and invisible world of microbes and its effects in each major system or organ of the body, and we present the current scientific understanding of how the systems' microbes might affect aging. We also offer lifestyle strategies and "Key Tips" that we can all take advantage of, whether we're eighteen or eighty, to grow old as healthfully and gracefully as possible. Leading medical professionals and scientific researchers lend their voices throughout to deepen our grasp of how knowledge of the microbiome is influencing their respective fields. Most are not microbiology experts–rather, they represent medical doctors, dentists, biomedical researchers, public health experts, and social scientists all grappling with their own well-being in addition to their work.

Both of us are scientists, and all the material presented in this book is based on the current scientific literature. Each chapter is founded on select scientific papers that helped shape our knowledge. These are not exhaustive–though we read over one hundred papers for each chapter–but the papers and reviews highlight major concepts in the chapters. If you are interested in looking further at the current scientific literature, we encourage you to use the PubMed website (ncbi.nlm.nih.gov/pubmed), which offers search options for biomedical literature and provides abstracts of peer-reviewed articles and reviews. Some articles are open to the public, while other journals charge for access to the full article, although libraries can usually get you access to the full articles for free.

We will cover several key concepts in this book. First, we will share exciting new data coming out in microbiology that will rewrite many chapters of modern medicine. However, the field is still extremely new–barely two decades old–which means that there are more questions than answers, especially when it comes to direct applications. And as with any new scientific field, the data can be full of conflicting findings and rather confusing results, making it harder to parse. This is especially true of microbiology because of the microbial differences found between individuals. However, there are also common themes that are emerging from all these studies that we highlight, such as beneficial health effects from having diverse gut flora, and how the microbiome influences inflammation at various body sites. Our goal is to synthesize this overwhelmingly large body of information and condense it into a digestible (pun intended) format that will be of use in your daily life.

Second, we focus our attention on the microbiome's effects on healthy aging–a perspective that has not as of yet been covered in popular literature. We believe this is a critical gap as there are many concepts in this book that can help you age with relatively good health by understanding the microbiome. At first, you might think this means only individuals who are over, say, the age of sixty-five. However, healthy aging spans one's entire life. What you do during your twenties can have effects decades later. Remember that ankle you sprained at twenty-two playing basketball, which is now giving you a hard time at seventy? This book is written for people of all ages who care about their long-term health.

Third, as we discussed above, there are microbes all over, inside, and around our bodies. Nearly all the attention so far has been on gut microbes. There is no doubt that they play a major role in all sorts of body functions. However, we are now beginning to realize that the microbes in different sites of the body also contribute in individually fascinating ways and play a large role in health, disease, and aging. Large microbial communities live happily in the mouth and oral cavity, the skin, and the urogenital tract–and, like the gut microbes, they busily make chemicals and do other things that can affect our body's functions. A recent study, for example, found that the microbiome contributed to over a third of the differences in people's high-density lipoprotein (HDL) cholesterol levels, and a quarter of the variation in body mass index (BMI). We can apply this knowledge toward developing effective personalized diets based on a person's unique microbe makeup.

Throughout the book we cover many areas of the body to better understand aging processes and consider specific lifestyle and nutrition interventions to enhance healthy microbiomes. There is some slight overlap between chapters when there are clear interactions among body sites, such as the gut microbiome's effects on the brain. We even discuss the microbes surrounding our bodies, such as those in your home or on your cell phone, which also immensely impact our own microbiomes. North Americans and Australians, on average, spend up to 90 percent of their time indoors. Cleaning and hygiene standards in private and institutional settings—especially hospitals and nursing homes—tend to promote multi-resistant pathogens instead of supporting diverse beneficial microbes. In the absence of contact with these key microbes, some dynamic microbial lineages have decreased in prevalence and abundance in today's humans. We want to stress the importance of all the body's microbiomes on healthy aging, not just the gut microbes we hear about every day.

By reading this book, you are about to embark on an exciting journey into a brand-new universe of human health and disease. The microbiome has been called the "newest discovered organ" and its many functions are only now being uncovered. It is our hope—and the hope of all the scientists working in this area—that we can use microbiome science to alter that top ten mortality list, or at least decrease the numbers of people with those diseases.

We guarantee you won't see the world the same way after you finish this book. You may pause and consider before shopping for groceries, eating lunch, brushing your teeth, sending a text message, washing your hands, or scrubbing the dirt off a freshly plucked carrot. We hope the journey is as fun and enlightening for you as it has been for us, and that we will all benefit from embracing microbes as long-life partners.

2

Microbe Mecca: The Gut Microbiome

Let's dive in and take a look at all the microbes we have in and on our bodies. While we have distinct microbiomes on various body parts (such as in our mouths and on our skin), by far the most numerous are those in the gut. When we talk about "the microbiome," we often refer specifically to the gut microbiome. The gut is the mecca of microbes–where they break down food, produce metabolites (by-products of metabolism) that enter the body's circulation to affect distant organs, interface with the immune system, and even "talk" to our brains. For all these reasons, we will start with the gut microbiome and then turn to other microbiomes in the body that also play a significant and underappreciated role in health and aging.

"Ridiculously healthy" elderly have the same gut microbiome as healthy 30-year-olds. This 2017 headline originating from the University of Western Ontario immediately drew our attention to research headed by Dr. Greg Gloor, principal investigator of a large human microbiota study. The study involved over one thousand "very healthy" Chinese people aged three to over one hundred. What researchers found is that the gut microbiota in the healthy older participants were similar to microbes found in healthy individuals decades younger. When kept in good health, it seemed the gut microbiome could remain robust for over a century. Is this a potential fountain of youth?

The gut microbes of our elders are full of clues in our search for lifelong health and vitality. We can look to the microbiomes of older adults (generally aged sixty-five and older), including centenarians and even semi-supercentenarians (over 105 years old). After the advent of large-scale microbiome DNA sequencing a decade ago, a series of studies suggested that the diversity of the gut microbiome in older people was diminished. Instead of health-promoting bacteria, scientists observed an increase in Proteobacteria, which are sometimes called "pathobionts" because of their ability to trigger inflammation. Prolonged low-grade inflammation (inflammaging) is strongly associated with the aging process—so this finding made sense. Scientists suggested that increased inflammation is partly caused by increased oxygen production, which, through reactive oxygen that accompanies inflammation, boosts the number of bacteria—known as aerobic bacteria or facultative anaerobes depending on how much they need or can tolerate such oxygen—including harmful Proteobacteria. As a result, some beneficial microbes that cannot tolerate oxygen (anaerobes) are killed by the oxygen. In our review of many studies conducted since then, we found that older adult populations do tend to have rather dysbiotic (imbalanced) microbiomes with a decrease in overall diversity. There is a distinct microbial signature among those older than sixty-five that includes marked decreases in beneficial microbes and increases in more harmful (inflammatory) bacteria.

In the incredibly old, however, this rule doesn't seem to hold, as diversity increases again. Centenarians' microbiomes, like those of younger populations, are dominated by a beneficial balance of Firmicutes and Bacteroidetes. These represent the two most predominant groups of bacteria in the gut, and while not perfect, the Firmicutes/Bacteroidetes (F/B) ratio is often used as a general measure of the gut microbiome's health. A balance between them is associated with good health, whereas an imbalance may indicate the opposite. For example, an increase in the F/B ratio is associated with obesity, and a decrease is associated with inflammatory bowel disease (IBD). Because semi-supercentenarians are quite rare as a population, it's harder to gather data about them. But from the data we've been able to gather, these individuals, too, have an increase in numerous beneficial microbes (*Akkermansia*, *Bifidobacterium*, and *Christensenellaceae*). We now see that the gut microbiome does not follow linear changes with age: The assumed "downward spiral" is actually a more complicated trajectory after the seventh decade of life. Since many people now live well beyond sixty-five years, there are ever-more opportunities to see why these changes occur in later life and to understand how we can nourish our microbes well before old age to help promote health and longevity.

Gut 101

While people often think of the gut as only the intestines, the gastrointestinal (GI) tract is in fact a long tube that runs through us from the mouth to the anus. It is divided into various sections including the stomach, small intestine, and large intestine. Although this bodily throughway is internal, the contents of the intestine are not technically inside us. Like the skin, a more obvious barrier between our insides and the external world, the lining of the gut serves as an external surface of the body–it simply runs through the middle rather than coating the outside. Also like the skin, the gut is an important permeable gateway between us and the world, including microbes.

Think of the gut microbiome as an ecosystem: Many different microbes live together harmoniously, most of the time, and can directly and indirectly influence each other. This ecosystem is characterized by a decrease in oxygen the deeper the descent down the intestinal tract (there is virtually no oxygen in the large intestine). Anaerobes are the predominant bacteria, especially in the colon (large intestine) where they make up 99 percent of the bacteria. Microbes that can tolerate some oxygen (facultative anaerobes) are found in larger numbers higher up the intestine. As in all robust ecosystems, the large diversity of microbial species in the gut is essential.

We can see how different parts of the GI tract have distinct environments, and correspondingly different microbes. As we will see, the stomach itself (close to the top of the GI tract and very acidic, with a fair bit of oxygen which is swallowed with food) contains very few microbes (about 10^3 to 10^4 bacteria/g). Next up (actually, down) is the small intestine, which has less oxygen and is more basic in pH. It is divided into three parts: the duodenum, jejunum, and ileum. The duodenum has about 10^4 to 10^5 microbes/g the jejunum about 10^5 to 10^6, and the ileum 10^8 to 10^9. Finally, we reach the finishing area, where we find the largest numbers of bacteria in–and on–the entire body; about ten trillion (10^{13}) in the lower bowel, better known as the large intestine. It is depleted of oxygen and has a basic pH. This remarkable concentration of microbes at the end of our digestive process explains why microbes make up about 30 percent of fecal matter. There are one hundred billion microbes in a single gram of feces—over ten times the entire population of humans on this planet. These microscopic gut microbes collectively weigh as much as two to five pounds. Given these staggering numbers of gut microbiota and their many functions, some scientists consider the microbiome the "newest discovered organ." How do we build up trillions of microbes in the intestinal tract?

The moment you are born, you receive your first and very best birthday present: a big dose of vaginal and fecal microbes. Although this isn't something you'd put on your birthday wish list any other time in life, these microbes are an essential part of health in early life as they kickstart your intestinal microbes and all their essential duties. See *Let Them Eat Dirt* by Brett and Dr. Marie-Claire Arrieta (or the video documentary online by the same name) if you are interested in the role of microbes in early life and how it affects child health and disease. Most new parents know how important a healthy digestive system is to their baby's well-being—and have likely seen firsthand what a "healthy" intestinal microbiome looks like. Remember diaper duty when you introduced solid food into your child's diet? This dietary change causes a major remodeling of the intestinal microbiome.

In the first years of life, we're exposed to many kinds of bacteria that can inhabit our gut microbiome. By adulthood, we harbor a multitude of diverse microbes, including bacteria, viruses, fungi (yeast), and protozoa. The microbial composition remains fairly constant for most of adult life unless you do something drastic, like become vegan or move to another country—more on that later. But our gut ecosystem isn't immune to change, and disturbances can have major influences on microbial composition similar to those in early years, when we first ate solid food. Antibiotics, for example, can decimate our microbiome like a nuclear bomb because they are not species-specific. They don't just attack the bacteria making us sick but many harmless resident bacteria as well. And like our nuclear analogy, the fallout effects are long-lasting: Recent research shows that the effects of a course of antibiotics on the microbiome can be seen at least a year after taking antibiotics. Some reports suggest that microbial changes up to four years later are apparent.

THE DOUBLE-EDGED SWORD OF ANTIBIOTICS

It is important to avoid the overuse and misuse of antibiotics for personal and societal health. Antibiotics treat infections caused by bacteria, not those caused by viruses (such as the flu, some ear and sinus infections, and COVID-19). Talk to your health care provider if they prescribe antibiotics to understand if and why it is necessary. The problem with antibiotics is that they don't just kill the pathogen causing the infection, they significantly alter your microbiome. Repeated courses of antibiotics seem to irreparably shift the microbiome, with detrimental effects. However, while it might be tempting to stop taking an antibiotic as soon as you feel better, it's important to take the full course to avoid contributing to antibiotic resistance.

The Gut's Microbial Village

Why is it important to protect the village of microbes in our gut? For starters, without them we'd have a hard time simply surviving, since gut microbiota play a huge role in breaking down food. The majority of the food we eat cannot be broken down without microbes. This is especially true of complex plant fibers–the polysaccharides found in grains, legumes, vegetables, fruits, and other plant foods–which are converted into short-chain fatty acids (SCFAs), which serve both as an energy source for intestinal cells and important signaling molecules. The beneficial effects of SCFAs produced by microbes are many. They help to decrease obesity and insulin resistance, shore up the gut barrier, serve as energy sources for other microbes, reduce inflammation, and send signals to our body to enhance immune response. Diet is a good way to boost your SCFA production. High-fiber diets with low amounts of fat and minimal meat are associated with much higher levels of SCFAs and other beneficial microbes. And not surprisingly, they are associated with increased overall health and longevity (see the MIND diet in chapter 4).

Another important role of gut microbes is competitive exclusion, or the outcompeting of pathogens. Research in Brett's and others' labs have shown that normal microbiota can be quite effective at preventing intestinal infections caused by *Salmonella* and pathogenic *E. coli*. In animal models, fecal transfers (which swap gut contents, including microbes, between hosts)–teeming with microbes of animals resistant to infections–into susceptible animals can enhance their resistance to infections. Some microbiota species even produce molecules that inhibit the virulence mechanisms of *Salmonella* and *E. coli* (i.e., diarrhea), thereby decreasing their ability to cause disease. Perhaps these resident microbes block diarrhea in order to prevent themselves from reaching the proverbial light at the end of the tunnel–thereby saving themselves.

Protecting the diversity and density of the microbes themselves is key to gut health, but there's another layer equally important to balanced digestion: the gut's thick mucus lining, which helps keep microbes inside our intestines where they belong. Mucus is composed of glycoproteins–a combination of complex sugars (carbohydrates) linked to proteins–that coat the intestinal wall. This lubricates it as well as provides a barrier between intestinal cells and the microbiome. By contrast, the mucus layer in the small intestine is thin, perhaps because there aren't as many microbes. The mucus lining has two layers in the large intestine: a very tight one nestled against the intestinal epithelial cells–the cells that make up the intestinal wall and form the intestinal barrier–forming a barrier to microbes, and a looser outer mucus layer that is embedded with microbes.

Some of these microbes are able to break down mucus and use it as a food source. *Akkermansia muciniphila* is one such microbe and is thought to be beneficial in preventing intestinal diseases that are associated with thinning of the mucus layer. By eating the mucus, this microbe triggers a feedback loop that actually increases mucus production and thickens the mucus layer, which promotes overall gut health. When the mucus barrier is thinner, intestinal permeability increases. More microbes are able to penetrate the gut barrier, resulting in intestinal inflammation and dysbiosis (the scientific term for a microbial imbalance consisting of less diverse and different microbes) that can also trigger increased tissue damage and, potentially, disease. As we will cover later in this chapter, many gastrointestinal diseases are associated with thinner mucus layers.

Your Body's Built-In Detox

In our journey through the body's microbiomes, we will see how intricately connected these discrete bacterial communities all are. The gut microbiome is no different, and because of its robust size of one hundred trillion bacteria, it influences–and can even improve–health conditions in sites quite distant from it.

Adjacent to the GI tract itself are two important organs that do their own kind of digestion, the liver and kidneys, which are heavily impacted by gut bacteria. The liver filters blood coming from the digestive tract before passing it to the rest of the body, metabolizes drugs, detoxifies chemicals, plays a role in fat metabolism, and produces proteins important to blood clotting. Healthy kidneys filter about half a cup (120 ml) of blood every minute, thereby removing wastes and extra fluids to produce urine. If either of these hardworking organs cannot function properly, it can wreak havoc on our bodies.

DRINK TO YOUR HEALTH–THE SKINNY ON RED WINE

Alcoholic liver disease (which encompasses fatty liver, alcoholic hepatitis, and chronic hepatitis with liver fibrosis or cirrhosis) is caused by chronic excessive consumption of alcohol. The risk for disease increases the longer one drinks and the more alcohol one consumes. While drinking alcohol in excess is unhealthy, moderate consumption of red wine has been associated with health benefits, including protection from cardiovascular disease and type 2 diabetes. Red wine is a component of the Mediterranean and MIND diets, which both lessen the risk of neurological diseases such as dementia (see chapter 4).

The major beneficial components in red wine are thought to be polyphenols, which are strong antioxidants that protect the body from reactive oxygen damage, found in the skin and seeds of grapes incorporated into the finished wine. White wines have fewer polyphenols than red wines: With one glass of white wine (120 ml, approximately 4 ounces), you would ingest about 30 mg of polyphenols, while a (recommended) glass of red wine would deliver about 210 mg.

It turns out polyphenols also have a beneficial effect on gut microbes, as about 90 to 95 percent of the polyphenols are metabolized in the colon. When patients with metabolic syndrome–a disease associated with obesity and diabetes–consumed one 272 ml (roughly 9-ounce) serving of red wine daily for thirty days, they saw large increases in the beneficial microbes Bifidobacteria and lactobacilli that decrease intestinal permeability. There were also increases in beneficial *Faecalibacterium prausnitzii*, which produce butyrate, an SCFA, and a decrease in the inflammatory Proteobacteria. Several other studies indicate similar beneficial changes in the gut microbiome associated with red wine consumption. In addition, it is thought that the microbial breakdown of polyphenols by gut microbes results in the production of beneficial metabolites, which positively affects human health. One more reason to raise a glass of red to your health!

Liver diseases are a broad category of conditions that damage the liver and prevent it from functioning well. The most common conditions include cirrhosis (chronic liver damage from a variety of causes, including alcohol consumption, that lead to scarring and liver failure); hepatitis A, B, and C (serious viral infections that attack the liver and lead to inflammation); hemochromatosis (an inherited condition caused by excessive iron absorption); and non-alcoholic fatty liver disease (the accumulation of liver fat in people who drink little or no alcohol). All types of liver diseases are associated with microbial dysbiosis, increased intestinal permeability–which, as discussed earlier, leads to an increase in the leakage of harmful inflammatory bacterial products into the body–and accompanying chronic inflammation.

Non-alcoholic fatty liver disease (NAFLD) is a catch-all for the spectrum of liver diseases including steatosis, non-alcoholic steatohepatitis (NASH), hepatocellular carcinoma, fibrosis, and ultimately cirrhosis (scarring of the liver) associated with liver failure. NAFLD is the most common type of chronic liver disease, affecting 32 percent of the adult population worldwide. The cause of NAFLD is unknown, but risk factors include obesity, gastric bypass surgery, high cholesterol, and type 2 diabetes. No standard treatment exists, so doctors usually try to treat the underlying condition(s) instead. Improvements have been shown from lifestyle changes such as increased exercise, weight loss, lowering cholesterol and triglycerides, controlling diabetes, and avoiding alcohol.

NAFLD patients have increased intestinal permeability and chronic inflammation. Because the liver clears the blood of potentially toxic compounds, it is thought that increased gut permeability exposes the liver to high levels of bacterial antigens such as lipopolysaccharide (LPS; a molecule found in the cell walls of Gram-negative bacteria) that trigger extensive chronic inflammation and resulting tissue damage. NAFLD patients have a dysbiotic microbial composition, an increase in Firmicutes and decrease in Bacteroidetes.

We may be able to use these marked differences in gut microbiome to better detect NAFLD, which typically is not identified until the disease is well advanced. Even then, diagnosis requires an invasive liver biopsy. Researchers at the University of California San Diego reported that in a small clinical trial the unique microbial makeup of a patient's stool sample (which is typically thought of as a "snapshot" of their gut microbiome) can be used to predict advanced NAFLD with 88 to 94 percent accuracy. The team found that more Proteobacteria and fewer Firmicutes were in stool samples from patients with advanced NAFLD than those with early-stage NAFLD. At the species level, a key difference was in the abundance of *E. coli*, a bacterium that has LPS in its membrane and can trigger inflammation: These bacteria were three times more common in advanced NAFLD patients than those in the early stage. Determining exactly who is at risk or has the disease is critically necessary for prevention and treatment. Stool-based tests may be key to detecting NAFLD simply based on microbial patterns.

FOODS THAT FIGHT NAFLD

A diet rich in fruits, vegetables, whole grains, and healthy fats can boost your microbes and reduce risk of NAFLD. Both green tea and coffee inhibit NAFLD progression, which may work through the microbiota. Experts also recommend limiting or avoiding alcohol and sugary drinks and maintaining a healthy weight.

As discussed previously, kidneys are essential to remove wastes and extra fluid from the body. They remove acid and maintain the balance of water, salts, and minerals, filtering our blood. Nerves, muscles, and other tissues cannot function normally if the kidneys are not able to maintain this essential balance. Chronic kidney disease (CKD) affects between 5 and

10 percent of the world's population, accounting for up to a million deaths worldwide per year. It is a nonspecific disease characterized by the slow deterioration of the kidneys over months to years. As the kidneys deteriorate and even fail, waste builds up in the circulation and tissues. Late stages of the disease, such as renal failure, often require a kidney transplant or dialysis, which warrants a machine to filter excess water, solutes, and toxins from the blood—the function healthy kidneys would normally perform.

Like so many of the chronic inflammatory diseases discussed in this book, CKD also appears to have a significant microbial contribution. Its progression is directly related to microbial composition and is correlated with high blood pressure, diabetes, and cardiovascular disease. The microbial effects are also similar to other conditions: marked dysbiosis in the gut microbiota, including fewer SCFA-producing bacteria (which dampen inflammation), accompanied by an increase in gut permeability. This results in substances produced by bacteria such as endotoxins (also known as LPS) entering the bloodstream, increasing the body's inflammatory responses and damaging the kidneys. Several studies suggest that repairing gut dysbiosis may improve CKD, including by following high-fiber diets; the use of some probiotics improved blood markers associated with CKD.

PAIN AND PANIC: KIDNEY STONES

Childbirth, a burst eardrum, kidney stones, a broken femur. Jessica once heard that these are the four most acutely painful events one can experience. She had the misfortune of experiencing all of these but a broken femur in one year. Then, during the writing of this book, Jessica awoke to an all-too-familiar sharp stabbing pain in the side of her lower back. Episodes of pain started to come and go, thankfully managed at home through pain relievers and a heating pad. Until they weren't—eyes widened as a vomiting, tearful, thirty-two-weeks pregnant Jessica hobbled into the emergency room at 3 AM. Jessica and her partner were rushed upstairs to the labor and delivery ward (even though she assured them it was not early labor), where she tried to pass a kidney stone with limited baby-safe medical options. Jessica endured multiple days of excruciating breakthrough pain while the baby bounced around excitedly and happily on the monitors. About a week later, she was completely shocked to pass a nearly quarter-inch (6 mm) stone!

Kidney stones are small, hard formations caused by minerals and acid salts (often calcium phosphate and calcium oxalate, sometimes uric acid) that stick together in concentrated urine in the kidneys. Up to 12 percent of Americans and about 10 percent of Australians are affected by kidney stones in their lifetimes. Once you've had one (which you will never forget), you're 50 percent more likely to get another within the next ten years. The stone-causing chemicals originate in our diets. It is thought that when microbes such as *Oxalobacter* and *Lactobacillus*, which normally break down oxalate salts, are in lower quantities, stones are more likely to form. A small study of twenty-three individuals with kidney stones and six controls found that those with stones had a markedly different gut microbiome. Those with kidney stones had higher Bacteroides and the controls had higher *Prevotella*. Focusing specifically on *Oxalobacter formigenes*, another study of 247 patients with kidney stones and 259 controls found a strong inverse correlation with kidney stones and this bacterium. In other words: People lacking this microbe had a much higher risk of kidney stones. In another study, three people were fed this bacterium once, along with a high-oxalate diet that is associated with kidney stones (foods including spinach, soy products, almonds, potatoes, legumes, and beets), which resulted in decreased urinary oxalate secretion, indicating that this bacterium may decrease oxalic acid, and thereby increase the risk of kidney stones. Antibiotic usage—and pregnancy!—are also associated with increased risk of kidney stones.

While we are still awaiting establishment of a direct causal relationship between gut microbes and kidney stones, these highly suggestive studies indicate that the gut microbiome is involved. This may present novel future solutions.

All Guts, No Glory

Certain specific digestive tract conditions, such as irritable bowel syndrome (IBS), are immediately and directly affected by the gut microbiome. IBS affects about 10 percent of the world population and is most common in women and younger people; however, it is also one of the most encountered functional GI disorders in older people. Its symptoms are vague and many—recurrent abdominal pain as well as changes in bowel habits and bloating—and while treatment can help ease symptoms, it cannot be cured.

IBS does not directly affect longevity, but it has a major impact on quality of life and can cause chronic pain for years.

IBS is a complex syndrome. Several lines of evidence indicate that the microbiome is involved through dysbiosis and/or decreased microbial diversity (no studies have yet been able to identify a characteristic microbial signal associated with the disease). One reason that researchers believe microbes have a role is because IBS often appears following gastroenteritis (post-infectious IBS) and, to a lesser extent, antibiotics. Fecal transfers of IBS patient feces into "germ-free" mice (animals without microbiomes, born and kept in germ-free conditions) transfer many symptoms of the disease, including diarrhea and anxiety. Like many intestinal diseases, there is an increase in intestinal permeability in patients and accompanying low-grade systemic inflammation. It is thought that this contributes to gut–brain signaling, perhaps by altering neuromuscular responses, gut motility, and pain perception.

Although there is no cure for IBS, pilot studies indicate that probiotics that decrease intestinal inflammation show some promise as a treatment to alleviate symptoms. In one study of forty-four patients with IBS, researchers found that *Bifidobacterium longum* NCC3001 reduced the depression often associated with IBS, but not IBS symptoms or anxiety. Other probiotics have shown promise in decreasing IBS symptoms, including *Bifidobacterium bifidum* MIMBb75 and *Lactobacillus plantarum* 299v, as well as a cocktail of three probiotics. Other therapeutic approaches to help manage symptoms of IBS include a high-fiber diet, physical exercise, stress management, diarrhea medication, laxatives, and other dietary supplements.

MYTH: Stress and anxiety cause irritable bowel syndrome (IBS).

FACT: Experts don't know exactly why people get IBS. While stress and depression can make symptoms worse, IBS is not solely a psychiatric illness. There is bidirectional communication between the brain and gut, so symptoms may be caused by dysfunctions predominantly in the central nervous system, the gut, or a combination of both.

A separate, and more severe, group of bowel conditions gaining increasing awareness in public conversations on gut health are inflammatory bowel diseases (IBD). They are often confused with IBS because they share similar names and some of the same symptoms, but these GI conditions are completely distinct. IBD results in the body's own immune system attacking parts of the digestive system. Nearly three million Americans and one hundred and eighty thousand Australians have been diagnosed with IBD, and 10 to 15 percent and 22 percent respectively were diagnosed at sixty years of age or older. Diagnosis may take longer and be more challenging in older people because of the large number of conditions common to aging that mimic the symptoms of IBD which doctors need to first rule out. Infections or certain medications, such as nonsteroidal anti-inflammatory drugs (NSAIDs) and antibiotics, can also complicate diagnosis in older people.

There are two IBDs in humans: ulcerative colitis and Crohn's disease. Although both cause inflammation of the intestinal tract, ulcerative colitis is limited to the colon, while Crohn's disease affects the entire digestive tract, from mouth to anus, leading to increased gut permeability, inflammation, tissue damage, and fibrosis (the thickening and scarring of tissue). As the name implies, both diseases feature an inflamed intestine that may result in diarrhea, rectal bleeding, abdominal cramps, pain, and other serious side effects. Given that they are lifelong diseases, many older people have lived with IBD for many years. The number of hospitalizations for those over the age of sixty-five account for approximately 25 percent (20 to 25 percent in Australia) of all admissions for IBD. As with IBS, unfortunately, there is no cure, and the exact cause remains unknown.

Researchers suggest that a combination of four factors leads to IBD: a genetic component, an environmental trigger, an imbalance of intestinal bacteria, and an inappropriate reaction from the immune system. There are over two hundred human genes associated with an increased risk of IBD, including many genes involved in inflammation and the control of microbial infections. However, together they account for only a small amount of the collective disease risk: about 13 percent for Crohn's and 8 percent for ulcerative colitis. This suggests that there are indeed other factors that contribute to the majority of the causes of these diseases.

The microbiome is now considered a major factor in these diseases, largely because of its interplay with the immune system, which ultimately affects inflammation in the gut (see chapter 3). Immune cells normally protect the body from infection, but people with IBD often lack normal immune responses that keep the gut microbes at bay. This allows microbes to penetrate through the gut barrier, which then triggers intestinal inflammation and tissue damage. IBD patients also tend to have a dysbiotic microbiome–more specifically decreased Bacteroidetes, Firmicutes, and the butyrate-producing *Faecalibacterium prausnitzii*; and increased inflammatory microbes such as Proteobacteria, and microbes that produce the harmful gas hydrogen sulfide, which damages tissue in the bowel.

There are two compelling lines of evidence that the microbiome is actually involved directly in IBD. First, fecal transfers can improve the disease symptoms, especially for ulcerative colitis. Second, studies show that if feces are taken from IBD patients and transplanted into mice without the disease, this causes intestinal inflammation and other symptoms associated with IBD. The current view of IBD is that it is not caused by a single microbe, but that it is a combination of certain risk factors, especially involving the immune system, plus enhanced microbial penetration of the gut, which triggers inflammation. Attempts to treat these diseases thus are now focused on dampening inflammation with anti-inflammatories and improving microbial balance with fecal transfers and other dietary and lifestyle methods.

Stool Transplants

The holy grail of the microbiota world is to identify specific beneficial microbes, grow them in culture, and put them into individuals to better treat diseases such as IBS and IBD and perhaps even promote overall health and longevity. While the process sounds simple enough, as we saw above, defining a healthy aging microbiome is still well beyond our abilities. However, there is one medical procedure that has changed the entire microbiome world, stimulating countless companies to think about microbial therapies: That is, transferring feces from one person into another.

The concept of fecal transfers–also called "fecal microbiota transplantation" (FMT), fecal bacteriotherapy, or duodenal infusion–is not new. As far back as the fourth century, people in China suffering from severe diarrhea were given oral fecal slurries ("yellow soup") as a treatment (thank goodness we've advanced beyond that method!). There are numerous similar reports of fecal uses throughout history. Our modern methods go back to 1958, when Dr. Ben Eiseman of Colorado led a group of surgeons in treating four patients with severe intestinal disease (pseudomembranous colitis) with fecal enemas–and remarkably cured their disease. Recently FMTs have garnered much attention in the medical field as well as the popular press, especially regarding infections caused by *Clostridium difficile* (colloquially known as "C. diff").

C. difficile is an intestinal pathogen that causes severe diarrhea by producing potent toxins in the gut. However, as pathogens go, it has trouble establishing itself in the gut if there is a healthy normal microbiome present. These infections are most often seen in hospitalized patients who are taking antibiotics for reasons such as hip transplants or other surgeries. Surgeons routinely give antibiotics such as clindamycin and other fluoroquinolones to decrease the risk of infections post-surgery. When the drugs wipe out the microbial ecosystem, *C. difficile* can more readily colonize people, triggering severe intestinal disease and, ultimately, even death.

It is now considered one of the most common health care-associated infections, with over a half million people per year infected in the United States and about eight thousand in Australia. It has a 9 percent mortality rate and between 3.5 and 8 percent in Australia. Because antibiotics created the conditions to cause infection, treatment with antibiotics such as metronidazole and vancomycin are often unsuccessful. Recurrent *C. difficile* infections, classed as two to three previous standard treatments with antibiotics failing, are common and medically challenging to treat.

Several well-designed clinical studies have shown that FMTs routinely cure more than 90 percent of these infections. It is groundbreaking that simply transferring feces from one person to another can cure a deadly disease. FMTs are now recognized as the clinical treatment of choice for recurrent *C. difficile* infections. About 300 to 500 grams (about a pound) of fecal slurry is given either by a nasogastric tube (a tube running down the throat to the intestine) or by an enema (injection of fluid into the lower bowel by way of the rectum). Donors are rigorously screened for potential pathogens and their history of antibiotic use, diarrhea, etc. Thus far this treatment seems safe and effective, although we still don't know all the short and long-term consequences. For example: A transplant from an obese donor into a lean recipient cured one patient of *C. difficile*, but the recipient also gained significant weight. More on the "microbial memory" later in this chapter.

Brett experienced the challenges of treating *C. difficile* firsthand a few years ago when he needed minor colon surgery. As per standard treatment to avoid infection complications, the surgeon suggested large doses of an antibiotic cocktail prior to surgery. When Brett told the surgeon that it would significantly increase his chances of getting *C. difficile*, he scoffed, so despite his hesitation, Brett took the antibiotics. The surgery went well. About ten days later, Brett came down with severe diarrhea, which his wife (a pediatrician) suggested was *C. difficile*. So, after sterilizing a jar and taking a fecal sample, Brett went off to the hospital. Within twenty-four hours, the test came back screaming *C. difficile*. He then started on the antibiotic vancomycin (which has a cure rate of about 31 percent), and the diarrhea went away. However, about two weeks later, Brett came down with diarrhea again. After the same hospital routine, it again was diagnosed as *C. difficile* (now called "recurring C. diff"). His doctors then turned to a very expensive special antibiotic that has a higher cure rate (that thankfully his health insurance covered), and the diarrhea went away. Given that the current clinical guidelines suggest an FMT following three rounds of *C. difficile*, Brett called up a colleague and friend who runs the FMT trials in Vancouver. His friend set aside a tube of a donor's feces that could be used on Brett if he had a third round of diarrhea. Fortunately, that never happened, and Brett is fine. Unfortunately, that means Brett never got his FMT, which would have made a wonderful end to the story given his profession!

MYTH: You can give yourself a fecal transfer from a healthy friend or family member.

FACT: Despite the simplicity of the procedure—and the numerous DIY YouTube videos featuring brown mixtures in blenders—do NOT attempt this at home. If the gut is ruptured, you can get sepsis and possibly die of complications. FMTs are to be performed only in regulated medical settings under careful medical observation.

If FMTs work for *C. difficile*, why not use them for other diseases such as IBD? There are literally dozens of FMT clinical trials underway for myriad diseases ranging from obesity to IBS and even autism. Thus far, in addition to recurrent *C. difficile* infections, the other disease showing significant promise for FMTs is the IBD ulcerative colitis (UC). However, the results are quite mixed among studies, with about 25 percent (30 to 60 percent in Australia) of IBD patients going into remission due to FMT. IBD is not as susceptible to microbiome competition as *C. difficile*, because in IBD, the gut is inflamed, and its microbiota are already dysbiotic. Incoming microbes from the fecal transfer have to displace the resident ones, dampen the inflammation, and reset the whole gut–which is a big ask. Different donors also seem to have different effects likely based on their microbiome composition. Some trials are experimenting with blending various donors' feces to provide an even more diverse microbiome. Experiments are also underway that give repeated fecal transfers, combined with pre-treatment antibiotics and/or anti-inflammatories to enhance the chances of the incoming microbes being able to establish themselves. There are initial reports coming from several diseases that FMTs hold promise as an intervention. In a preliminary small trial, FMTs were able to increase insulin sensitivity, which is important for treating type 2 diabetes and obesity. Unfortunately, patients weren't followed long enough to measure an effect on body weight.

Further establishing the safety, efficacy, and validity of FMTs could positively translate into broader usage with gut-related ailments including IBS, IBD, obesity, type 2 diabetes, and colorectal cancer. We might even reset the gut microbiota of an older person with microbes from a thirty-year-old to combat a specific disease or boost overall healthy aging. But given that gut microbiota and intestinal environments vary significantly between individuals, a lot more research is needed to precisely define and validate which microbes are considered "healthy" and "ideal" for everyone, and how to fill in the gaps where individual needs are concerned. In either case, research progress will hopefully allow for earlier detection and prevention of these diseases, so that our guts–and the rest of us–are happy for longer.

If the idea of an FMT slurry turns your stomach (or your gut), there is hope on the horizon. Work is underway to pack feces into pills (although you would have to swallow a lot of pills to consume a pound of feces). Even more encouraging is the concept of growing a defined population of human microbes in the lab to give directly to patients. This decreases the risk of unknown viruses and other blood-borne diseases. Dr. Emma

Allen-Vercoe and her team at the University of Guelph piloted and successfully treated two *C. difficile* patients with this synthetic microbe mix. She affectionately calls the procedure "rePOOPulating," and we shall discuss it in greater depth in chapter 16. As we further define certain microbes associated with particular benefits, we should be able to move away from fecal material into clinical-grade cultured organisms. Companies such as Vedanta Biosciences, Inc. are working on specific combinations of live microbes (Live Microbial Products, or LBPs for "live biotherapeutic products") that can be used instead of crude fecal transfers. They used a combination of eight microbes taken orally (after antibiotics) that worked nicely in Phase II clinical trials and are being developed as a "drug" for recurrent *C. diff.* Stay tuned!

PASSING GAS

Although flatulence (farting) is frowned upon in most societies, it is a natural process in which microbes play a key role. The term *flatulence* comes from the Latin word flatus, which means "blowing, act of breaking wind." Whenever you ingest and swallow food or drink, a small amount of air also enters the gastrointestinal tract. Once inside, it has to go somewhere—usually expelled as either a burp or fart. Drinking carbonated drinks or chewing gum increases this air intake. The average person passes gas ten to twenty times per day, expelling between 500 and 1,500 ml daily, or roughly two to six cups. About 99 percent of the gases expelled are odorless, and include nitrogen, oxygen, carbon dioxide, hydrogen, and methane.

The real problem with flatulence is its smell, for which we have microbes to thank. In addition to odorless gases, microbes also produce hydrogen sulfide (which smells like rotten eggs—and is the main culprit for smelly farts), methanethiol (rotten vegetable smell), and dimethyl sulfide (cooked broccoli odor). The smelly compounds are produced in the colon by microbes breaking down complex oligosaccharides (think: plant fiber), which the body is unable to metabolize on its own. Thus, eating broccoli, beans, cauliflower, and other plant fibers can increase the odor of our farts. Vegetarians have increased flatulence given their plant-based diets. Regular flatulence, however, is a good sign, as it indicates good consumption of fiber and a healthy, gas-producing microbiome.

Nourish Your Microbes, Nourish Yourself

The diet of the Western world has shifted drastically over the past fifty years—to the detriment of our waistlines and our microbiomes. On average, Americans eat about 23 percent more calories per day in 2010 than in 1970 according to the US Department of Agriculture. Nearly half of these calories come from just two food groups: flours and grains, and fats and oils. Chicken has topped beef as the most-consumed meat (as in Australia), while in the dairy aisle we drink 42 percent less milk compared to 1970, but eat more cheese (21.9 pounds, or 9.9 kg, per year, nearly three times the average consumption in 1970). Americans now eat 29 percent more grains, mostly in the form of breads, pastries, and other baked goods. In 1999, the average American consumed an average of 26.7 teaspoons of caloric sweeteners per day. This number went down to 22.9 teaspoons per day by 2014 (13 teaspoons in Australia)—although, remember that these figures don't include noncaloric sweeteners such as aspartame. While most of the sweetener consumed in 1970 was refined sugar, we now eat a lot more corn-derived sweeteners, including cheap and readily available high-fructose corn syrup.

When you alter your diet, such as switching to a high-fiber/low-fat diet, changes in the microbiome can be detected within three days. Changes in diet may account for over half of the variation in a person's microbiome (57 percent), while genetic variation accounts for 12 percent. One great example of how the gut microbiome adapts to diet comes from Japan. We know that a specific microbial enzyme, beta-porphyranase, is found in marine microbes and breaks down a component of seaweed (glycans). This enzyme is also found in a certain microbe called *Bacteroides plebeius* in the gut microbiomes of Japanese people, but not in North American microbiomes. Eating unsterile seaweed, as many Japanese do, enabled the transfer of the gene encoding the enzyme of an ocean-dwelling microbe to resident members of the Japanese human microbiome and passed this around Japan, thereby enhancing the population's digestion of seaweed.

The case of seaweed is a specific illustration of how food consumption uniquely altered a community's microbiome. By extension, there is concern that broad dietary changes across the general population will cause us, as humans, to lose the microbes that we evolved with since we no longer eat the foods that allowed for our evolution. In a series of intriguing experiments, Dr. Justin Sonnenburg from Stanford University showed that we may be doing serious, irreparable damage to our collective human microbiome. First, he fed "humanized" mice (i.e., germ-free mice colonized with human fecal microbes from a Westerner) a diet rich in plant fiber for six weeks. Next, he fed half of those mice a low-fiber (Western) diet for seven weeks, followed by a high-fiber diet for another six weeks. The control group remained on the high-fiber diet the whole time. The mice were bred, and this was repeated for each subsequent generation. What he and his team found was quite disturbing. At first, the changes in the gut microbiome accompanying the diet change were partly reversible in a single generation (one third of the original species did not fully recover). But then, with each subsequent generation, a low-fiber diet caused a further decrease in microbial diversity. After four generations, no length of time on a high-fiber diet could recover the microbes that break down fiber. Interestingly, however, researchers could restore the high-fiber microbes by a fecal transfer of normal microbes to the depleted animals.

Collectively, this suggests we are driving the microbes that digest high amounts of fiber (which then produce SCFAs and many other beneficial effects) to extinction as society continues its low-fiber/high-simple-sugar diet. This effect could compound over just a few generations to the point of becoming irreversible, thus ending our relationship with the beneficial microbes that were so integral to our successful evolution. Losing the diversity and abundance of our ancestors' gut flora could negatively impact health and well-being if our species has fewer and less diverse microbes, making us more susceptible to gastrointestinal disorders, other diseases, and dysbiosis. Perhaps the diverse gut microbiomes characteristic of centenarians and semi-supercentenarians will become impossible to achieve in the future, which could detrimentally affect our prospects for longevity. Scientists are now even considering the possibility that we biobank feces from our grandparents for the health of future generations.

The Obesity Epidemic

Obesity was once considered a cosmetic issue caused by overeating or lack of self-control. But now, multiple national and international medical and scientific societies, including the WHO, recognize obesity as a chronic progressive disease resulting from multiple environmental and genetic factors. Obesity is common, serious, and very costly worldwide: One report estimated the global cost of obesity at two trillion dollars annually. More than one third (36.5 percent) of adults in the United States (31.7 percent in Australia) are obese–a massive increase from 13 percent (about 10.7 percent in Australia) in 1962–and over two thirds (69 percent) of American adults are overweight (65.8 percent in Australia). An estimated 2.5 billion adults are overweight worldwide, which includes around one billion adults who are obese. The disease has a greater cost on our longevity and quality of life, as it leads to other life-threatening diseases, including heart disease, stroke, and, most especially, type 2 diabetes.

Obesity has surpassed smoking as the top preventable cause of cancer death. The disease raises mortality risk for adults of all ages, but this relationship is nearly twice as strong for people under the age of fifty. Obese middle-aged people are more than twice as likely as normal-weight persons to die prematurely. Being slightly overweight in later life is in fact associated with lower mortality risk, but obesity raises mortality risk–especially for coronary heart disease.

The prevalence and severity of obesity is a major cause of attention on the microbiome. In the mid-2000s, pioneering work by Jeffrey Gordon's lab at Washington University revealed that the microbiome plays a key role in body weight. The studies showed that germ-free mice consumed many more calories than normal mice yet gained less weight, and that transferring microbiota from obese mice to thin mice through FMTs was linked to significant weight gain, while transferring microbiota from thin mice to obese mice caused weight loss. This profound finding suggests that the microbiome affects not only weight but also metabolism rates and calorie production.

Fast forward a decade: We have learned even more about these crucial connections but, as with all things in science, also realize that it's more complex than we originally thought. We know that the microbiome breaks down much of our food into energy products such as SCFAs that feed the body. If you consume an obesity-inducing Western diet–including processed sugars and refined carbs–that is low in fiber and high in calories, your body selects a less diverse microbiome. This is because most of the processed food is readily absorbed in the small intestine, since it is already broken down, thereby starving the fiber-munching large bowel microbes.

Hence why obese individuals have a different microbiome than those of normal weight: There is a higher ratio of Firmicutes, which are very efficient at energy extraction from food, to Bacteroidetes, which are enhanced by a fiber-rich plant-based diet. It seems like we need the Bacteroidetes to balance out the Firmicutes. Multiple studies confirm the association of obesity with gut microbiota composition by studying the Firmicutes/Bacteroidetes (F/B) ratio, although others point out it isn't quite so straightforward. Weight gain and loss is a multifaceted lifestyle process that cannot be reduced to gut microbiota composition alone.

Recalling the link between the microbiome and inflammation, we see how the microbial dysbiosis observed in obese individuals leads to increased intestinal permeability, which allows microbial substances to seep into the body and trigger chronic inflammation. This can lead to insulin resistance (type 2 diabetes), cardiovascular disease, cancers, and dementia. Diets with higher fiber and fewer processed products are thought to help prevent this gut permeability, as well as decrease excess energy production from SCFAs, which helps weight control.

Several recent studies indicate that foods rich in fiber are beneficial for microbiome composition, and also contribute to weight loss. In one study where young healthy participants were either fed a standard Western diet or a Microbiome Enhancer Diet (lots of dietary fiber and less processed foods), they found that following the microbiome diet resulted in 116 kcal (485 kilojoules)/day lost in feces. This means that there was less energy available for the host, which would lead to a predicted long-term weight loss. There was also a robust remodeling of the microbiome in favor of fiber-degrading (beneficial) microbes, and increased SCFA production.

Because of the complexity of the microbiome, there are currently no magic combinations of microbes you can take to create the right ratio of microbes and help you lose weight (although there is a lot of work underway in this area). However, many studies suggest that dietary fiber helps in weight loss. Personalized diets hold significant promise in tailoring food intake to your microbiome, and there is hope that approaches incorporating the microbiome can be used to help combat obesity.

STOP YO-YO DIETING

We know all too well that losing weight is really hard. How many of us have made a New Year's resolution to shed pounds, achieved some weight loss after lots of effort, only to gain back the weight we lost—if not even more—a few months later? So, we try again the next year and the cycle repeats.

This pattern of yo-yo dieting is extremely prevalent in our society. About 80 percent of people with long-term obesity who lose weight through dieting gain it back within a year, often even more weight than they previously started with. Six years after participating in *The Biggest Loser*, a dramatic weight-loss reality television show where contestants undergo intensive, monitored dieting and exercise regimens, most participants were back where they started. On top of that, their metabolism had slowed so much that they were in fact burning fewer calories per day than before appearing on the show. Our bodies fight hard against weight loss, which may have served as a buffer in our evolutionary past by helping our bodies cope with a feast-and-famine existence.

Renowned microbiologist and gastroenterologist Dr. Eran Elinav, a scientist at the Weizmann Institute of Science in Israel, experienced the effects of a yo-yo diet firsthand, telling us, "One of the lab's projects started because of my screwed-up lifestyle. I was drinking lots of artificial sweetener drinks and dieting. I suffered from recurrent obesity." Partnering with Dr. Eran Segal and other researchers at the Weizmann Institute, he devised a mouse model to mimic yo-yo dieting in humans. They fed mice one of three options: 1) normal food, 2) a high-fat diet, or 3) cycled between these diets about every five weeks. Mice on the yo-yo diet cycles experienced major problems: They incurred massive microbiome changes (researchers identified 773 bacterial genes that were affected) that lasted about one quarter of the mouse's lifetime; and those mice gained weight much faster than even the mice who remained on high fat diets (or the controlled regular food).

"The pattern of recurrent obesity seems to have an inherent capability of exaggerating from cycle to cycle," explains Dr. Elinav. "This is why, over the years, we gain a little bit and then a little bit more." These results suggest that there is "microbial memory" in the gut that sabotages weight loss efforts (at least in mice) because of its "memory of previous episodes of obesity—one that is a very disturbed, obesogenic configuration." Even though weight fluctuated drastically up and down, the mice's microbiome memory configuration was highly persistent.

Using fecal transfers, Elinav and Segal showed that, amazingly, these effects could be transferred into germ-free mice. Fecal matter of the cycling-diet mice promoted faster weight gain in the germ-free mice, which also supports the theory of microbial memory. Although the exact mechanisms of this process remain undefined, researchers found decreases in the flavonoids apigenin (found in artichokes, parsley, and celery) and naringenin (found in grapefruits) in the yo-yo diet mice. These flavonoids are associated with high energy consumption, which can help stave off weight gain. By feeding flavonoids to the mice, their energy consumption rates returned to normal.

Although exciting in theory, we still know very little about how this might apply to humans. Dr. Elinav explained: "We studied mouse weight gain and loss over six months, which is a quarter of mice's lifetime in captivity. A quarter of a human's life is much more complicated to study given that humans live much longer than two years." The data are still to come. Dr. Elinav and colleagues are now following a cohort of humans to study their microbiomes through recurrent obesity behavior over the course of a year. Our best takeaway is that in order to maintain healthful changes in the microbiome structure, we have to aim for long-term maintenance of the diet changes that produce it, not cycle on and off, otherwise our microbes rapidly revert to their previous composition. Moving forward, we can work with our microbes to, hopefully, develop more successful, long-term, and healthful diet strategies to maintain a healthy weight.

Diabetes

Approximately thirty-eight million Americans (two million Australians) have diabetes, and one in five (one in three Australians) don't realize they have it. Diabetes remains a leading cause of death in the United States and Australia, and direct medical costs were $306 billion in 2022 (about $3.4 billion in Australia). The disease is caused by a lack of response to insulin, which stimulates the body to absorb glucose. This results in elevated levels of glucose in the blood (hyperglycemia), which then causes tissue damage, blindness, and circulatory issues (e.g., diabetic foot ulcers, which can result in lower limb amputation). People who are overweight or obese have added pressure on their bodies' abilities to use insulin to properly control blood sugar levels, which makes diabetes more common among this population. There are three types of diabetes:

- **Type 1 diabetes:** Also called "insulin-dependent diabetes," this autoimmune condition often begins in childhood. The body attacks its own pancreas with antibodies to the point that the damaged pancreas cells cannot make insulin.

- **Gestational diabetes:** This form occurs only during pregnancy, and researchers do not know why some women develop the disease. Women with gestational diabetes develop high blood sugar levels, which can be managed with help from doctors, as well as dietary and lifestyle adjustments. After delivery, gestational diabetes usually disappears.

- **Type 2 diabetes:** Most people with diabetes have this condition. Over 10 percent of Americans have type 2 diabetes, and another 8.5 million have prediabetes (their blood glucose levels are abnormally high). People with type 2 diabetes make insulin, but their cells do not use it as well as they should (insulin resistance). Being overweight is a major risk factor for type 2 diabetes, because the more fatty tissue in your body, the more resistant your cells become to insulin. However, you do not have to be overweight to get the disease.

Given the close linkages between obesity and type 2 diabetes, the microbial involvement in this disease is very similar to that in obesity. The shift toward increased Firmicutes, decreased Bacteroidetes, and increased gut permeability contributes to the body becoming increasingly unresponsive to insulin (insulin resistance). Just as with obesity, there are studies indicating that modulating the microbiome improves glucose homeostasis and decreases disease effects. Although not clinically proven, there are reports that prebiotics and probiotics such as *Lactobacillus reuteri* GMNL-263 can decrease the inflammatory responses and improve metabolic control and insulin sensitivity in type 2 diabetes patients.

Beneficial diets rich in fiber also improve insulin sensitivity, probably by restoring the helpful microbes and decreasing inflammation. In a small study using fecal transfers, obese people with type 2 diabetes who received feces from healthy donors had improved insulin sensitivity after six weeks, although there was no observed weight loss. Not surprisingly, multiple courses of antibiotics (two to five, taken over years) were associated with an increased risk of type 2 diabetes, although a single course was not.

Metformin is the most commonly used drug to treat type 2 diabetes and works by lowering blood glucose to inhibit liver glucose production. Several studies indicate that the drug works at least partially through the microbiota, which may be why it must be taken orally (think access to the gut microbiome). In fact, it doesn't work if injected directly into the bloodstream. There are two main mechanisms that may be at work in metformin. First, particular members of the microbiome may modify the drug into a more beneficial molecule that the body responds to positively. Second, several studies support a theory that metformin affects the microbiome composition by pushing it toward a more beneficial anti-inflammatory composition, which then helps improve insulin sensitivity. This beneficial microbial effect can even be transmitted by fecal transfer from metformin-treated patients (with their metformin-altered microbiota) into germ-free mice.

ARE PREBIOTIC SODAS GOOD FOR YOUR GUT?

Grocery aisles now abound with fun, colorful cans of pop that advertise gut health benefits by including starchy substances and dietary fibers as a source of prebiotic fiber. However, there is limited scientific research on these beverages and the Food and Drug Administration (FDA), or Food Standards Australia New Zealand (FSANZ) has not approved any health claims. There are current legal disputes about whether there is enough prebiotic fiber in these products to cause meaningful gut health benefits. While this might be a tasty addition to your diet, you would likely benefit more from consuming a variety of prebiotics in fiber-rich foods.

You (and Your Microbes) Are What You Eat

Sugar, maltodextrin, corn flour, wheat flour, whole grain oat flour, degerminated corn flour, corn bran, oat hull fiber, hydrogenated coconut and vegetable oil, salt, concentrated carrot juice, anthocyanin, annatto, turmeric, concentrated watermelon juice, concentrated blueberry juice, concentrated huito juice, stevia leaf extract, iron, niacinamide, zinc oxide, thiamine hydrochloride, D-calcium pantothenate, cholecalciferol, pyridoxine hydrochloride, and folic acid. These are the contents listed on a box of popular breakfast cereal. The box also touts the cereal as a source of eight vitamins and minerals, made with whole grains, and natural fruit flavors. Is this a healthy food? It has some healthy ingredients, but they are also highly processed.

The above is a good example of what are now called "ultra-processed foods" (UPFs). We don't mean to pick on sugary cereals (heck, any kid will tell you they taste great, and they *do* have healthy additives including minerals), but the past few years have seen an explosion in data suggesting that UPFs are not good for general health. Humans have been processing food for centuries to make it safer, longer lasting, and tastier. The term UPF was introduced in 2009 to define highly modified food products created through industrial processes which contain multiple additives, preservatives and artificial ingredients. They include sugar-sweetened beverages, packaged meats, processed breads, canned soups, flavored yogurts, packaged snacks, and cereals, and are found throughout any grocery store. Take an apple for example. On its own, it is an unprocessed food. Apple juice on the other hand is considered a processed food (minimal processing and additives), while store-bought apple pie is regarded as a UPF (including the crust and pie filling). UPFs also encourage eating: the high carbohydrate and fat content is associated with a dopamine surge in the brain, which is comparable to nicotine, resulting in "UPF addiction."

Consumption of UPFs is increasing throughout the world, with the US and UK having the highest rates (just below 60 percent of food consumed; 40 percent in Australia). While convenient and tasty, UPFs are increasingly being associated with many Western diseases. For example, a UPF diet results in about five hundred more calories per day and links to obesity. A study of mother-child pairs found that offspring of mothers who consumed UPFs were at 26 percent higher risk for obesity. There are also strong links to type 2 diabetes and other metabolic diseases. A recent meta study (compiled findings of multiple studies) showed that higher consumption of UPFs increased the risk of Crohn's disease by 71 percent. Similarly, high UPF consumption is associated with a 20 percent higher risk of irritable bowel syndrome (IBS). UPFs are also associated with higher cancer rates, and conversely, substituting 10 percent of UPFs with unprocessed foods lowered overall cancer rates by 4 percent and some specific cancers by over 25 percent. They are also correlated with higher risks of cardiovascular disease, strokes, and cognitive impairment. The depressing list goes on, but the bottom line is that UPFs are strongly associated with poor health outcomes.

As we will see throughout this book, all these diseases have strong ties with the microbiome. We know that diet changes are closely associated with changes in the microbiome. There have been four studies which show what one would expect with a UPF (low fiber) diet: some decrease in microbial diversity (although not consistent across the studies), and an increase in microbes associated with obesity, diabetes, and other adverse health conditions. Because of the limited data, direct conclusions with UPF consumption and microbiome are still lacking. However, it is well established that diets that emphasize plant-based fibers and less-processed foods, such as the Mediterranean and DASH (Dietary Approaches to Stop Hypertension) diets, all have a profound beneficial effect on the microbiome. A recent study of more than twenty-five thousand women over twenty-five years showed that following a Mediterranean diet resulted in a 23 percent decrease in mortality, including from both cancer and cardiovascular disease, as well as decreased blood pressure.

Common food additives are emulsifiers. These are chemicals which allow oil and water to mix. Some emulsifiers include lecithins, modified fatty acids, carboxymethylcellulose, and polysorbate, and they are found extensively in processed food. But are they bad for us? This has been a hard question to answer as they are so ubiquitous in food, and the conclusions are not as strong as for UPFs. There are hints that they increase risk of IBD and cancer, and a large study of French adults found an association with increased risk in type 2 diabetes for various emulsifiers (but of course they urge more studies be done). Current health guidelines do not suggest avoiding emulsifiers. Again, correlations with these diseases hint at microbiome involvement. A 2015 study in *Nature* showed that two emulsifiers, carboxymethylcellulose and polysorbate 80, caused a detrimental change of the microbiome in mice and increased weight gain and inflammation. However, as this study was in mice, and the doses used were higher than most humans normally consume, the jury is still out with humans.

Another common food additive is salt. While salt is essential, too much causes significant cardiovascular problems (see chapter 7). A healthy adult should consume about 2,300 mg of sodium (about a teaspoon) a day, but the average American consumes 3,400 mg (3,500 mg for the average Australian). While some comes from a saltshaker, about 70 percent of our salt intake comes from UPFs such as breads, chips, packaged meats, and canned soups. And, of course, it impacts the gut microbiome. One study showed that decreasing salt increased beneficial bacteria and SCFAs, thereby decreasing inflammation, as well as lowering blood pressure. High salt intake caused reductions in beneficial microbes such as *Lactobacillus* and increases of pathogenic/inflammatory bacteria in the gut—one more reason to avoid UPFs.

ARTIFICIALLY SWEET

Noncaloric artificial sweeteners are used extensively in diet drinks and foods, and widely touted as safe substitutes in weight loss programs and diabetes management. Six artificial sweeteners are currently approved by the FDA for use in humans: acesulfame potassium (also called "acesulfame K"), aspartame, saccharin, sucralose, neotame, and advantame. Also approved by the FSANZ, they are used to sweeten food with fewer calories and carbohydrates than sugar—the sweetening power of most low-calorie sweeteners is at least two hundred times more intense. With the exception of aspartame, none of these sweeteners can be broken down by the body, so they pass through our systems without being digested—hence, no added calories.

But are these products really the panacea for excessive sugar consumption? The question is a contentious one with many differing opinions, and studies on them offer mixed results. A recent study called their safety into question due to effects specifically on the microbiome. Dr. Eran Elinav and his team in Israel gave mice three sweeteners in their drinking water (saccharin, sucralose, and aspartame) for eleven weeks. They found that they developed marked glucose intolerance, yet the control group of mice given normal sugar had normal glucose tolerance. They also found that treating the mice consuming the artificial sweeteners with antibiotics on either lean or high-fat diets blocked the increase in glucose intolerance, suggesting that this intolerance has microbial involvement.

Moving from mice to humans, they found that in 381 nondiabetic subjects, those who consumed artificial sweeteners had increased metabolic syndrome parameters, including impaired glucose intolerance. When a group of individuals who normally do not use artificial sweeteners consumed saccharin for seven days, there was a marked shift in the gut microbiome of four of the seven subjects who responded to the sweeteners in that time. Their microbiomes resembled those found in type 2 diabetics (i.e., not good): increased Bacteroides and decreased Clostridiales. When feces from these responders were placed into germ-free mice, the recipient mice had significant glucose intolerance compared to those that received the non-responder feces. This one study suggests that the products we use to control glucose tolerance, obesity, type 2 diabetes, and metabolic disease may actually aggravate risk and symptoms due to their microbial effects. Further studies are needed in humans to better understand short and long-term effects of artificial sweeteners.

The Ozempic Revolution

We have witnessed a recent explosion in drugs that lower blood sugar, and moreover cause significant weight loss, resulting in what many call the "weight loss drug revolution." Glucagon-like peptide-1 (GLP-1) is a natural hormone (incretin) that causes insulin release and sugar uptake, thereby lowering blood sugar levels. Several companies have made drugs, including Ozempic and Wegovy, that mimic the action of GLP-1 (called "GLP-1 Receptor Agonists," or GLP-1 RAs). Moreover, another drug, tirzepatide (brand name Mounjaro or Zepbound), mimics both GLP-1 and another related hormone, glucose-dependent insulinotropic peptide (GIP), and seems to work even better in clinical trials. These drugs have been remarkably effective at controlling type 2 diabetes, although they are costly. They have also caused a decrease in cholesterol and blood pressure, a decrease in cardiovascular disease, and, as became obvious very quickly, remarkable weight loss of upward of 15 to 20 percent of total body weight. Given that over a third of the world's population is overweight or obese, these drugs have become incredibly popular for weight loss—so much so that it has caused drug shortages for those with diabetes. We should note that these drugs come with side effects including nausea, vomiting, diarrhea, and constipation (as well as a few rare serious side effects), and they aren't tolerated by everyone.

Although their mechanism for stimulating insulin release and blood sugar control is well understood, what remains a puzzle is *why* they cause weight loss. They seem to delay gastric emptying (the draining of stomach contents into the small intestine) and even decrease hunger signals in the brain. However, many recent studies suggest that part of their effect may be due to mediating the gut microbiome, which in turn can affect body weight. Several studies in people with type 2 diabetes taking these drugs show major shifts in their microbiome, including an increase in the Bacteroidetes to Firmicutes ratio and increased diversity (obese individuals have less microbial diversity and more Firmicutes). They also have an increase in microbes associated with leanness, and an increase in *Akkermansia muciniphila* (which promotes gut barrier integrity and is decreased in obese individuals). The increase in the Bacteroidetes levels would result in increased SCFAs including butyrate, which are known to increase GLP-1 levels (at least in mice). Although it has yet to be fully proven, given the systemic effects of these drugs that are associated with changes in the microbiome, it seems that one of the major ways these drugs work is by shifting the microbiome.

The Personalized Microbe Diet

Perhaps the most exciting promise in gut microbiome research is developing personalized diets based on each person's unique microbial composition. This could help us answer burning questions about why people respond differently to foods and why certain diets seem to work well for some people but not others.

One way we've been able to address this question is by comparing individuals' microbiome compositions to the foods they consume. From there, we can assess corresponding glucose spikes, which contribute to obesity, type 2 diabetes, and metabolic syndromes. In a landmark paper published in 2015, the team led by Drs. Eran Elinav and Eran Segal followed eight hundred people for a week, monitoring all foods consumed (close to fifty thousand meals), tracking glucose levels, and characterizing each person's gut microbiome throughout. They found that particular foods caused different levels of glucose spikes in different people (hinting that standard diets may not work for all). Using machine-learning algorithms, they were able to predict which foods might cause glucose spikes in particular individuals based on their microbiome composition. They then confirmed their predictions in a cohort of one hundred people in a double-blind controlled trial (neither the participants nor the scientists knew which group any one participant belonged to).

These results suggest that each of us responds differently to different foods based on our microbiome composition. It is now possible to predict which foods cause glucose spikes in a person and thereby design a personalized diet to avoid such spikes. Dr. Elinav explained: "We are now engaged in long-term studies to directly compare gold-star diet recommendations with personalized microbiome diets. In diabetics and pre-diabetics, for example, we can hopefully ameliorate, or even prevent, disturbances in blood sugar control. The jury is still out on long-term benefits of this approach, but in the short term, we're already seeing great success."

In a recent study confirming this, researchers compared the effects of such a personalized diet to those of a Mediterranean diet (which is currently recognized as the best diet for controlling blood sugar) in 225 people. Remarkably, they found that the personalized diet improved glycemic (blood sugar) control significantly better than the Mediterranean diet, and these beneficial changes were maintained for a year.

Case Study: Inside Brett's Gut

Given that Brett has spent his life studying microbes, he was curious to know which in particular are in his body. And thanks to our current technology, he decided to experiment with commercial gut microbiome analysis to find out. (Disclaimer: Brett has no financial interest in this company but does know the founder given his research in the field.)

Run by Rob Knight, a well-known microbiota researcher, American Gut Project was set up primarily for data acquisition. By using vast amounts of data provided by clients, they hoped to better understand the human microbiome–think of crowdsourcing for microbes. Brett ordered a kit to be sent to him in Canada, but after several weeks, no kit arrived. After much back and forth with their helpful team, it turned out that FedEx did not like shipping sterile swabs to Canada.

Finally, after another six weeks, a kit arrived. Brett placed a small amount of his feces in a solution in a tube (usually swabbed off toilet paper) and mixed it up (this preserves the microbial DNA during shipping). You can also get skin and oral microbiota analyzed for additional fees. Fortunately, the post offices in Canada and the US had no problems shipping feces across the border. After two more months (which is a normal wait time for this type of analysis), the results were ready for viewing via a website.

The results are basically a snapshot readout of your gut microbiome at the time of sampling. You get a long list of the gut microbes that are in you, and various graphs of how your microbes compare to those of others. This is great if you are a curious microbiologist like Brett, but there are no actionable items that can be taken from the results. They do provide lists of certain microbes that are more prevalent in you than in others, your most abundant microbes (Brett had 17.7 percent *Faecalibacterium*), and some moderately interesting dot plots comparing your sample to others, including Amerindians and Malawians (non-Western populations that, guess what, have different microbes). Their website also offers some generic information on the analysis and the human microbiome. If you would like to sponsor microbiome research, then getting a test with American Gut will help those efforts. However, unless you are a serious microbial geek, the information is not particularly enlightening other than at a general interest level.

SHOULD YOU TEST YOUR MICROBIOME?

The short answer is no, unless you are truly curious about what is in your gut. There are thirty-one companies worldwide (seventeen are based in the US, and two in Australia) that offer direct-to-consumer microbiome testing, with 45 percent of them offering recommended supplements based on your test results, and actionable information. The problem is that these companies are not regulated, there is no standardization to their testing, and they use proprietary software for the analysis. There are many examples of people sending samples to two or more companies and getting different results or sending the same sample under more than one name to a company and getting different results for the same sample. They also often encourage you to send in repeated samples for continued monitoring. Finally, they ignore the fungal and viral microbiome components, which we are only starting to discover. Even if one could get a standardized reliable analysis, we still don't know what exactly a healthy microbiome looks like, and it is probably different for every person. One can gauge general trends in the composition (more beneficial short-chain fatty acid producers, for example), but one cannot currently get a microbiome analysis that then provides a detailed diet or probiotic to alter the microbiome in a defined way. There are no clinical guidelines for microbiome testing, and it is not used routinely in the clinic—partly because of the tests' non-standardization and partly because there are no clinical actions that can be taken based on test results (hence insurance companies will not reimburse for the tests). So, while everyone recognizes the importance of health and disease, microbiome testing is not currently at the stage where it can be used clinically. There is hope that in the future, microbiome diagnostic tests will become standardized, and their application can be adopted to the clinical setting.

Intermittent Fasting and Microbes

Intermittent fasting (IF) means purposefully limiting caloric intake (i.e., not eating) for anywhere from twelve to forty-eight hours at a time. There are many different variations, from alternating IF, where you eat every other day, to 5:2 IF, which means that you eat normally for five days out of the week and fast for two. Time-restricted fasting means limiting caloric intake to only a six- to twelve-hour window each day. Whichever pattern we follow, some studies show that IF has potential health benefits, including improving heart health, regulating blood glucose levels, and promoting weight loss. IF may also help achieve the kind of caloric restriction a large number of animal studies show promotes longevity, but this is nearly impossible to maintain in humans because of the severity of the restrictions (about a 40 percent reduction in calories) needed to see improved longevity.

Recent studies show that IF has temporary beneficial effects on the gut microbiome, which may help explain its benefits. An interesting study followed Islamic individuals during Ramadan. These individuals fasted on average for sixteen hours a day for thirty days. Researchers found a significant increase in the butyrate-producing bacterium *Lachnospiraceae*, along with improved blood glucose levels and BMI. However, upon stopping their fasting, their microbiomes returned to pre-Ramadan composition. Other studies have found that IF increases microbial diversity in lean and obese individuals, but for some reason these changes were not seen in those with metabolic syndrome (conditions that increase the risk of heart disease, stroke, and diabetes). The evidence suggests that IF is beneficial for metabolic health, and that this is mediated by beneficially altering the microbiome, as well as by the promotion of anti-inflammatory bacteria (increase in Firmicutes, *Lactobacillus*, *Akkermansia*) in the short term.

However, a new preliminary study suggests that IF may actually have a detrimental long-term effect. Researchers followed twenty thousand US adults who limited their eating to eight hours per day (thereby fasting for sixteen hours) for seven to seventeen years. Worryingly, the study found that this IF increased the risk of dying of cardiovascular disease by 91 percent. Those who limited their eating to between eight and ten hours per day had a 66 percent higher risk for heart disease or stroke. They also found that IF did not reduce the overall risk of death by any cause, and an eating duration of more than sixteen hours per day was associated with lower cancer mortality among those who had cancer. Thus, it seems that although IF may have short-term benefits, there may be significant long-term detrimental effects. Given these results, there are at present more established and safer ways to enhance your microbiome, such as eating a healthy diet.

In Pursuit of Longevity, Trust Your Gut

At the start of this chapter, we saw that the microbial composition of extremely healthy older people resembled the gut microbiomes of healthy individuals many decades younger. Whether this is cause or effect remains unknown: Did the "ridiculously healthy" ninety-year-olds have diverse gut microbiomes because they were active and ate well? Or was their healthy aging predicated by the bacteria in their guts? Either way, there is a robust correlation between a healthy gut and healthy aging–your microbiome is a biomarker of healthy aging.

We coevolved with our microbes to mutual benefit. Minimizing disturbances to your gut's microbial ecosystem is thus essential to health and longevity. Disruptions can have devastating consequences, including increased risk for chronic GI diseases (e.g., Crohn's disease, ulcerative colitis, IBS) and metabolic disorders (e.g., type 2 diabetes, obesity). There are significant efforts underway to identify specific "core" gut microbiota that mediate precise disease mechanisms. Diet is a major and controllable environmental factor that influences microbial composition. We're looking at new ways to influence that with personalized diets and advanced probiotics and prebiotics that may help us reestablish "keystone" species. We are even examining methods of isolating probiotic strains from healthy older people or centenarians to develop therapies intended for healthier aging. We can envision a standardized cocktail of beneficial microbes obtained from healthy centenarians' feces.

KEY TIPS

Eat plenty of dietary fiber, especially probiotic and prebiotic-rich foods: Foods that include high amounts of fiber include nuts, seeds, beans, oats and other whole grains, cooked and cooled brown rice, and unripe (green) bananas and plantains. Maintain your gut's rich microbial diversity as much as possible throughout life by eating probiotic-rich foods (e.g., kimchi, sauerkraut, kefir, tempeh, yogurt, kombucha), and prebiotic foods (e.g., asparagus, Jerusalem artichokes, bananas, oatmeal, red wine, honey, maple syrup, legumes; see more on these in chapter 16).

Don't yo-yo diet: Cycling between diets is bad for your waistline and for your microbes, since they likely remember their unhealthier composition when at a heavier weight, making a sustained weight loss more difficult.

Avoid intermittent fasting: While purposeful periods of calorie deprivation may temporarily benefit your gut microbiome, emerging studies indicate that intermittent fasting may have detrimental long-term impacts on your longevity.

Eat fewer ultra-processed foods (UPFs): Studies overwhelmingly show that UPFs are associated with increased risk of obesity, diabetes, cardiovascular disease, cancer, IBD, and other conditions. What to do? Shop in the outside aisles of the grocery store where you can find more unprocessed foods such as vegetables, fruits, eggs, and fish. Limit your shopping in the middle aisles where most processed foods are found.

Think of fermented foods as their own food group: Fermented foods such as kimchi, sauerkraut, kombucha, tempeh, and miso contain live microorganisms (with the exception of cooked fermented foods like sourdough bread). Try to eat them regularly—ideally every day—to support the diversity of your gut microbes.

Skip the stool test: Because the information is not currently actionable, don't bother getting your microbiome tested unless you are truly curious and want a long list of your microbes.

Take antibiotics only when necessary: While antibiotics save lives, they aren't always the answer. Common viral infections including the cold, flu, and COVID-19 won't respond to antibiotics. If you may need them, talk to your health care provider to determine whether the benefits outweigh the risks and side effects.

Talk to your doctor about a fecal transfer: If you or a loved one suffer from recurrent *C. difficile* infections (and potentially if you have IBD), talk to your doctor about a fecal transfer instead of another round of antibiotics. Exciting clinical studies suggest that simply transferring feces from one person to another can potentially cure recurrent *C. difficile* infections. But remember, do not try this at home!

3

Microbe Tug-of-War: The Immune System

Every second of your life, you are under attack. Trillions of bacteria, viruses, and fungi are trying to make your body their home. In response, we have developed a complex army with sentinels, guards, soldiers, intelligence, weapons, factories, and communications called "the immune system." A finely tuned fighting machine, it protects us from the dangerous world of deadly microbial pathogens, scours our body for tumors, and remembers previous dangers–even from decades ago. In a book about the microbiome, why do we have a chapter on the immune system so early on? Because microbes have a tremendous influence on the immune system from the moment we are born, which can have major effects on both lifelong health and aging. A key concept is inflammation, a normal part of the body's immune response to injury or infection. While inflammation is fundamental to fighting off infections, too much inflammation can harm our bodies. As we age, we experience increased low-grade inflammation, which causes general tissue damage. This is called "inflammaging," and represents a fundamental cornerstone of the aging process that we will encounter throughout this book. Limiting chronic low-grade inflammation is critical to a healthy longer life.

So, how does the immune system work? Let's say you're out for a hike on a beautiful summer day, and you trip on a wooden bridge crossing a stream and scrape your leg on a rusty nail. The immune system's first line of defense–your skin–has been penetrated. Nearby bacteria seize the opportunity to enter through your open wound. They multiply inside your body's warm, moist environment, at first flying under the radar. No alarm bells go off. But then the bacteria become so numerous, they start to attack your body. The immune system kicks in, trying to stop them as quickly as possible.

Your sentinel guard cells, known as macrophages, are the first to intervene. These cells patrol and protect every crevice of the body. Most of the time the macrophages alone can stop an attack by devouring and breaking down (i.e., killing) the intruders. On top of that, they muster the release of cells in the blood vessels, summoning them and other infection-fighting molecules to the battlefield; this process is what we see and feel as inflammation in the form of redness, swelling, warmth, pain, and–in certain cases–fever. An entire immunity army coordinates to attack foreign objects, stabilize your body, and prevent illness. It is a smart, efficient, and wonderfully complex system. This doesn't happen only when we trip and fall, however. The immune system is constantly in tune with the environment regardless of acute injury: It adjusts inflammation levels up and down depending on how much of a threat is encountered and how successfully it can control the invaders. Because microbes are such a key part of environmental exposure, they are intimately intertwined with the immune system and its function. The first interactions between microbes and the immune system occur immediately–when you are born. Maternal vaginal and fecal microbes encountered during birth jumpstart the immune system, and in our first few months, contact with our mother's microbes shapes our immune system, ultimately determining whether allergies, asthma, and eczema may arise years later.

Microbes and the immune system are in a constant tug-of-war throughout our lives. How do we prevent microbial pathogens from entering the body, yet tolerate the trillions of harmless and often beneficial gut, mouth, and skin microbes? In this chapter, we will explore how the body achieves that balance, as well as the startling effects that microbes can have on the immune system to both our benefit and detriment.

IMMUNOLOGY CHEAT SHEET

Discussing the immune system involves many complex components. Here are the most frequent terms we use throughout the chapter.

Antibody: These protective proteins, also called "immunoglobulins," are produced by the immune system in response to the presence of a foreign substance such as a pathogenic microbe (an antigen). Antibodies latch onto antigens to remove them from the body.

Antigen: Any substance foreign to the body that stimulates an immune response, ranging from pollen to infectious microbes. Antigens are targeted by antibodies.

B cells: A type of white blood cell, also known as B lymphocytes. They help the adaptive immune system by binding to a specific antigen, against which it will initiate an antibody response.

Cytokine: These small proteins are especially important to cell signaling during inflammation. They aid cell-to-cell communication in immune responses and stimulate the movement of cells toward sites of inflammation, infection, and trauma.

IgA: Immunoglobulin A is an antibody that plays a critical role in the immune function of mucous membranes. These specialized antibodies selectively target and kill invading microbes.

Immune cell: The overarching category of cells that make up the immune system, including types of white blood cells—lymphocytes (T cells, B cells), neutrophils (one of the first cell types to travel to the site of an infection), and monocytes/macrophages.

Lymphocyte: A type of white blood cell that responds to foreign invaders in the body; some lymphocytes work alone, while others coordinate with other cells.

Macrophage: A type of large immune cell whose job it is to engulf and destroy any invading microbes. They are some of the first immune cells to be recruited to the site of infection.

Pathogen: Any biological agent that causes disease or illness to its host, such as a bacterium, virus, or fungus.

T cells: Also known as T lymphocytes, T cells play a central role in determining the specific immune response to antigens. Types include:

- **Cytotoxic T cells:** Destroy virus-infected cells and tumor cells.
- **Regulatory T cells (Treg):** Act to control immune reactions, including dampening inflammation.

T Helper cells: Assist other white blood cells in immune system processes, and include T helper 17 cells (Th17), a subset of pro-inflammatory T helper cells.

Microbes and the Immune System

Since microbes are part of what triggers our immune systems, would we be able to live without microbes in a blissful, pathogen-free existence? Although possible (with some caveats), it is certainly not ideal, as was seen in an experiment undergone by David Vetter, who was born in Texas in 1971. Prior to birth, David was diagnosed with severe combined immunodeficiency (SCID), a hereditary disease that severely compromises the immune system. Patients with SCID die very young because they are abnormally susceptible to infections, and exposure to typically harmless microbes can be fatal.

Vetter's parents and doctors unfortunately knew what to expect because David's older brother had been born with SCID but died at seven months old. The only way for David to survive was to keep him in a sterile environment from birth and hope that a donor could be found for a bone marrow transplant to reconstitute his immune system (many of our immune cells originate in bone marrow). David was born by C-section to keep him sterile and immediately placed in a sterilized cocoon bed designed especially for him. A plastic germ-free environment would be his home for twelve years.

David occasionally ventured out into the world in a transport chamber, six times to be exact, wearing a NASA-provided space suit. Eventually he received a bone marrow transplant from his older sister, who was born without SCID, but he died a few months later from an undetected virus in his sister's bone marrow. David's story emphasizes just how critical an immune system is for survival in this world.

Although David was the only human on whom this experiment was performed, scientists have conducted similar exercises on animals since the 1950s. These required the invention of germ-free mice, who remain sterile from birth. Through various experiments using both these germ-free mice and antibiotic-treated mice, we realized that microbes are critical for normal development of the immune system. The experiments revealed a specialized immune tissue in the intestine called the "gut-associated lymphoid tissue" (GALT). GALT is the immune system's first line of defense in the gut. In germ-free animals, the GALT part of the immune system is poorly developed. The animals have fewer helpful immune cells in the intestinal wall. Similarly, mesenteric lymph nodes (where immune cells drain to) are smaller and fewer in number. Even intestinal epithelial cells have fewer receptors that recognize microbial products. Overall, germ-free animals have fewer antibodies and immune cells. What all this information suggests is that microbiota are critical for normal immune system development and function.

MYTH: Airplane air makes you sick.

FACT: The recycled cabin air on airplanes is filtered by high-quality filters and is not the direct source of you catching a cold. What could make you sick is being packed on a plane (or in a crowded airport) with other people—who have a cold or other viral infection—coughing, sneezing, or even talking nearby. Those up to six feet away could make you sick if droplets containing a virus such as COVID-19 become airborne. Fatigue, which many of us experience while traveling, may also dampen your immune system: Think sleep deprivation from jet lag, crack-of-dawn early flights, and the elusiveness of sleep when crammed into a tiny transoceanic seat. When traveling, wash your hands frequently with soap and water, potentially wear a face mask, and prioritize sleep to help your immune system. (See "Jet Lag and Snowbirds" on page 99 for more about how traveling affects the microbiome.)

We are only beginning to understand which microbes are needed for particular immune system functions. In many cases it may not be a specific microbe, but rather the presence of typical common surface molecules (especially lipopolysaccharide [LPS] and peptidoglycan) that trigger immune system development early in life. In a particularly ambitious and expensive experiment, investigators colonized individual germ-free mice with fifty-three different microbiota species normally found in the human intestine. They found that each of the different species had different effects on immune system development and activity. To contemplate the various permutations and combinations found in a normal microbiome (which contains several hundred different types of species), sorting out individual effects is extremely difficult. However, as we will see, particular microbes that affect key cells of the immune system, including regulatory T cells (Tregs) and Th17 cells, have now been identified. Clues about the critical role microbes play in controlling the immune system should allow us to better address numerous immune diseases that have become so prevalent in the world today, including allergies, asthma, autoimmune diseases, and inflammatory disorders.

Microbial Conversations with the Immune System

The intestine was historically understood as a major part of our immune system's defense system against invading pathogens. It acts as a major physical barrier inside our bodies, offering multiple ways to attack microbes before they can cause an infection, similar to a "demilitarized zone" with extremely high security surrounding a nearly insurmountable barrier. Should a microbe attempt to penetrate this zone, it is met with an arsenal of antimicrobial responses from the immune system. First, the intestine has a nearly impenetrable mucus coating. Second, it secretes antimicrobial peptides (short chains of amino acids) and specialized antibodies called "IgA" that selectively target and kill invading microbes. Third, immune cells such as macrophages patrol the gut, searching for hidden microbes to destroy. Fourth, the intestinal cells have microbial sensors that immediately recognize microbial signature molecules to trigger inflammatory responses.

As we've learned more about the gut immune system, our concept of how the immune system works in the gut has changed. Given that the immune system evolved in a sea of microbes, animals had to figure out ways to differentiate between ubiquitous harmless and potentially beneficial microbes and the few that could kill them. We now realize that there is a constant but small microbial seepage across the gut barrier. Previously, we thought that this occurred only during infections. In fact, the immune system is in continual surveillance mode. It does not turn on and off–instead, it is always idling, sometimes revving up as needed. That way it can immediately put its full force behind eradicating serious microbial threats should they arise.

A major question still dogging scientists is how the microbes "talk" to the immune system. Although there are some examples of certain microbes having close contact with epithelial and/or immune cells, the method of choice is for bacteria to make molecules that diffuse to receptors on host cells, which recognize these signals and trigger defined effects. By far the best-studied class of molecules are the short-chain fatty acids

(SCFAs). They are mainly acetate (a small two-carbon molecule), propionate (three-carbon chain), and butyrate (four-carbon chain), which have major effects in the body. These molecules are produced by certain members of the microbiota that break down dietary fiber and produce SCFA as a result. SCFAs have a variety of important functions. First and foremost, they are absorbed by intestinal cells and used for energy by the body's cells. Second, they are "anti-inflammatories" that dial back excessive inflammation, which they achieve by affecting the size and function of the network of regulatory T cells (Tregs)–the specialized immune cells that balance the immune response. This, in turn, dampens effector T cells that generate inflammation. We will see the microbiome's important anti-inflammatory benefit derived from fiber consumption and resultant butyrate production throughout this book. Third, SCFAs communicate with various cells in the body to improve tissue resiliency. We now realize that microbiome-derived SCFAs are central to most aspects of the immune system and its responses, tightly linking microbes to the immune system via these potent molecules.

On the flip side, we also now realize that the immune system has some control over shaping microbial composition. Under abnormal conditions such as an inflamed gut, where there is excessive inflammation in the intestine, or in an immunocompromised host lacking a normal immune system, there are major effects on the microbiota composition in the gut. How exactly the immune system achieves this is not well understood. Some, but not all, microbes are tagged with IgA antibodies, which would hasten their clearance by the immune system, while antimicrobial peptides that kill bacteria target certain groups of microbes, which could also influence the microbial composition.

Inflammaging: A Key to Aging

Although inflammation is needed to defend against invading pathogens, as is true most of the time, too much of a good thing can be harmful. Chronic low-grade inflammation negatively impacts the long-term health of our tissues and organs, and thereby how we age.

The efficiency of our immune system starts to wane after approximately age fifty, a process called "immunosenescence." Although the exact mechanisms of this process are not known, one thought is that long-term overloading with various antigens may in part trigger immunosenescence–i.e., over the years, our bodies get tired of constantly responding to microbial molecules. Furthermore, as we get older, we may not produce enough new immune cells to be able to continue controlling microbes. A decrease in antibody-producing cells (B cells) and other immune T cells, as well as a decreased ability to process antigens, results in a less efficient immune system overall. This is why vaccines do not work as well in older people, and why older people succumb to infections such as pneumonia that would otherwise not be as dangerous in young healthy adults.

Although the immune system wanes with age, ironically there is also a marked increase in low-grade inflammation in aging populations. This process is aptly named inflammaging. One thought is that as the immune system's efficiency decreases, it cannot keep the microbiota and other foreign bodies contained as well. These microbes seep into the body to trigger inflammation. As one ages, two major events happen: the gut becomes more permeable, and the gut microbiome becomes dysbiotic, containing more proinflammatory microbes and less inflammation-reducing microbes. This allows more microbes and their inflammatory-stimulating molecules to enter the body, causing increased inflammation throughout. Such immune stimulators trigger inflammatory responses which, through a complex series of pathways involving an increase in pro-inflammatory cytokines and a decrease in anti-inflammatory cytokines, result in low-grade inflammation. Older people (generally over the age of sixty-five) typically have significantly higher levels of pro-inflammatory cytokines in their blood than younger populations. Measuring inflammatory cytokines is an excellent prediction for determining risk of death within ten years, as well as predicting susceptibility to most age-related diseases.

What is the effect of inflammaging on health and disease? In both mice and fruit flies (the favorite animal models of scientists), limiting such inflammation both maintains healthy gut microbiota and extends the organism's lifespan. Because cytokines circulate throughout the body, inflammaging affects most tissues and organs. It is associated with atherosclerosis (the hardening of arteries, which results in heart attacks and strokes), metabolic diseases of the liver and kidney, obesity and type 2 diabetes, muscle and bone loss, cancer, autoimmune diseases, and neurodegeneration associated with depression and dementia. There are other degrading consequences to the body as this low-grade inflammation causes tissue damage. Inflammaging is at the center of nearly all degenerative processes associated with aging. The key to a healthy longer life is to limit this chronic low-grade inflammation.

Still, we cannot help but question: If inflammaging is so bad for us and our longevity, why did evolution allow it to exist? The simple answer is that inflammaging mainly occurs later in life, long after we have reproduced, so there is no evolutionary pressure to select against it. Evolution has selected traits that increase our likelihood of living long enough to reproduce, but how long we live beyond our child-producing years is irrelevant genetically. Further, inflammation is critical to our ability to survive infections and other diseases during our earlier reproductive years. That survival itself is key to longevity. So, there is no evolutionary reason to get rid of this protective mechanism, even though it becomes detrimental later in life.

What do microbes have to do with inflammaging? As you've probably guessed, everything. Scientists are uncovering major differences between the microbiomes of older people, particularly centenarians, and those of younger people. Overall diversity decreases around age sixty-five (less diversity is generally a bad ecological sign), and there is a decrease in the beneficial Firmicutes (including *Faecalibacterium prausnitzii*) that lessen inflammation. One of the processes associated with inflammation is the production of toxic reactive oxygen species (ROS), which increases overall oxygen levels and probably contributes to the decline in oxygen-intolerant Firmicutes. This also causes a bloom in the pro-inflammatory microbes that produce inflammatory molecules such as LPS. These are facultative anaerobes (meaning they can tolerate oxygen, and hence survive in the modified gut environment) and include *Enterobacteriaceae* (such as *E. coli*). A combination of the gut having fewer beneficial microbes and more proinflammatory ones, along with increased intestinal permeability, a characteristic associated with aging, collectively results in low-grade inflammation and, ultimately, tissue damage throughout the body.

INFLAMMAGING: THE BANE OF LONGEVITY

Way back in 1908, Élie Metchnikoff, the famous biologist who is considered the father of immunology, proposed that the gut microbiome was the driver of ill health associated with aging. He also believed that if he used microbes (those now found in probiotics such as lactobacilli), they would restore gut health and subsequently increase longevity and health. He believed it so strongly that he personally consumed significant quantities of probiotic-rich foods like yogurt and fermented foods. Needless to say, his ideas were severely ridiculed at the time. It has taken over a century to scientifically prove him right.

In a neat set of experiments done at McMaster University, Dr. Dawn Bowdish's team demonstrated that microbes are at the center of aging and longevity in mice. In older mice (which, like humans, had increased intestinal permeability compared to younger mice), researchers could find gut microbes outside the intestine, as well as their products such as LPS. When they tested old germ-free mice, however, as expected, these products were not found. Germ-free mice are known to live longer than normal mice. They do not develop inflammaging, have less tissue damage, and do not have increased intestinal permeability. Bowdish's team demonstrated that aged regular mice's microbiota, when transplanted into younger germ-free mice, triggered inflammaging and intestinal permeability in the younger mice. They also showed that macrophages from old regular mice were not as effective at engulfing and killing invading microbes when compared to old germ-free mice. The macrophages in old germ-free mice still worked normally and were similar to young mice's macrophages in their ability to kill microbes.

One of the most exciting studies from this team showed that blocking TNF (one of the inflammatory cytokines associated with aging) could reverse microbial dysbiosis. In other words, reducing TNF levels to help limit inflammation also returned the microbes to a healthier balance. Collectively, these experiments suggest that a lifetime of exposure to microbes and their products leads to a gradual increase in intestinal permeability and inflammaging. This also affects microbial dysbiosis and macrophage dysfunction, which in turn lead to more inflammation and subsequent tissue damage.

Knowing that inflammaging is central to the aging process, is there anything we can do to try to counter inflammation at the right time (i.e., when it becomes detrimental in old age, but not when we need it in youth)? At present, we think so but don't yet have any scientific proof.

All data suggest that inflammaging could be a reversible process, so there is certainly hope. Studies in older adults following Mediterranean diets versus control diets have shown that this diet reduces inflammaging, increases longevity, and decreases frailty, as well as many other benefits. The Mediterranean diet is also associated with keeping the microbiome in a healthier, less inflammatory state, mainly by keeping the anti-inflammatory SCFA producers that eat the fiber well-fed (and producing anti-inflammatory butyrate). Also, if probiotics help to maintain a healthy gut microbiome and decrease intestinal permeability, perhaps probiotics that reduce inflammation and gut permeability may help decrease inflammaging. When we embrace the microbes' role in immune function, as Metchnikoff pointed to over a century ago, we see many novel possibilities to control and reduce inflammaging. Sometimes science takes an awfully long time to get it right.

Microbes and Advanced Immunity

Immunologists were among the first non-microbiologists to embrace the microbiome and realize that it plays a central role in normal body function. This started with germ-free mice, which as we saw previously, had poorly developed immune systems. Soon, experiments started to show surprising results; using antibiotics, fecal transfers, or cohousing mice with mice that had different microbes (enabling behaviors like licking each other and eating other mice's feces) changed the animals' microbial composition, yielding remarkable immune effects. Nowadays, most immunology meetings contain significant microbiology components as the two fields tightly intersect, providing much excitement and a new way to look at the immune system and its functions.

Typically, immunologists concern themselves with the two main parts of the immune system: innate and acquired immunity. Innate immunity refers to nonspecific defense mechanisms that are ready to act immediately or within hours of an invading microbe's appearance in the body. These defenses include physical barriers such as the skin, antimicrobial chemicals in the blood, and immune system cells such as macrophages that attach to foreign microbes. This system is found in nearly all multicellular organisms, from flies to humans. Innate immune responses are activated by the conserved microbial signatures of invading microbes, including the potent activators LPS and peptidoglycan.

Because the innate immune system works to defend all animal and plant life, its response to invading microbes is more generic. In the gut, specialized intestinal epithelial cells called "goblet cells" secrete copious amounts of glycoproteins (proteins that have large sugars attached to them) to form the all-important protective mucus layer. As already mentioned, we have two layers of mucus in the colon: The inner layer forms a near-impenetrable barrier, which contains relatively few microbes, keeping them separated from the intestinal barrier. The outer layer is looser and contains several microbes that happily eat mucus as a food source. This provides both the microbes and their host (us) with energy. In the small intestine, where there are fewer microbes, the mucus layer lacks clear inner and outer layers. Embedded within the mucus are antimicrobial peptides produced by specialized underlying epithelial cells called "Paneth cells." These tiny molecules kill bacteria in general, or major subsets of them, much like a broad-spectrum antibiotic. The underlying intestinal epithelial cells also have a set of molecules that are designed to detect microbial signatures in case microbes penetrate this barrier. If activated, they send out messages (cytokines) that trigger inflammatory responses to further help control invading microbes.

In most cases, the innate immune system does most of the hard work to keep us alive. But if this line of defense is insufficient or should fail, acquired (adaptive) immunity comes in with reinforcements. Because of its complexity, only vertebrates (animals higher on the evolutionary ladder) have this added level of protection–simpler organisms have to rely on their innate immune systems alone to survive. Acquired immunity recognizes specific molecules on specific microbes by using antibodies (made by B cells) and particular T cells that target certain microbes. Although it takes at least a week for this system to boot up (we rely on the innate system to keep us alive that long), the adaptive immune system can create a long-term strategy for the army of immune cells and antibodies to specifically seek out and destroy incoming pathogenic microbes.

This slick structure also has the ability to remember previous encounters with a specific pathogen. After the first encounter, our body does not need to design a new defense but can refer to the previous all-out assault tactic. It happens because of the B cells, whose antibodies recognize particular molecules on microbes and neutralize the microbe expressing it. T cells then orchestrate the immune response by secreting cytokines to modulate inflammation. Subsets of T cells (cytotoxic T cells) also directly kill host cells that harbor viruses and other intracellular microbes that are inaccessible to antibodies. Having this additional layer of immune complexity allows jawed vertebrates like humans and other mammals, birds, and reptiles much more flexibility when dealing with pathogens, vaccines, etc. Acquired immunity also gives us a "backup" in case the innate system can't handle it.

VACCINES

No chapter on the immune system is complete without a discussion on vaccines, which exploit the immune system to give us further protection against some of the deadliest infectious diseases. It is highly recommended that you get your yearly influenza vaccine. Yet reports indicate that over half of Canadians do not get the flu vaccine each year, and just 57 percent of children and 47 percent of adults in the United States and 30 percent of Australians get theirs. Unfortunately, since the COVID-19 pandemic, there has been a major increase in vaccine hesitancy for various reasons (discussed in chapter 15). In mouse models, regular flu vaccines decrease inflammation, which in turn leads to less inflammaging, cardiovascular disease, and dementia. Mice that were vaccinated against the flu early in life were less likely to get chronic diseases as they aged. Unvaccinated mice got chronic diseases earlier, and when they got the flu, it accelerated the appearance of chronic diseases.

Discovery Mode

In the past two decades, we have come to realize that microbes have a profound effect on shaping the acquired immune system. Even more exciting, there are now at least three examples that identify particular microbes or their products as critical to shaping the immune system. This suggests that in the future we can use this knowledge to attempt to harness and shape immune responses.

The first major leap in our knowledge of microbes influencing T cells came in 2005, when Drs. Sarkis Mazmanian and Dennis Kasper showed that a common gut microbe, *Bacteroides fragilis*, could shape the ratio of T cells. *B. fragilis* affected the ratio that balances the immune system (called the "Th1/Th2 balance"), which is critical for a normal immune response. Germ-free animals make increased Th2 cells (which increase allergic responses), and by colonizing these animals with *B. fragilis*, the T cell ratio normalized. Even more surprising was that one of the microbe's surface molecules, a capsular polysaccharide called "Polysaccharide A" (PSA)–a sugar on the outside of the bacterium–could repair T cell balance all by itself. *B. fragilis* without PSA colonized mice, but were unable to restore this T cell defect, suggesting this molecule alone could correctly balance the immune system. We now know that PSA also triggers the production of IL-10, which is an important anti-inflammatory cytokine that dampens excess inflammation. For example, PSA can protect against experimental colitis–a disease with similarities to inflammatory bowel disease (IBD)–by decreasing gut inflammation via the T cell response. These findings were a major paradigm shift in the field of immunology as they identified a particular microbe, and its molecule, that affects T cell functions. It was the first link between microbes and the acquired immune system.

Around 2006, there was another leap forward in this field, which we discussed with Dr. Dan Littman, professor of molecular immunology at the New York University School of Medicine, where he is also professor in the Department of Pathology and the Department of Microbiology. It came about when a postdoctoral fellow in Dr. Littman's lab, Ivaylo Ivanov, was looking into recently discovered Th17 cells. These cells were found to be critical in promoting inflammation, particularly in autoimmune diseases. They play important roles in the immune response and comprise 30 to 40 percent of the T cells in the gut. Germ-free animals lacked Th17 cells (three groups simultaneously showed this), but nobody knew what might trigger their formation.

Ivanov had a hunch that microbes might influence Th17 cells since these cells are particularly abundant in the intestine. To investigate this hypothesis, he treated his mice with various antibiotics and successfully demonstrated that antibiotics could influence Th17 cell levels. Different antibiotics had different effects, hinting that a particular microbe or group of microbes could be involved.

Dr. Littman recounted that Ivanov then made yet another surprising and completely accidental discovery: "He noticed that genetically identical mice from two different standard mouse suppliers had very different levels of these cells. The differences were five to tenfold!" Ivanov even showed that if mice from one supplier were cohoused with mice from another, the levels of Th17 cells changed (mice are coprophagic and swap microbes through eating each other's feces). This finding had profound implications for immunologists. Until then, it had been common practice for scientists to order a special gene-mutated mouse (a "knock-out mouse") from one supplier, and the complementary strain with no mutation (the "parental" strain) from another supplier, assuming they would be identical except for the mouse gene mutation. Or scientists could even compare newly arrived special mice to regular ones that had been in the lab for years. Ivanov's hunch forced immunologists to cohouse mice in cages to normalize their microbiota, and to recognize that the microbiome has profound influences on the immune system. It has also called into question fifty years of immunology results based on mouse immunology!

Once Littman's group had shown that microbes are involved in the production of Th17 cells, the quest began to identify which one(s) were responsible. However, this was easier said than done. In those days, the tools to identify particular microbes were in their infancy and not wholly reliable. In an effort to address this, Brett's own lab used particular microbe DNA sequences coupled to fluorescent probes to make microbes visible under a microscope, thus enabling the researchers to get a general idea of the types of microbes that were present. This technique may have been crude, but it provided an indication of the general microbial composition. Brett will never forget the day when Dr. Littman excitedly called him up and asked for help identifying the guilty microbe. Littman's lab had stained the microbes, so in the animals that had Th17 cells, they could see long, skinny, segmented microbes that were lacking in those animals missing Th17 cells. Way back in 2000, the Finlay lab had studied rabbits that carried these segmented filamentous bacteria (SFBs) and were more resistant to pathogenic *E. coli* infections, but the lab had no way of studying them other than looking at them under powerful microscopes. So, the scientists rolled up their collective lab coat sleeves and showed that, yes, these SFBs seemed to be associated with Th17 cell production.

A year later, Ivanov and Littman, along with Dr. Kenya Honda, proved that SFBs were responsible for Th17 cell production, and that they were buried in the mucus, in intimate contact with underlying epithelial cells, in the small intestine. We now know that SFBs are a gram-positive spore-forming bacterium called *Candidatus Savagella.* These microbes are now grown in labs around the world, and intensive studies are underway to determine exactly how they shape the immune system.

The third chapter in the microbiome/T cell story came out of Dr. Honda's lab in Japan in 2011. Using similar techniques with germ-free mice, the team showed that a collection of microbes (forty-six in all) belonging to the genus *Clostridium* were needed for the proper balance of Treg cells. Even more importantly, they showed that seventeen specific human isolates (but again not a single strain) of Clostridia had the same effect in germ-free mice. This group of human microbes is now being commercialized as a potential way to modify the immune system to treat various diseases such as IBD and other immune diseases.

Collectively, these three breakthroughs (and many more) demonstrate that microbes heavily influence T cell development and function (one of the two main arms of the acquired immune system). Dr. Littman recounted that it is an exciting time as we begin to understand how different bacteria generate different types of immune responses. We are beginning to turn to animal models of autoimmune diseases to see that certain bacteria can amplify–and even cause–symptoms of disease. In a study on rheumatoid arthritis, for example, mice did not get sick if they were treated with antibiotics or were germ-free, depleted of all the microbiota. The take-home message is that contact between bacteria and the immune system in the intestine can lead to systemic (whole body) reactions via the immune system. This in turn can contribute to autoimmune diseases in sites distant from the gut.

In addition to T cells, the other major component of the acquired immune system, B cells and the antibodies they produce, is also affected by microbes. Germ-free animals are defective for IgA antibody production.

IgA is an antibody type that is secreted into the gut (and is even in breast milk) and has been shown to influence the microbiome composition by recognizing specific subsets of microbes. If a host animal (e.g., human, mouse) makes IgA in response to a particular microbe, it means that the microbe has breached the mucus barrier and triggered an immune response–meaning the immune system has been alerted to its presence, which also indicates it is in intimate contact with the body, not just hanging around the lumen (the hollow space in the intestine) of the gut. This is a way of stopping invading microbes from entering the body, and also a useful way of identifying microbes that directly contact the immune system.

When germ-free animals are transplanted with microbes, IgA production increases markedly. On the other hand, we see that IgA-deficient people naturally have more "inflammatory" microbes as part of their microbiota, and IgA-coated microbes transferred into animals seem to trigger inflammatory responses. We hope that such techniques can be used to further home in on the inflammatory microbes in diseases such as IBD, as the IgA gives clues as to which microbes the body is responding to.

The current paradigm shift in the field of immunology makes for exciting times in microbiology. As Dr. Littman put it: "What is now clear is that there are particular microbes we evolved with that are necessary for everyday functioning. Our microbes can lead to very beneficial results given their interconnections with the immune system. I think we can harness this knowledge to treat autoimmune and other diseases." While we still do not know all the mechanisms at work, Dr. Littman eats a yogurt every morning with his microbes in mind: "Hopefully we'll be able to make better yogurt soon to keep us young for a lot longer!"

Autoimmune Diseases

The immune system is designed to detect and destroy foreign microbes and particles, and as we've seen throughout this chapter, for the most part it does a terrific job. However, to function properly it has to be able to tell the difference between friend and foe: a foreign organism versus one doing no harm, happily hanging out in our body. In the case of autoimmune disorders, the immune system mistakes internal body molecules and tissue for intruders and then organizes an attack on these supposed external threats. This causes the body to attack itself for no apparent reason, the phenomenon behind a series of often-serious diseases. They are quite varied in nature, and we will go through some of the most common conditions below: rheumatoid arthritis, ankylosing spondylitis, lupus, and multiple sclerosis. Now that we know microbes' intimate connection to immunity, we have increasing evidence of how the microbiota plays a role in many autoimmune diseases. This might lead to promising new treatments for these patients.

RHEUMATOID ARTHRITIS

Rheumatoid arthritis is a chronic inflammatory disorder that affects the joints, including the hands and feet. The body makes autoantibodies that attack joint components; this leads to inflammation in synovial joints (the lubricated movable joints, such as elbows, wrists, and ankles), deforming damage to cartilage and bone, and eventual disability and increased mortality. Age is a major risk factor for this disease–it usually starts in forty to sixty-year-olds–but there are also genetic and environmental factors that we do not yet fully understand. We think that in the disease's development, the equilibrium between pro- and anti-inflammatory pathways may become unbalanced. An increase in Th17 cells, coupled with a decrease in Treg cells, would result in increased B cell production. This leads to increased autoantibodies produced by the B cells, which seems to lead to rheumatoid arthritis.

Several lines of evidence point to microbial involvement in rheumatoid arthritis. In animal models, germ-free mice remain healthy while the introduction of gut bacteria triggers the disease. Antibiotic treatment in animal models alters the outcome of disease, either worsening or improving it, depending on the antibiotic. Given that segmented filamentous bacteria (SFBs) trigger the production of Th17 cells (as discussed earlier in this chapter), putting SFBs into germ-free animals triggers the disease in a mouse arthritis model. Recent studies have shown that autoantibodies can react with common gut bacterial species, and one study identified *Subdoligranulum didolesgii* as a potential gut microbe involved in autoantibody formation–when tested in a mouse model, it caused rheumatoid arthritis, hinting that gut bacteria may trigger the disease. There is also a strong correlation between periodontal disease and rheumatoid arthritis, a recognized link being the dental pathogen *Porphyromonas gingivalis* (discussed in chapter 6). Several studies have shown that patients with rheumatoid arthritis have dysbiosis of both their oral and gut microbiota. In a study of 114 individuals, the presence of *Prevotella copri* strongly correlated with rheumatoid arthritis.

The awareness of microbial involvement has increased hope that additional therapies can be designed to help treat and control rheumatoid arthritis. However, like most things microbiota-related, we await more studies and information before we can put new therapies into practice. Diet can impact pain outcomes. People who eat high inflammatory diets have a more severe pain trajectory over ten years, and patients who adhered to a lower-inflammatory Mediterranean diet were at lower risk of worsening pain. There are no data for probiotic use in humans to treat rheumatoid arthritis.

ANKYLOSING SPONDYLITIS

Ankylosing spondylitis (AS) is another autoimmune arthritis and is characterized by long-term inflammation of the spine. It eventually results in a curved spine and stooping posture. Over 90 percent of those with the disease are positive for HLA-B27 (a human gene marker found in only a fraction of the population), although there are hints that environmental/microbial factors may also be involved in this disease. Patients with this disease have documented dysbiotic gut microbiota. They also have increased gut permeability and local and systemic inflammation. Inflammatory microbes such as *E. coli* and *Prevotella* increase in the ileum area of the small intestine, which presumably promotes further inflammation. Similar to inflammaging, scientists propose that dysbiosis increases gut permeability, which then allows inflammatory bacterial products to enter the bloodstream. This, along with altered host genetics, triggers the inflammation associated with AS. In terms of altering inflammation, probiotics were trialed but did not have an effect. Similarly, the Mediterranean diet has been proposed as a way of controlling inflammation, but there are no trials yet that have tested this. Low fiber intake has been associated with increased incidence of AS, indicating that diet may be a way to help control the disease.

LUPUS

Lupus (systemic lupus erythematosus) is an autoimmune disease caused when the immune system attacks its own tissues in the body. It can affect the joints, skin, kidneys, blood cells, brain, heart, and lungs. It is more prevalent in women: Studies show a ratio of up to 9:1 that women are more likely to have lupus than men. A red face rash, a common symptom, gave the disease its name back in the thirteenth century. Lupus means wolf in Latin, and the face rash apparently resembles a wolf bite. People with this disease will have periodic flare-ups of such symptoms, including fatigue, joint pain, rash, and fever. Like all the autoimmune diseases we discuss, there is a strong genetic factor to this disease, in addition to an environmental–microbial–one. Some studies indicate that lupus patients' gut microbiota are less diverse, with an increase in Proteobacteria (inflammatory microbes) and a decrease in Firmicutes (which are generally anti-inflammatory). Interestingly, patients also had an increase in *Prevotella copri*, which also had a strong signal in rheumatoid arthritis patients. Also similar to rheumatoid arthritis was an increase in Th17 cells, the primary immune cell responsible for the inflammatory responses and tissue destruction. In addition, there is evidence that an impaired intestinal barrier may be a factor in lupus. These are clues that correcting and restoring the gut microbes to improve T cells (increased Tregs and decreased Th17 cells) may provide new tools to help treat this disease. Future microbial therapies may be applied to reshape the immune system of lupus patients.

MULTIPLE SCLEROSIS

Multiple sclerosis (MS) is a disease in which the immune system eats away at the myelin sheath, a protective covering around the nerves, and is thus considered both an immune and neurological disease. The resulting nerve damage disrupts communication between the brain and the body. Treatments such as physical therapy and medications to suppress the immune system can help with symptoms and slow disease progression, but it cannot be cured. Symptoms can include vision loss, pain, fatigue, and impaired coordination.

Animal models have shown that changes in T cells–including increases in Th17 cells and decreases in Treg cells–result in changes in autoimmune inflammation, including autoantibody production by B cells. Germ-free mice are markedly less at risk for the disease. However, if SFBs are added to germ-free mice, Th17 cells increase, and this is sufficient to trigger disease. There are at least eight human studies comparing microbiota composition in MS patients and healthy controls. The details of microbes vary between studies, but general themes emerge. There is a decrease in short-chain fatty acid producers including *Faecalibacterium prausnitzii*, which decrease the anti-inflammatory effects of butyrate, as well as an increase in pro-inflammatory microbes such as *Enterobacteriaceae*. More recently, *Akkermansia muciniphila* and *Acinetobacter calcoaceticus* were associated with MS patients and shown to cause pro-inflammatory responses in both human blood and when added to germ-free mice. Further, there was a decrease in *Parabacteroides distasonis*, an anti-inflammatory microbe that is known to induce Treg cells. When feces from MS twin patients were transplanted into germ-free mice, these mice showed more symptoms of MS than those that were transplanted with non-diseased twin human feces. This observation is striking because MS is not an infectious disease–we cannot directly transmit it. So, the fact that transplanting microbes can affect immune system function is a big deal. A recent study suggests that a probiotic might be useful in MS. Forty MS patients were fed the probiotic *Saccharomyces boulardii* for four months. The researchers found improvements in inflammatory markers, oxidative stress indicators, pain, fatigue, and quality of life in the MS patients. An anti-inflammatory diet was tested on one hundred relapsing-remitting MS patients, and there was a significant improvement on several MS scores. Studies such as these significantly raise the hope that in the near future microbiota can be used not only as a predictor of disease, but potentially as an immune modifier for MS.

Diet and the Immune System

Although we have presumed for a while that healthy diets can impact the immune system, we are now seeing studies that definitively prove this. And of course, at the center of it all is the microbiome: diet rapidly changes the microbiome, which then influences immune response through factors such as the anti-inflammatory SCFAs produced from fiber. A couple of recent studies show that there are swift changes in the immune system following dietary changes, and most excitingly, that eating fermented foods improve your immune system.

In the first study, they used twenty people of diverse backgrounds and fed them a vegan diet (plant based, low fat, high carbohydrate, high fiber) for two weeks, then a ketogenic diet (high fat, very low carbohydrate) immediately after for two weeks, and another set of people who ate the two diets in the reverse order. Because diet studies are notoriously difficult (people are not good at honestly describing what they eat), the volunteers were kept in a research center for the month, and their immune responses monitored. The researchers made several interesting observations: First, they saw rapid changes in the subjects' microbiomes; second, that both diets affected the immune responses, with the vegan diet enhancing the innate responses, including antiviral effects, while the ketogenic diet affected the acquired (T and B cell) responses; and third, it didn't matter in which order the diets were fed. These effects were seen throughout the subjects, despite their diversity. This study nicely shows that a rapid response in both the microbiome and immune responses occurs following diet changes, and there is hope that this knowledge can be exploited further for treating other diseases.

A second recent study finally provides concrete evidence that certain foods (fermented) can be used to decrease inflammation in adults. In this study, thirty-six healthy adults were randomly assigned to follow a ten-week diet either high in fiber or rich in fermented foods that included yogurt, kefir, fermented cottage cheese, kimchi and other fermented vegetables, vegetable brine drinks, and kombucha tea. Both diets altered the immune responses. What the researchers found that was really encouraging is that those on high-fiber diets saw a marked increase in microbial diversity (good), and when fermented foods were consumed, nineteen markers of inflammation (cytokines) were decreased. Thus, if one wants to decrease levels of inflammation, this study nicely demonstrates that consuming fermented foods is one such practical way.

IS SOURDOUGH BREAD A FERMENTED FOOD?

During the COVID-19 pandemic, many more households began to make sourdough bread. Sourdough is touted as being good for you as a fermented food. Because the starter contains yeast (over twenty species of *Saccharomyces* and *Candida* have been identified in sourdough starters) and bacteria (over fifty species of lactic acid bacteria, mostly *Lactobacillus*) that ferment the flour and water, sourdough bread is indeed a fermented food. (Conventional bread has only one of three strains of *Saccharomyces cerevisiae*, and no added bacteria.) However, the baking process destroys the bacteria and yeast, so there are no live bacteria in sourdough bread, unlike other fermented foods such as yoghurt or kimchi. That said, it is considered to contain prebiotics, since the breakdown products from the fermentation contain beneficial ingredients that make it more nutritious than conventional bread. These nutritional benefits include more soluble fiber, improved mineral and vitamin bioavailability, higher levels of resistant starches (which take longer to break down and help manage hunger and weight), higher glycemic index, and decreased gluten (which makes it easier to digest, although not gluten free).

Because sourdough starters are initiated by exposure to air, each one has a unique microbiome. When analyzed, most of the yeasts and bacteria come from the flour, but some come from the baker's hands. Also, it was found that the microbial composition of starters can change over time. So yes, sourdough bread is a fermented food, but it lacks live bacteria (due to baking). That said, it does contain many prebiotics and other beneficial products from the fermentation process, and is better for you than commercial bread.

Probiotics to Enhance the Immune System?

Wherever one looks, whether online or in the scientific review literature, there are extensive claims that probiotics boost or enhance the immune system. However, when one digs deep, there is currently little data to support these widespread claims, even in the scientific reviews. There is some evidence that lactobacilli strains can prevent pathogens such as *E. coli* colonization in the gut. Similarly, these probiotics have been shown to increase mucin production and strengthen the gut barrier (which would decrease systemic inflammation). In the lab, lactobacilli strains have been shown to decrease inflammatory cytokines, but studies to assess the beneficial immune modulatory effects of probiotics in humans are sparse. One probiotic, *Bifidobacterium lactis* HN019, has shown in two clinical trials to have beneficial immune effects in older adults when consumed both orally through capsules and in milk, although there are few other trials published for other probiotics.

In This Together: The Cooperative Future of Microbe Immunology

There are two main takeaways from this chapter: 1) the microbes and the immune system are intertwined, and 2) inflammaging is a bane of longevity. We know that the immune system shapes microbial composition in and on our bodies, but we also now realize that microbes actively shape the immune system. This can affect everything from controlling infections to triggering autoimmune diseases.

Even though the immune system quiets down in later life (called "immunosenescence"), inflammatory microbial products leak into the body to cause low-grade inflammation. Years of inflammaging cause tissue damage, which results in the breakdown of the body's systems. As we understand more about how inflammaging contributes to aging, fascinating new ways of countering this process through the microbes will become available. There is significant hope that we can exploit these new findings to decrease the overall incidence of autoimmune diseases and slow down the natural degradation of body tissues that contributes to illness as we age.

KEY TIPS

Eat high-fiber and fermented foods: To help decrease unnecessary and chronic inflammation, keep your microbes happy with plenty of dietary fiber. Fermented foods contain natural probiotics, as well as prebiotics to enhance digestion and decrease inflammation.

Aid arthritis symptoms through food: If you have rheumatoid arthritis, follow a low-inflammatory diet to help with the pain. Anti-inflammatory foods include green leafy vegetables, tomatoes, olive oil, nuts, fatty fish, and fruits. Minimize inflammatory foods such as red meat and processed meats, refined and deep-fried carbohydrates, trans fats, and foods high in added sugars.

Consider probiotics for multiple sclerosis symptoms: If you are navigating MS, consider trying *Saccharomyces boulardii* probiotics. As with arthritis, an anti-inflammatory diet may also help.

Keep your vaccinations up-to-date: Getting vaccinated (including a yearly flu shot each fall) helps your immune system fight off viruses. A healthy diet can improve vaccine responses, and perhaps avoid antibiotics prior to vaccination. Don't bother with probiotics to improve your vaccine response, since there are no significant data that they work.

In general, maintain as robust and diverse a microflora as possible: Help diminish gut permeability, low-grade inflammation, and inflammaging by making dietary choices that increase SCFAs—namely eating plenty of fiber. High-fiber foods include legumes, berries, and cruciferous vegetables. Dark-colored grapes, blueberries, red berries, nuts, and dark green veggies are examples of antioxidant-rich foods.

4

Mind Your Microbes: Microbes and the Brain

The brain is key to your sense of self. It provides you with a unique identity, different from every other human, and yet our brains are what bring us all together, as the most intellectually advanced species. We didn't always have such a big head about the importance of our brains to the human species. Historically, it was thought that the gut could be a source of reasoning, hence the common expressions "gut feeling" and "go with your gut." Over the past 150 years, however, scientists came to understand that we operate with a much more top-down approach, with the brain controlling every part of the body. The process seems simple: Upon receiving signals from the brain via connecting nerves, the body obeys. But not so fast. Nerves are not doing all the work, it seems; rather the microbes in the gut have something to say about all this, too. They are in constant communication with the brain, either directly or through other mechanisms that alter the brain. This connection is turning into one of the most fascinating and complex areas of microbiome research.

We spoke to Dr. Brian MacVicar, a distinguished neuroscientist at the University of British Columbia and former codirector of the Djavad Mowafaghian Centre for Brain Health. He studies glial cells, which surround and interact with our neurons to control everyday behavior and internal functioning. His research led him to a transformation in thinking—specifically about the microglia, one of two classes of glial cells. As he told us, "We knew that the microglia were involved in infections and reactions, that they were part of the immune system. We thought they were just sitting there, and that they slowly transformed with diseases after several days." But using new technology, he and his team saw that these microglia were moving all the time, actively checking on the health of brain tissue. This groundbreaking discovery was the first step that led him to consider microbial connections to the brain.

When he first suggested pursuing gut-brain research at scientific meetings in 2012, Dr. MacVicar faced widespread skepticism and doubt. But since then, the entire neurobiology field and research climate have changed. An influential paper from Germany showed direct communication between the brain and microbiome. The researchers studied germ-free mice, which lack a microbiome, and discovered that the microglia cells in their brains were different from mice with microbes. This was a pivotal moment that demonstrated interaction between the brain and microbiome. As Dr. MacVicar explains, the discovery has huge implications for dementia, Alzheimer's, Parkinson's, multiple sclerosis, and other brain diseases.

Microbiome-brain research, he says, is now the "flavor of the week–or hopefully decade; maybe even the flavor of the next generation!" It is so trendy that the number of speculative articles about it in every major neurology journal is far greater than the handful of actual data-based, peer-reviewed papers currently published. Dr. MacVicar acknowledges that while there is much enthusiasm, lots of work and questions lie ahead for scientists to address: "We know that there is definite communication between the microbiome and brain, but how exactly do they communicate? We don't have a clue about the mechanisms yet." Understanding this process would represent a huge step in society's ability to leverage the microbiota and promote brain health.

The Gut-Brain Axis

Control of the gut's functions specifically occurs via the brain, but the communication is reciprocal and happens along what is often called "the gut-brain axis," a pathway along the vagus nerve. This major throughway in the body runs down from the brain, winds through the nerves in the gut (vagus means "wandering" in Latin), and hooks up the gut neurons (enteric neurons) with signals from the brain. The number of neurons in the gut is second only to the number in the brain, so together these two systems form a powerful communication hub.

So, how might the gut microbiota affect the brain? Increasing data indicate that microbes use three major routes to "talk" to the brain. The first involves the main conduit on the gut-brain axis, the vagus nerve. By influencing gut neurons directly hooked up to the vagus nerve, gut signals, which the microbes can also influence directly, can be communicated to the brain. The second route involves microbes making chemicals (neurotransmitters and hormones such as dopamine, norepinephrine, and serotonin) that can signal the brain through other nerve networks. The third route involves influencing the immune system, which interfaces directly with the nervous system throughout our entire bodies. And as we saw in chapter 3, microbes love to tweak the immune system.

There are two major barriers that physically separate the gut and the brain and complicate communication. The first is the intestinal wall, a tube passing through our entire body that keeps undigested food and microbes confined and transports nutrients from the gut into the body to use for energy. Although it sounds counterintuitive, what's inside the intestinal tract is actually considered outside our bodies, since this tract is really just a tube that runs through us. Several animal studies have shown that holes in this tube–aka a leaky gut–have a major impact on the brain. If microbial products leak into the body, it immediately responds with inflammation. As covered in chapter 3, inflammation does a lot of damage to our body, even as it seeks to protect it. This can result in brain conditions and many other diseases.

The second major barrier is aptly named the blood-brain barrier, or BBB. It is formed by the special endothelial cells that line blood vessels in the brain. So, although there are lots of blood vessels running throughout the brain, their contents are kept separate (except for specific nutrients and oxygen that are transported). The BBB is incredibly efficient at keeping most things out of the brain; this is why delivering chemicals/medicine to the brain via drugs is so difficult. Several animal studies have shown that microbes are needed to fully develop this barrier. Germ-free animals have a more permeable BBB because microbes influence the expression of key proteins that form seals between endothelial cells, gluing the cellular joints together to make the barrier.

Amazingly, if these germ-free adult animals with leaky BBBs are then colonized by intestinal microbes, their BBB permeability goes down (i.e., the barrier reseals itself).

Describing all the pathways and mechanisms that microbes use to influence brain activity is a large, complex, and still confusing proposition. So, instead of trying to tackle the work of future scientists, we will focus the rest of this chapter on key brain issues associated with aging–there are many! And we will explore how the microbiota might influence these major geriatric diseases. While we are still determining the extent to which we can use this information to improve cognitive health (the ability to learn, think, reason, remember, pay attention, solve problems, and make decisions), the field is a fast-moving one. For example, a study of over fourteen thousand women over the age of fifty found that those with at least two months of antibiotic use in midlife had lower cognitive function scores seven years later.

BUGS AND BUD

A larger percentage of American adults now use daily cannabis (marijuana) than daily alcohol, according to a recent national poll, and the same applies in Australia. Cannabidiol (CBD) products abound through an ever-growing menu of options, including vaping and smoking products, gummies and candies, seltzer drinks, tinctures, oils, ointments, and lotions,though these require a valid prescription in Australia. CBD is used by many for its believed health and wellness benefits, including help with chronic pain, epilepsy, anxiety, and insomnia; however, it can have side effects and isn't regulated by the FDA.

Given its rising national popularity, we wanted to see if CDB has any effects on the microbiome. A quick search of the scientific literature suggests that it may have some effect, but evidence is limited. One study showed that CBD use impacted the oral microbiome differently than tobacco or cocaine use. A metareview of nine studies looking at marijuana users found that CBD was linked to changes in the gut, oral, and vaginal microbiomes. However, in both cases we do not know yet whether observed microbiome changes are good or bad.

The Aging Mind

We've all misplaced keys, blanked on the name of a person or place, or forgotten a phone number. When we're young, we don't often pay much attention to these lapses; however, as we grow older, we increasingly worry about what they could mean. Close to four in ten people over the age of sixty-five experience some form of memory loss, known as "age associated memory impairment." There is no underlying medical condition for this; it is considered a normal part of aging, since getting older means all parts of our bodies–including the brain–can slow down. Dementia involves the loss of mental function (namely thinking, memory, and reasoning): i.e., losing one's unique source of personhood. One new case of dementia occurs every three seconds in the world, and naturally, we fear falling victim to its gradual and relentless march: to memory loss, confusion, irritability, wandering, and even the inability to speak or recognize common things.

But people frequently mix up normal age-related memory loss and dementia. Dementia involves cognitive impairment that is severe enough to interfere with a person's daily functioning. It is not a normal part of aging, and it is not itself a disease; rather, it comprises a group of symptoms of mental loss caused by a number of different diseases and conditions such as Alzheimer's disease, Lewy body disease, cerebrovascular disease, and other cognitive impairments. Nor does old age cause dementia. Age is, however, the biggest risk factor. In other words, dementia can happen to anyone, but it is more common after the age of sixty-five (four in one thousand people aged sixty to sixty-four are diagnosed with dementia, in comparison to 105 in one thousand people aged ninety and older). It costs billions of dollars for treatment and care; if global dementia care were a country, it would be the eighteenth-largest economy in the world!

Alzheimer's disease is an irreversible illness that slowly and progressively damages nerve cells in the brain. Most people's first symptom is forgetfulness–which seems harmless–but symptoms gradually worsen as more brain cells are destroyed, to the point where some people can no longer form coherent words or feed themselves. Over the past ten years, Brett and Jessica have witnessed the disease's devastating impact among multiple older family members.

The disease is increasingly common. According to the CDC, Alzheimer's represented the seventh leading cause of death in United States in 2021 (nearly 120,000 deaths), and is the leading cause of death in Australia, and is expected to increase threefold (and double in Australia) by 2050. Sadly, it is the only disease on the CDC's list for which there is no way to meaningfully prevent or cure its progression. There were over fifty-five million people worldwide living with dementia in 2020, and this number will almost double every twenty years, reaching 139 million in 2050. A person with Alzheimer's disease tends to live three to eleven years after diagnosis, although some may live as long as twenty years.

What do microbes have to do with dementia and Alzheimer's? There are several indications that the microbiota may have an impact–direct or indirect–on these brain diseases. We know that the microbes in people with Alzheimer's are unbalanced and less diverse. The rate of Alzheimer's is higher in high-income countries and communities (though predicted to rise in low- and middle-income countries given population aging and development)–a hint that increased hygiene and the Western diet, and their microbial side effects, could be contributing factors. In addition, urban areas can have up to ten times more cases of Alzheimer's than rural areas where all sorts of good microbe-rich stuff lives.

High levels of circulating sugars are not healthy for the body and brain, and as we have seen, gut microbes play a major role in both diabetes and blood sugar levels. Diabetics, who often have high levels of sugar in their blood, are twice as likely to develop Alzheimer's disease; indeed, Alzheimer's is sometimes unofficially called "type 3 diabetes."

Chronic low-grade inflammation, or inflammaging, is an especially significant risk factor for Alzheimer's disease. Alzheimer's patients have up to three times the amount of lipopolysaccharide–or LPS, a predominant surface molecule that is found on many bacteria–circulating in their blood than normal controls. LPS and other bacterial molecules trigger inflammation in our bodies, our immune system's 911 response to these bacterial signals, thinking a nasty pathogen is invading. Both dementia and Alzheimer's patients have increases in many of the normal markers of inflammation–such as cytokines, which indicate inflammation is occurring–circulating throughout the body. It is thought that this long-term inflammaging is the link between microbes, aging, and Alzheimer's disease.

Scientists know that the gut barrier and the blood-brain barrier become more permeable with age, making them less capable of keeping less beneficial microbial products out. When they seep across these barriers, we experience low-grade chronic inflammation. Gut microbes in Alzheimer's patients are different than in controls without the disease, and this dysbiosis may contribute to the increased inflammation, including increased LPS release. We also see Alzheimer's patients with increased permeability in the blood-brain barrier, which would allow inflammatory microbial products to cross into the brain and trigger more inflammation.

Certain cells in the brain respond to inflammation by increasing the production of a molecule called "amyloid beta." This forms the tangle of intertwined protein that makes up the characteristic spider webs seen in the brains of Alzheimer's patients–plaque that builds up between nerve cells. This neuroinflammation also causes other brain damage, contributing to overall learning and memory impairment, and cognitive decline. Multiple studies have shown that taking anti-inflammatories for more than two years to decrease inflammation can significantly decrease the risk of both Alzheimer's and Parkinson's diseases.

Perhaps the strongest evidence of a microbial connection with Alzheimer's comes from a traditional Alzheimer's model using mice. In this model, diseased mice have a very different microbiota than normal control animals. Several studies have shown that when germ-free animals were raised without microbes, their brains did not develop normally but they had much less neuroinflammation. When these microbially sterile mice were recolonized with feces from diseased mice, they had a much higher rate of damage than if they were recolonized with feces from normal mice.

In the Alzheimer's field, controversy rages over the claim that certain infections are associated with increased risk of Alzheimer's disease. These are infections caused by a virus–Herpes Simplex Virus (HSV-1)–or by certain bacteria; *Chlamydia pneumoniae*, which causes pneumonia and eye infections; and *Borrelia*, which is associated with Lyme disease. Although this connection has not been proven, people with a genetic susceptibility to Alzheimer's have more frequent infections from these organisms. Again, the concept is the same: increased brain inflammation from infection may trigger increased amyloid production and plaque formations, thereby triggering Alzheimer's.

Delaying Dementia

Identifying the exact ways microbes may influence the brain is a big step forward, but the bigger question remains: How can we use this information to keep our brains healthy? Although there is currently no effective pharmacological cure for Alzheimer's disease and other forms of dementia, treatments are available to alleviate symptoms. Medications such as donepezil, galantamine, memantine, and rivastigmine slow the progression of neurodegenerative diseases, and recently medicines have been approved that target plaques (although their approval process and efficacy is controversial). But you can also do a lot by proactively modifying your lifestyle and diet to minimize the risk for dementia and reduce your symptoms if you already have a condition.

There are fourteen risk factors across the lifespan that could theoretically be reduced to delay or prevent 45 percent of dementia cases worldwide, according to the *Lancet Commission*. Risk reduction starts with early life education to boost your cognitive reserve (your brain's agility and ability to improvise to solve problems and cope with challenges). But it's never too late: You can continue to "brain train" throughout all stages of life through continued education, intellectual stimulation (pursuing creative and complex activities), social engagement, and curiosity.

In midlife, it is important to protect your hearing (e.g., wear hearing protection, minimize blasting music through earbuds) and prevent traumatic brain injury (e.g., always wear a seat belt in a vehicle; helmet during contact and extreme sports; take precautions to avoid falls). Midlife hypertension, cholesterol, and obesity, which have microbial links (see chapters 2 and 7), are both risks for dementia. So too is heavy drinking (see chapter 7): More than twenty-one units of alcohol per week increases risk for dementia. Tobacco and smoking are big risk factors, which deprive your brain cells of oxygen and important nutrients. Depression, physical inactivity, and diabetes are additional risks for dementia that also involve our microbiomes. Approaching later life, social isolation and air pollution increase the risk. As you'll see in chapters 8 and 14, these are linked to the billions of microbes all around and inside our bodies.

THE MIND DIET: MIND WHAT YOU EAT

Given the links between diet, inflammation, and the microbiota, there is growing and compelling evidence that an anti-inflammatory diet affects the health of our brains via the microbiome. Two randomized trials of the Mediterranean diet and DASH (Dietary Approaches to Stop Hypertension) found that following these diets had protective effects against cognitive decline. Researchers at Rush University Medical Center in Chicago took this information and developed a new diet specifically tailored to protect the brain: the MIND diet (Mediterranean-DASH Intervention for Neurodegenerative Delay). MIND includes mainly natural plant-based foods and limits meat and food high in saturated fat.

The researchers purposefully included foods in the diet that have been shown by compelling evidence to protect the brain against dementia. For example, a number of studies have observed that people who consume high amounts of vegetables, especially green leafy vegetables, have slower declines in cognitive abilities. One large study using animals showed that berries may also protect the brain; in another study, rats fed grapeseed extract (grapes are scientifically considered a berry) digested the micronutrients and produced phenolic acids via their intestinal microbiota. This increased the accumulation of two key acids in the brain—3-hydroxybenzoic acid and 3-(3′-hydroxyphenyl) propionic acid—that are known to protect against Alzheimer's disease.

Overall, the MIND diet clearly shows a promising approach to protection against cognitive decline (and also works against Parkinson's, as discussed later). In a 2015 study, the MIND diet lowered the risk for Alzheimer's disease by 53 percent in participants who carefully adhered to it (regardless of other factors such as lifestyle and heart health). Even modest adherence to the diet reduced Alzheimer's risk by 35 percent. So, following this diet is currently among the best ways to decrease your risk of developing Alzheimer's disease. Besides, the MIND diet has components that are already proven to reduce risk for hypertension, heart disease, and stroke.

As you can see in the chart below, the diet is fairly easy to follow. Have a green salad and another vegetable every day, and snack on nuts. Enjoy a glass of wine once a day to keep your taste buds and brain happy. Here is a list of fifteen foods to include and to avoid for brain-boosting meals.

THE MIND DIET

Include these

- Green leafy vegetables: every day
- Other vegetables: at least once per day
- Whole grains: 3 times per day
- Nuts: every day
- Wine: 1 glass per day
- Beans: every other day
- Berries: at least twice per week, especially blueberries and strawberries
- Poultry: at least twice per week
- Fish: at least once per week
- Olive oil

Limit these

- Red meats: less than 4 servings per week
- Butter and stick margarine: less than 1 tablespoon per day
- Cheese: less than 1 serving per week
- Fried or fast food: less than 1 serving per week
- Refined sugars and carbohydrates (e.g., pastries and sweets): limit as much as possible

The beauty of the MIND diet is that it benefits your brain even if you are not following it to the letter, so enjoy what you like most from this list and you can still boost your microbiota.

Along with a healthy diet, it's essential to exercise your body regularly throughout your life. When you get your heart pumping, blood flow to the brain increases, providing additional nourishment. Regular physical activity reduces risk factors for dementia including high blood pressure, diabetes, and obesity. Exercise also affects microbes, as we will see in chapter 11. A growing and convincing body of evidence shows that regular aerobic exercise not only helps protect your brain from Alzheimer's and dementia but also improves your quality of life if you already have the disease. Results from several randomized controlled trials (randomly selected groups compared to a control group, the gold standard of science experiments) showed that people with Alzheimer's on aerobic exercise programs achieved higher cognitive scores, improved memory status, and felt more alert and organized and less anxious, irritable, and depressed. To boost results–and to find that much-needed motivation to get out the door–consider physical activities that are also mentally and socially engaging. Walk or jog with a friend, join a group exercise class, volunteer in a local animal shelter or garden–whatever you do, make sure it's something that you enjoy.

Parkinson's Disease

Brett has been a serious classical clarinet player since his school days, but during an early forties midlife crisis, he decided to become a "cool" jazz sax player. He began playing tenor saxophone and other woodwinds in what became known as the Oscar Hicks Jazz Sextet. The bass player in the group, Rod, is an outstanding musician who breathes, sleeps, and eats jazz. He patiently transformed the group from neophyte, classically trained jazzers (read: improvisation was not on their theory syllabi) into a reputable jazz band with actual paying gigs. The close-knit group is still together, in a slightly different iteration, many years later and actively plays in Vancouver at various venues, rehearsing and drinking good single malt whiskey every Wednesday night. Not bad for a midlife crisis, right?

About seven years ago, in his early sixties, bandmate Rod noticed that his left hand shook and twitched when it was resting. His gait also became a bit more rigid, and his face seemed tighter when he smiled. When he finally saw a neurologist, he was diagnosed with Parkinson's disease. In addition to the tremor, he struggled with fine motor control. The disease made his hand "feel like a club," and playing bass became extremely difficult. "The subtlety and nuance required for smooth technique disappears and makes playing feel lumpy, primitive, and no fun at all," he said. Rod had to quit playing bass.

Luckily, Parkinson's is a slow-acting disease. Although not curable, there are ways to control the symptoms so that "Parkies" (a self-proclaimed label) can function in society for many years. Rod used to eat a lot of meat and would often buy fruit only to let it spoil. Since his diagnosis, he has become much more aware of his diet and its potential impact on the microbiota. He makes fruit smoothies with raspberries, strawberries, bananas, and mango for breakfast; in general, he has decreased his meal sizes and meat portions. Rod previously had a sedentary desk job, but now he walks his dog twice a day and rides his bike more often. He also takes Sinemet (the brand name for carbidopa and levodopa) three times daily. Sinemet is a medication that the body converts into dopamine—the neurotransmitter that is lacking in Parkinson's and affects motor control. His symptoms are under control. As a Canadian, he's also able to experiment with high-CBD medical marijuana, which is prescribed by his doctor and which he feels helps to reduce his tremor, elevate his mood, and enhance his sleep. But as he says: That's another story for another time. To everyone's delight, Rod is back to playing strongly and reunited with everyone for gigs and practices (and whiskey tasting). There is an expression in jazz that seems appropriate as an end to Rod's story: "Play and solo like there is no tomorrow."

Parkinson's disease is the second most common neurodegenerative disease (after Alzheimer's) and affects 1 to 2 percent of the population over the age of sixty-five, and 5 percent of people over age eighty-five. It is a neurological disease with symptoms that include those Rod experienced: tremors, rigidity, slow movement, and facial stiffness. Although the symptoms first present as a neurodegenerative disease, Parkinson's may start twenty to thirty years earlier in the gut. The two most common early clues of Parkinson's are constipation in the gut and loss of sense of smell, both of which hint at microbe involvement. In addition, red meat consumption is also a big risk factor. People usually live for many years after onset, and the motor symptoms can be controlled to a fair extent by dopamine for several years. High profile people affected by the disease such as Muhammad Ali and Michael J. Fox have increased public awareness and are examples of how it's possible to continue most aspects of one's daily routine for years before the symptoms become too severe.

A protein called "alpha-synuclein" plays a key role in Parkinson's disease as the substantia nigra (a specific area of the brain that helps coordinate muscle control by producing the neurotransmitter dopamine) is slowly destroyed. The gut also expresses alpha-synuclein, which can become misfolded in the gut—think of a ball of knitting yarn that becomes tangled into a knot. Scientists think that these misfolds have a domino-like effect on misfolding synuclein moving up the vagus nerve into the brain, causing plaques to build up similar to those seen in Alzheimer's, and ultimately leading to the destruction of the dopamine-producing cells. Think back to that ball of yarn: If you just tug and pull at the knot haphazardly, the knot gets bigger and bigger until you have a giant tangled mess.

As with Alzheimer's disease, there are currently no ways of reversing the damage to the substantia nigra. Researchers have tried to use stem cells but were not successful. Healthy eating, exercise, and diet modifications (see the box on the MIND diet on page 87) seem to slow the progression of Parkinson's to some extent, and dopamine can be used to help manage symptoms.

With the realization that the gut and perhaps, due to loss of smell, the oral-nasal route, are involved early in Parkinson's, attention has recently shifted to exploring how our body's microbiota may contribute to this disease. There are no causal data yet, but there are several smoking guns hinting at gut and microbe involvement, which we'll explore here. Collectively, all the recent data point to Parkinson's disease being associated with gut microbes before brain symptoms are noticed. This constitutes a paradigm shift in thinking about the disease.

Remember the vagus nerve, or the main "telephone line" connecting the gut and brain? One line of evidence comes from a medical procedure seemingly unrelated to Parkinson's: cutting the vagus nerve to help with peptic (stomach) ulcer pain. In a fascinating study conducted between 1977 and 1995, researchers in Denmark tracked over five thousand people whose vagus nerve was cut. Five years later, researchers examined the group's Parkinson's rates. What they found was startling: Patients who had the nerve severed completely had less risk of Parkinson's than those who either had the nerve partially severed or had it left completely intact. Another Swedish study involving close to ten thousand patients who had this nerve cut supports the Danish finding, showing that complete, but not partial, cutting of the vagus nerve had a protective effect against Parkinson's. It could be that severing this nerve blocks misfolded synuclein from reaching the brain (which has actually been shown in rats), or that gut signals, including those from microbes, are blocked as a result.

A recent animal study provides even more compelling evidence that Parkinson's may start in the gut. A model of this disease used mice that overexpress alpha-synuclein, and therefore develop motor disabilities and synuclein aggregates. Researchers showed that if these mice were raised without microbes, they showed significantly fewer motor disabilities and alpha-synuclein aggregates. If researchers added short-chain fatty acids—which are produced by gut microbes—to these germ-free mice, the mice had more disease symptoms. The most remarkable part of this study is that researchers placed feces from Parkinson's patients in the mice, and the feces from the Parkinson's patients increased symptoms of the disease. Feces from the controls did not increase disease symptoms.

A common theme emerging in our discussion about aging and its associated diseases is increased chronic inflammation in the body—inflammaging. Inflammatory microbial products such as LPS—lipopolysaccharide—are a key component of this effect. As with Alzheimer's, Parkinson's patients have been shown to have increased gut permeability. The resulting dysbiosis of gut microbiota to become more inflammatory (perhaps caused by constipation) and leakage of microbial products into the body triggers inflammation in the gut as well as in the rest of the body. It is currently thought that this inflammation may occur many years before any appearance of brain symptoms and may lead to increased misfolding of alpha-synuclein throughout the enteric nerve system, including the vagus nerve, therefore moving all the way up to the brain.

So, what starts this process of inflammation? We have clues that the intestinal microbiota may play a significant role. The general idea emerging from various studies is that gut microbes in Parkinson's patients have shifted to include more microbes that produce the inflammatory molecule LPS, and fewer microbes that dampen inflammation. This causes increased inflammation, which is associated with Parkinson's.

Several human studies show that there is a difference in microbiota between those with Parkinson's and the controls without. One study found a staggering 77 percent decrease in *Prevotella* among Parkinson's patients. They found that just by measuring the decrease in this bacterium, they could distinguish between patients and controls. This is important, as there is currently no good biomarker to identify Parkinson's early, meaning doctors normally have to wait until the neurological symptoms appear in order to diagnose. *Prevotella* has been associated with promoting a healthy gut by increasing short-chain fatty acids (SCFAs) that decrease inflammation and by making vitamins. Researchers also know that the prevalence of this bacteria increases in people who follow diets rich in fiber, fruit, and vegetables. Sound familiar? The study found that bacteria thought to be more inflammatory (*Enterobacteriaceae*, which produce LPS) were associated with patients who had increased severity of motor defects. Similar differences between these microbes have been reported for another neurological disorder: autism. A further study found that Parkinson's patients had lower levels of "good" microbes associated with anti-inflammation, and higher levels of "bad" microbes associated with inflammation. Although the exact microbes differ between studies, a general theme has emerged that microbiomes in people with Parkinson's have less anti-inflammatory bacteria (less SCFA production), and increased inflammatory microbes. Both of these point to the key role that chronic inflammation plays in this disease.

Constipation is another risk factor for Parkinson's, with up to 80 percent of diagnosed patients reporting this gastrointestinal issue. The reason may have to do with the fact that due to slower transit time, constipation can lead to alpha-synuclein accumulation in the gut–which, as we know, causes it to misfold and trigger the disease like that knotted ball of yarn. Similarly, constipation could precede the microbial dysbiosis; or the microbial imbalance could trigger it, resulting in increased intestinal permeability and inflammation.

There are two rather surprising lifestyle traits associated with reduced risk for Parkinson's disease. The first is smoking, which has been documented to decrease the risk by 36 to 50 percent; the second is regular coffee consumption, which decreases risk by about one third. There are lots of ideas, and of course no concrete answers, as to why this is the case. One involves the gut. As any morning coffee drinker knows, coffee stimulates bowel movements–within four minutes, according to studies. Perhaps coffee keeps one regular, which deters the constipation so often associated with Parkinson's. Coffee also has antioxidants that could decrease inflammation, and thereby protect the misfolding of alpha-synuclein.

What can one do to decrease risk of Parkinson's or slow its progression? The answer is remarkably like that we saw with Alzheimer's, which makes sense given the role of inflammation in both diseases. Several studies indicate that regular exercise decreases Parkinson's risk and progression. A remarkable result came from Brett's scientific lab during the COVID-19 pandemic. Like everywhere, the lab shut down overnight and everyone was stuck at home. One of Brett's PhD students, who is gifted with bioinformatics, asked if there was something he could do while at home as he was bored (we all were!). We decided to look at a group of Parkinson's study participants we had been analyzing for microbial composition, but to now focus on their diets. We already know about the profound impact of the MIND diet on Alzheimer's, but nobody had looked at Parkinson's. Amazingly, we found that following the MIND diet delayed the onset of Parkinson's by over seventeen years in females and nearly ten years in males! This was a startling result, especially given that Parkinson's usually presents after age sixty-five when you are at increased risk of dying from other diseases. Additional studies are under way, but it seems that the anti-inflammatory effects of the MIND diet significantly delay the onset of Parkinson's. This provides a concrete solution to postponing the disease, as all other medications just treat the symptoms once the disease starts.

Mental Health

Depression is one of the most frequent causes of emotional suffering in later life, yet it often goes undiagnosed and is inadequately treated. Many people think that as health problems occur and loved ones pass away, it is inevitable for older people to become depressed. Not true! According to the experts, older adults who live independently (i.e., not in a care facility) have a low rate of clinical depression: 1 to 5 percent in large-scale US and international studies, in comparison to over 8 percent in the general American population. However, depression rates do greatly increase, to over 30 percent, with hospitalization and medical illness (patients with stroke, heart attack, or cancer have rates over 40 percent). As many as 50 percent of nursing home residents have depression. More than half of older adults with depression have their first episode after the age of sixty. Stress and anxiety go hand in hand with depression–as in younger adults, anxiety typically precedes depression and at least 50 percent of older adults with depression also have anxiety disorders. However, in other respects, the condition often looks different in older adults compared to younger adults; for example, older adults with depression do not generally report sadness or worthlessness. Instead, their symptoms may include insomnia, apathy, decreased energy, loss of appetite, agitation, poor memory and concentration, and physical aches and pains.

No one knows exactly what causes depression, which can make it difficult to diagnose and treat. Making the situation worse, late-life depression (especially in men) is often undiagnosed or misdiagnosed, including being confused with the effects of multiple health conditions and the medicines used to treat them. Undiagnosed depression can result in severe harm—even suicide. The latter is especially troubling, as suicide rates are higher in older people—white men aged eighty-five and older have the highest rate of suicide in the US and Australia. Just as depression has no single cause, there is no one treatment that works for everyone. Typical treatments involve some combination of therapy, medication, and lifestyle interventions.

As we've seen, the gut microbiota appears to have a large influence on brain function, much more than we ever imagined. Some recent compelling animal studies have shown that behavior, anxiety, stress, and depression are all linked to the gut microbiota. There are strong data that early-life microbiota play a major role in mood disorders. More evidence is also emerging concerning adult microbiota; for example, germ-free mice have very different behaviors than germ-filled controls, as they become more daring (like many "prey" animals low on the food chain, mice are normally pretty cautious). Even more remarkable: transfers of feces from stressed, anxious, or depressed rodents into normal laboratory animals cause the control group to exhibit stress, anxiety, or depressive behavior. The fact that these behavioral issues can be altered by simply modifying gut microbiota has profound implications for the potential of altering these diseases in humans. Many indications increasingly support this.

Two small studies recently pointed to a conclusion that people with mental health conditions have an altered gut microbiota. One looked at the fecal microbiota in thirty-four patients with depression, compared to seventeen controls, and found significant differences: Patients with depression had increased levels of the "inflammatory" microbes, such as Proteobacteria and Bacteroidetes that make LPS, and decreased levels of less-inflammatory Firmicutes, a group of bacteria including some that produce anti-inflammatory effects. The scientists also found that levels of a small molecule called "isovaleric acid," which is produced by microbes, were increased in patients with depression. Isovaleric acid–a compound that chemically resembles the neurotransmitter gamma-aminobutyric acid (GABA), which works to balance mood–can cross the blood-brain barrier, where it can affect neurotransmitter function by competing with the GABA receptor. Think of this as a microbial interference with the chemical messaging sent from our brain throughout our body. In the second study, which was of a similar size, a different group of researchers found increases in Bacteroidales and decreases in *Lachnospiraceae*–but the correlation between species was "complex" (a scientific term meaning: "we just don't know what it means yet…"). In 2022, a larger study of over three thousand people in six different ethnic groups really drove home the link between the microbiome and depression. They identified sixteen types of bacteria they called "predictors" of depressive symptoms, including the depletion of *Eubacterium ventriosum*, and the presence of *Eggerthella*. Many of the bacteria identified produce neurotransmitters involved in depression such as glutamate, butyrate, serotonin, and GABA. They also found that consuming less fiber was associated with a decrease in bacteria that produce butyrate (the anti-inflammatory SCFA). This excellent study lays the foundation for microbial involvement in depression, and much additional work needed to identify mechanisms and solutions is underway.

By far the most compelling line of evidence that gut microbes may affect depression comes from studies on antibiotic use. A massive retrospective study looked at antibiotic usage in over two hundred thousand people with depression in the UK. The researchers followed people who had been treated with a single course of an antibiotic over a year previously and found that those treated with any of the seven different classes of antibiotics had an increased risk for depression. Those who were treated with more than five courses of penicillin had a 50 percent increase in the risk for depression. They also found that antibiotics increased the risk for anxiety. The researchers found no correlation with antivirals, and only a small one with one course of anti-fungals, but not with repeated courses. This all points to the involvement of bacteria in depression, but not viruses or fungi. It also serves as a reminder that antibiotics can be harmful in ways we're only just beginning to understand. Overuse of them can affect not only our physical health, but our mental health as well.

Chronic stress can have a number of negative health effects, ranging from insomnia to weight gain, increased risk of heart disease, and disrupted immune and digestive systems. Stress increases gut permeability; scientists have measured this by stressing individuals through public speaking and cold-water treatments. A study of seventy-three Norwegian soldiers, who, on strict rations and carrying a hundred-pound (45 kg) pack, cross-country skied 31 miles (51 km) over four days, showed that stress does indeed increase intestinal permeability and inflammation, as well as producing significant changes in the intestinal microbes. As we have seen, increased gut permeability leads to an increase in the leakage of inflammatory bacterial products such as LPS into the body. Anti-LPS antibodies (which protect the body) are higher in number in patients with depression, suggesting increased LPS leakage. Further evidence for this comes from diet studies, where we see that unhealthy diets significantly correlate with chronic inflammation and depression. Strict adherence to the Mediterranean diet correlates with decreased risk of depression.

One of the ways probiotics are thought to work is by decreasing gut permeability, which may impact mood. Extensive studies in animals show that probiotics can indeed decrease depression, anxiety, and stress. There are similar models for neurodegenerative and mood disorders. However, the data in humans are only just starting to emerge, and we need more studies on large numbers of people with diverse health backgrounds. In one study of fifty-five healthy people, researchers administered either the probiotics *Lactobacillus helveticus* and *Bifidobacterium longum R0175* for thirty days or a placebo control. When the subjects were subsequently evaluated for anxiety, depression, stress, and coping mechanisms, they found that the people on probiotics fared much better. A similar study of twenty healthy people who were given a mix of probiotics showed that probiotics reduced negative thoughts associated with sad moods. But remember, these were healthy individuals to begin with. There are potentially many ways probiotics could affect the brain, including making chemicals that have direct or indirect effects on brain health (including inhibiting neuroinflammation). The above studies suggest that further investigations are certainly worth trying.

Strokes

Imagine being trapped inside your own body–paralyzed physically but still mentally "you." This is what happens in a stroke, one of the most feared health problems among older people, along with dementia. And rightly so: Strokes are the fifth leading cause of death in the United States (third in Australia) and remain a major cause of adult disabilities.

A stroke occurs when blood flow to the brain is either blocked or ruptured. The lack of blood supply causes cell death within the brain and subsequent numbness, paralysis, loss of speech, and other symptoms depending on which area of the brain is affected. Early treatment and therapy can minimize brain damage and restore function, but there is usually some residual damage to brain cells and less than complete recovery.

There are two general types of strokes. The most common are ischemic strokes, which cause blockages within blood vessels that feed the brain. Hemorrhagic strokes are less common but more fatal; they result from the rupture of a vessel in the brain and subsequent bleeding and are often caused by high blood pressure. Fatty cholesterol deposits in blood vessels are a major contributor to both kinds of strokes, as they restrict blood flow. Controllable risk factors–including high blood pressure, diabetes, obesity, high cholesterol, excessive alcohol, and smoking–account for half the risk of stroke. The uncontrollable factors that account for the other half include age (older than sixty-five), gender (men have more strokes, although women tend to have more deadly strokes), and family history.

Just like blood supply to the heart, blood flow to the brain is critical for all functioning, so cutting off the blood supply will have other major implications for the body besides strokes. The health of the arteries that supply the blood is critical for both the brain and heart–and the rest of the body. Plaque–consisting of cholesterol and fats–can build up and plug the arteries, which causes cardiovascular disease (CVD), and blocked arteries directly affect the brain through strokes. We'll discuss heart attacks, strokes, CVD, and the microbiota in much more detail in chapter 7.

The microbiota has major effects on blood vessel health, which affects CVD and, by extension, strokes. When you eat red meat, the microbiota in the meat itself convert its components into specific compounds (trimethylamine, or TMA); the liver then converts these compounds into a derivative compound (trimethylamine N-oxide, or TMAO) which then causes plaque accumulation and CVD. Without red meat and its accompanying microbes, these compounds don't form, which drastically reduces the incidence of CVD and stroke. Eating red meat enriches the microbiota that produce these problematic compounds, and the differences in microbiota (and TMAO levels) can, in a crude sense, be used to provide an indication for risk of stroke.

There are easy ways to decrease the risk of CVD, including reducing red meat consumption and increasing fiber intake. The latter seems to be an especially good way of decreasing stroke risk; we can look to studies involving vegans and vegetarians–who consume a lot of plant-based fiber–and germ-free mice, which have no microbes. All have little to no CVD. Most likely, this has something to do with the microbiota, since fiber has profound effects on microbiota composition. A recent meta study (a compilation of the findings of many studies) found an inverse correlation of stroke risk and fiber intake. Increasing dietary fiber by just 7 g per day lowered the stroke risk by 7 percent. To put this in perspective, the average fiber intake in the US for women is 13 g per day (recommended is 21 to 25 g), and for men it is 17 g per day (recommended is 30 to 38 g). In Australia, it's 21 g for women (recommended is 25 g); and 25 g for men (recommended is 30 g). Seven g of fiber roughly translates into a 70 g serving of whole wheat pasta (approximately two thirds of a cup) along with a fruit and a serving of tomatoes.

In addition to affecting CVD and resulting strokes, the microbiota may also play a role in poststroke recovery. When the microbiota is measured in poststroke patients, it shows signs of dysbiosis within twenty-four hours of the stroke, and the worse the stroke, the larger the change in microbiota composition. This is an interesting finding, but we have no idea what the implications are. However, there are some more concrete clues that the microbiota may affect the outcome of the stroke. We know that the microbiota has a large impact on the immune system and resulting inflammation (see chapter 3). Tissue damage following a stroke frequently occurs due to inflammatory damage by the immune system. Here, antibiotics can play a positive role, as stroke victims are often given antibiotics to control poststroke infections. In animal studies, treatment with antibiotics reduced the brain injury, due to the decrease in the activation of key immune pathways. This included an increase in cells that dampen inflammation (regulatory T cells), and a decrease in those that cause more tissue damage (delta gamma T cells, a subset of T cells that promote inflammatory responses). Antibiotics can't be used to prevent strokes in people for many reasons, including general antibiotic resistance and the profound upsetting impact of antibiotics on the microbiota. However, other tools are becoming available to identity the microbes involved in stroke and, accordingly, manipulate the microbiome to curtail strokes and/or improve recovery.

JET LAG AND SNOWBIRDS

A dream retirement often includes visions of long periods of luxurious, exotic travel. Without the burden of work or dependent family members, you may finally have the time to explore some of the many wonders and corners of the world. In Canada, a major national pastime is called "the flight of the snowbirds," referring to the many retirees who flee their snowbound home cities to spend the winter on a warm beach, returning like clockwork only when spring has sprung. However, long-distance travel comes with a major discomfort: jet lag. Groggy head, lack of energy, severe sleep deprivation, random junk food cravings, and increased appetite . . . yuck, you know the feeling! For the first few days, it is hard to really enjoy the beach; you may even fall asleep midday and get a severe sunburn to help you painfully remember the trip. Jet lag and other disruptions of the body's internal clock, or circadian rhythm, are not just associated with these short-term changes, but also with higher rates of obesity, diabetes, and cancer. These diseases all have a microbial link. What has become apparent in the last couple of years is that the microbiota is tightly linked to jet lag and other body-clock rhythm disruptions in ways we never previously dreamed of.

Circadian rhythm is under the rule of the hypothalamus, an area of the brain that is regulated by light and other factors to control sleep, appetite, and similar daily rhythms. However, we now know that other parts of the body also have their own molecular clocks that sync up to the brain. For example, there is a clock that causes the liver and intestine to "wake up" when it is time to digest a meal during the day, or slow down while we are asleep. In 2014, scientists discovered that the intestinal microbiota underwent circadian rhythms of their own. The scientists engineered genetic mutations in some of the molecular-clock genes of mice, which impaired the rhythmic oscillations of their microbiota. They found that the body's clocks actually control the microbiota, with cyclical changes occurring in about 15 percent of the microbial species. The scientists could even recognize characteristic "time of day" microbial species. These changes could be overridden by regular feeding hours, meaning that the mice could get back to normal daily body rhythms with regular mealtimes—just as we humans get over jet lag after a trip. If irregular feeding times were implemented, the main brain clock of the mice became uncoupled from the more local clocks, such as the intestinal clock, which causes the intestine to "wake up" to digest a meal and slow down when asleep. This study affirms what we already suspected, that mucking up the biological clock affects many biological processes, including digestion and the gut microbiota.

Any such changes in metabolic activities—how we break down molecules to get energy—can also lead to obesity and diabetes. For example, scientists transferred feces from a jet-lagged mouse—or from humans (in this case, graduate students flying around the world to attend a scientific meeting)—into germ-free mice. If you're curious how a mouse gets jet lag, you don't actually fly the mouse around the world—just shift the lights in the mouse-house by eight hours for three days, then shift them back again. Researchers found that the metabolic symptoms of jet lag (think carb and junk food cravings) associated with obesity and diabetes could be transferred to the newly colonized mice. The infusion of jet-lagged feces disrupted the mice's microbiota enough to affect their metabolism and make them more prone to diabetes and obesity. The scientists also found that feeding mice high-fat diets was detrimental to their circadian rhythms (and microbiota and expanding waistlines). Other mouse studies showed that female mice were more susceptible than male mice to jet-lag changes in the microbiota, that alcohol worsened the changes in both sexes, and that even intestinal infections were increased given disruptions to normal sleep and rest time.

So, how can we use this information to ensure we enjoy our next transatlantic holiday to its fullest? Unfortunately, we are still at an early stage of understanding, and since most of the studies have been done in animals, we can't draw human connections. However, some themes are becoming apparent. High-fat diets and alcohol both worsen jet lag. Both eating at your regular at-home mealtimes and exposure to daylight help you and your microbes adjust more quickly to your current beach time. The hope is that as we understand these complex interactions more, we can develop a probiotic or a prebiotic to lessen the sleepless nights that follow travel.

The Future

Of all the body sites discussed in this book, the brain stands to gain the greatest future potential improvement in lifelong well-being and healthy aging thanks to microbiome findings. We've seen that Alzheimer's, Parkinson's, dementia, anxiety, stress, depression, and strokes all have microbial aspects. Through more studies, we'll gain a clearer idea of how well the MIND diet works and be able to design even better diets for our brains. With advances in testing, we'll hopefully be able to accurately profile gut microbiota to identify individuals at risk for cognitive diseases, and in some cases, even make an early diagnosis before the damage is done. And with the next generation of probiotics–scientifically engineered "cocktails" of beneficial microbes–we anticipate benefiting from "mind-altering" microbes, thereby gaining more control over–or even preventing–depression and other mental health conditions. There may be drugs that target microbial enzymes in order to prevent strokes and cardiovascular disease, and probiotics that can be used to reconstitute good microbes following antibiotics and to help with recovery from strokes. All in all, we can expect to leverage our microbes to fight cognitive decline and hopefully diminish some of the greatest fears associated with aging.

KEY TIPS

Know your risk: If you're concerned about Alzheimer's, you may consider getting tested for the gene ApoE4. A single copy of the faulty gene doubles or triples your risk (it doesn't mean you will get it for sure, it just increases your risk), while having two copies increases your risk eight to twelve-fold. Knowing if you are at increased risk may be added motivation to take all possible lifestyle steps to protect your brain.

Avoid unnecessary antibiotics: Using antibiotics only when necessary may help lower your risk of depression and other mood disorders, in addition to Alzheimer's disease.

Give your brain a workout: The brain is no different from the rest of your body—it needs exercise to stay healthy. Aerobic exercise gets your heart pumping, which boosts blood flow to the brain. This improves brain function and protects your brain from Parkinson's, Alzheimer's, and dementia. Exercise also decreases stress, improves mood, and has positive impacts on your microbes.

Trade your T-bone for a turnip: A diet high in fiber like the MIND diet is associated with significantly lower risk of stroke, Parkinson's, and Alzheimer's, while red meat increases risk. High-fiber foods good for the brain and intestinal microbes include whole grains, fruit (e.g., berries, pears, apples), vegetables (e.g., leafy greens, root vegetables), beans, nuts, and seeds.

Get plenty of sleep: Sleep is essential for brain health—not to mention its impact on the microbiota. Lack of regular, solid pillow time (such as when you're jet lagged) can cause problems with memory, thinking, and mood.

Enjoy your morning cup of java: Besides helping with constipation and keeping you regular, coffee may also decrease risk for Parkinson's and Alzheimer's.

5

Your Microbes Are Glowing: The Skin Microbiome

We all want to live long, healthy, and fulfilling lives. But we don't exactly want the long part to show on our face and skin. From hair dyes and anti-wrinkle creams to Botox and surgical facelifts, it seems that there is no limit to the ways we try to preserve our appearance. With age, the skin becomes more fragile and more vulnerable to damage. Despite the staggering number of commercial products and DIY skincare concoctions available, anti-aging therapies often lead to mixed results. Attempts to "turn back the clock" on sun damage and minimize wrinkles and age spots in general have plateaued. Retinoids–considered among the best anti-aging products available–have been around since the 1980s, and the pace of innovation for other topical products such as moisturizers and serums has slowed. A new approach to aging skin and its care is sorely needed.

Inflammatory skin disorders such as eczema (also called "atopic dermatitis"), skin allergies, and dry or irritated skin are also rapidly on the rise. This increase is largely attributed to Western lifestyles, complicated by sealing ourselves away from beneficial microbial exposures in climate-controlled buildings, destroying skin microbial communities through overuse of antibacterial hand sanitizers and antibiotics, and eating highly processed diets that starve our microbes. Inflammatory skin disorders are linked to a decrease in the diversity of the skin microbiome and an increase in skin pathogens.

For years, conventional wisdom dictated that we use antibacterial agents (e.g., topical antibiotics, rubbing alcohol, hydrogen peroxide) to blast "bad" bacteria, which was partially the cause of blemishes, aging, and illness of the skin. However, researchers are discovering that these toxic antibacterial products are, in many cases, far more dangerous to overall skin health than any bacteria they are designed to kill. We now realize that microbes have a critical, and most often positive, role in skin health. They can reduce wrinkles, dryness, sun damage, resistance to infections, acne, and even body odor. Compared to the killing effect of antibacterials, microbes keep our skin healthy and strong: They alter and educate our immune system, enhance the skin's ability to keep out foreign invaders, and even help in wound healing. They outcompete certain disease-causing pathogens, meaning that the resident microbes occupy any potential colonization site available to pathogens and block those incoming pathogens to nutrients and places to bind. As a result, there is a lot of potential for microbial strategies to rejuvenate our skin in adulthood, even after the damage is done. A better understanding of how these microbes work offers new ways to age gracefully inside and out.

The Best Foundation Is Healthy Skin

We are completely coated in microbes. There are approximately one million bacteria composed of hundreds of species on every square centimeter of our bodies. They predominantly live on the skin's surface, with smaller numbers deeper down in our pores. Skin contains the body's fourth-largest collection of microbes after the gut, oral, and vaginal areas, although it is less studied than the gut microbiome. Have a look at your hand–there are over 150 species on one palm alone. Although we tend to think of our skin as homogeneous, from a microbial point of view it comprises immensely different environments: both the moist, warm areas–the "tropics" of your groin, armpits, navel, and between the toes–and drier surfaces; the "deserts" of your forearm, buttocks, and hands. Although we don't know why, the dry areas of the skin have the most diverse composition of microbes but lower microbial numbers. (Just like plants, microbes need moisture to grow.) There are even microbial differences between the sides of our bodies. One study found that we share 68 percent of microbes between the left and right forearms, but only 17 percent between the left and right hands. While alarming at first, this difference makes perfect sense: In the last five minutes, which hand did you use to pick up a pen, scratch your head, or scroll on your phone? The things our two hands touch vary wildly, whereas our forearms are used in a much more even capacity.

What do these teeming colonies of surface microbes do to us? In addition to outcompeting harmful microbes, they also produce molecules that counter specific pathogens. For the most part, they go about this business silently, breaking down fats and other molecules produced by our skin for food so that they can be our strongest first line of defense. To do this well, they also train and educate our immune system by reporting on the state of our skin surface, so the immune system can better recognize, respond to, and defend against foreign invaders.

One microbe that illustrates these concepts is *Cutibacterium acnes* (*C. acnes*, previously known as *Propionibacterium acnes*), so named for its involvement in acne. This microbe breaks down the triglycerides (fats) in sebum, an oily secretion that is produced by our skin glands. Breaking down these molecules produces fatty acids, which in turn acidify the skin. This acidity is important and necessary to block pathogens such as *Staphylococcus aureus* (*S. aureus*) from causing infections on the skin, as the bacterium prefers a more neutral pH. In fact, people with atopic dermatitis (an inflamed skin disease) have lower levels of beneficial microbes, and higher levels of pathogenic *S. aureus*. Another common skin inhabitant, *Staphylococcus epidermidis* (*S. epidermidis*), works for our benefit by lowering the pH and secreting molecules that kill pathogens like *S. aureus* and group A *Streptococcus*—pathogenic bacteria that can cause a variety of illnesses, ranging from minor skin infections and medical conditions such as pimples, cellulitis, atopic dermatitis, abscesses, and strep throat to life-threatening diseases such as pneumonia, endocarditis, and sepsis. A recent study showed that certain normal skin microbes, including *S. epidermidis*, secrete these antimicrobial peptides in order to kill off the competition vying to live on the skin. The researchers found that when these beneficial microbes were added to the skin of patients for twenty-four hours, the number of *S. aureus* (the pathogen) decreased. The takeaway from all this seems to be that we can actually benefit from this ongoing microbial warfare on our skin. But if we lose the beneficial microbes, we also lose their protection.

A MICROBE-FRIENDLY TREATMENT FOR MINOR CUTS AND BURNS

With three children crawling and running around, Jessica constantly hears, "Mom! I have an owie!" While it might seem logical to apply an antibiotic cream or ointment to a minor cut, burn, or other wound, these products may actually irritate your skin and contribute to antibiotic resistance (when microbes develop the ability to survive the drugs designed to kill them). Infections caused by antibiotic-resistant microbes can be difficult—and sometimes impossible—to treat.

The Australasian College of Dermatologists recommends washing the cut gently with clean water or saline, after stopping bleeding by applying pressure with a clean cloth or bandage for about five minutes. Carefully pat the area dry with a clean towel or pad and cover with a non-stick dressing. Antibiotic creams are generally not recommended unless prescribed.

Most minor cuts and wounds (even from surgery) do not require antibiotics. For minor burns, the Australasian College of Dermatologists recommends not using ice, creams or alternative treatments, and protecting the burn with a clean, non-stick dressing to reduce pain and stop infection. Seek immediate medical attention if you notice any signs of infection such as pus, increased redness, swelling or warmth, or fever.

Beauty Is Skin Deep

While you wouldn't want to go around guessing people's ages by their faces, from a microbial perspective, it's completely possible to do so. Because microbes are our essential companions as we age, and respond to our ever-changing internal and external environments, we can tell someone's age within a decade just from analyzing a microbial swab of the forehead. Remarkably, people over the age of fifty have distinctly different microbial signatures than younger adults. Scientists are just beginning to uncover exactly how and why the skin's microbiome shifts and loses diversity as we age. No matter the reason, this phenomenon speaks to the critical need to enhance and maintain your skin microbiota as a robust ecosystem throughout life. Cosmetic companies have picked up on this fact: You can now find commercial skincare products that incorporate emerging microbial scientific discoveries into topical applications. L'Oréal, for example, patented several bacterial treatments for dry and sensitive skin; Estée Lauder patented a skin application with *Lactobacillus plantarum*; and Clinique sells a foundation with *Lactobacillus* ferment (a probiotic extract). Products such as La Roche Posay Lipikar Baume AP, used to treat eczema and other dry skin issues, likewise include bacterial additives to help restore a healthy skin microbiome and to stop itching. Keep an eye out for these and more emerging microbial skincare lines.

Despite this progress, Dr. Greg Hillebrand, a recently retired senior skin scientist at Amway, a major health and beauty corporation, believes there is still a serious need for new methods and treatments for aging skin. "The pace of innovation in the anti-aging category is slowing. Conventional topical products like moisturizers, serums, and essences contain active ingredients aimed at preventing or reversing the signs of aging. Retinoids [a class of active ingredients] remain the gold standard, yet they have been around since the 1980s. The skin microbiota represents an exciting new focus area for us, and it's the next best opportunity to solve many of the challenges associated with aging skin." Dr. Hillebrand's enthusiasm for the use of microbes goes back to 1995. He was sent to Japan by his former employer, Procter & Gamble, to figure out exactly how skin care products worked by studying a prestige skincare line that consisted of a concentrated fungi ferment cultivated, processed, and filtered down into an essence product. "Many of my colleagues at the time did not actually believe it did anything; they all thought it was 'foo-foo dust.' I was only there for a few months when my director from the US came over to see how I was doing. I was excited to share my progress and ideas and met with him and my VP. I told them that I thought it might be possible that the fermented filtrate worked in part by favorably modulating the bacteria on the face in a way that we didn't yet understand. Basically, I was proposing that the use of the product might shift the bacterial composition, perhaps maintaining the good ones and not the bad ones on the face." In 1995, we didn't yet appreciate the concept of "good" and "bad" bacteria on the skin–it simply wasn't conceivable that the skin microflora were important, and we certainly didn't culture bacteria specifically to benefit the skin–so it was not surprising that the reaction of Dr. Hillebrand's director to this novel idea was less than enthusiastic.

Thankfully, Dr. Hillebrand followed his hunch. Flash forward to the present day and Amway now explicitly focuses on microbes. Much of their efforts involve data gathering to better understand this emerging area. Amway set up a clinical test site during a major art event in Grand Rapids, Michigan, where they figured there would be a large variety of patrons of all ages in attendance. The Amway team measured the skin microbiome of hundreds of festival-goers via swabs of their scalps, foreheads, forearms, and nasal/oral areas. The samples showed fascinating differences in microbial communities, especially associated with people's ages. Describing this particular sampling, Dr. Hillebrand grew animated at the prospects of how we can use these microbial differences to enhance appearance and health of aging skin. While gaining traction, he admits that the concept of embracing, rather than eradicating, bacteria on skin remains as foreign today as the discovery of groundbreaking topical products was thirty years ago. But he remains optimistic: "With the microbiome, we can actually *do* something. The challenge now is to figure out exactly how to leverage science into more effective skin products for real innovation."

MYTH: Antibacterial soaps are necessary to sanitize your hands.

FACT: You do not need to use antimicrobial soap to get the job done: Using regular household soap with a proper handwashing technique is generally a better way to remove germs.

Skip the Antibacterial Soap

One of the few certainties we have when it comes to the microbiome–and a common theme throughout this book–is that we need to become *less clean* in our everyday practices and allow a diverse microbiome to flourish. A fine line exists between being hygienic and over-sanitized. When caring for sick or older people, hand sanitization is a common, and often mandated, practice. This became even more prevalent during the COVID-19 pandemic (see chapter 15). Hand sanitizer dispensers dot the halls and carts of nursing homes, hospitals, and clinics, where spreading bacteria could wreak havoc on patients who have a variety of serious illnesses and compromised immune systems. Every day in the United States, about one in thirty-one hospital patients (about one in a hundred in Australia) has at least one health care-associated infection—while they're being treated for something else.

But we're often, and unnecessarily, encouraged to use antimicrobial cleaning supplies and disinfectants in daily life to prevent the spread of infection. Visit any high-traffic tourist area, grocery store, or restaurant and you'll be blasted with squirts of astringent hand sanitizer. According to a US Food and Drug Administration (FDA) statement on the safety and effectiveness of antibacterial soaps, hand sanitizers do not uniformly prevent the spread of germs, as we all thought. In fact, the FDA ruled that companies can no longer market "antibacterial" washes containing certain ingredients (the most common being triclosan and triclocarban) because manufacturers did not sufficiently demonstrate that the ingredients are effective for long-term daily use. Repeated antibacterial handwashing seriously disrupts the skin microbiota, which can result in various skin irritations, disorders, and infections. Some data even suggest that these antibacterial ingredients may do more harm than good over the long-term—for individuals and the whole population—by creating hardier, more resistant bacterial strains.

Alcohol-based hand sanitizers kill most of the microbes on your hands, good and bad. However, they cannot kill spores of *Clostridium difficile* (*C. difficile*), a common pathogen in health care settings that causes severe diarrhea and other potential complications (as we saw in chapter 2). To ward off these bacteria, regular soap and water is all you need! With a *C. difficile* infection, a health care provider should wear gloves to examine patients and wash his or her hands before and afterward; wearing gloves alone is not enough to prevent the spread of infection. Surprisingly, according to the Centers for Disease Control and Prevention (CDC), health care providers clean their hands less than half of the times they should. Patients and loved ones can play a role by both politely reminding health care providers to clean their hands and serving as a good example by doing so themselves. This simple step is generally the best way to avoid getting sick and spreading germs to others.

THE CDC RECOMMENDS HANDWASHING

- Before preparing or eating food
- Before touching your eyes, nose, or mouth
- Before and after changing wound dressings or bandages
- After using the bathroom
- After blowing your nose, coughing, or sneezing

If soap and water is not an option or you have to use a hand sanitizer—such as in a senior care home where this practice is mandated for employees—the CDC recommends that it be an alcohol-based hand sanitizer containing at least 60 percent alcohol. Put the product on your hands and rub them together, covering all surfaces until the hands feel dry. This should take approximately twenty seconds. The FDA's antibacterial soaps ruling does not apply to health care settings, so be sure to inquire about the use of these products when in these locations.

An Eye for an Eye

Why are contact lens wearers at risk for frequent eye infections? It may have something to do with the delicate balance of our ocular microbiome and what happens when it comes into contact with the skin. If we displace the eye's microbiota through bacterial organisms introduced on contact lenses, this could affect the eye's ability to fight off infection. Brett conducted such an experiment in grad school: He washed one of his contact lenses with the usual cleaning solution, containing enzymes that break down proteins and other gunk on the lenses, and put the contact lens under a powerful scanning electron microscope. It was a terrifying sight! Instead of having a nice pristine lens surface, the contact was coated in a thick blanket of microbes. To top it off, this was the first biofilm Brett had ever seen; needless to say, it's an image he will never forget—especially when putting his contacts in every morning.

There is also a practical link between contact-related infection and age. Because eyesight shifts with age, and many of us rely on contact lenses instead of glasses to correct vision, our microbe-coated hands and eyes have more chances to swap bacteria. In an experiment of twenty volunteers, researchers found the ocular microbiota of contact-wearers more closely resembled that of the body's skin rather than the standard eye microbiota. In other words, constant blinking and tears–which contain natural antimicrobial substances–keep our ocular microbiota load low most of the time. Regularly touching our eyes can shift this balance.

The take-home message is to be aware of the microbes living in the moist biofilm of contacts. Under normal conditions, the eye's surface can overcome these pathogens; however, trauma, surgery, disease, and, notably, age make eyes more vulnerable. Washing your hands before applying or removing contacts helps immensely, as does cleaning the contacts and storage case thoroughly with contact lens solution (which contains substances that inhibit microbial growth). Don't think you're off the hook if you are only an occasional contact wearer: Organisms transferred to the lens from the skin during removal that are not destroyed by the disinfecting solution can proliferate over time in a static lens case. Since learning this, Jessica (an occasional contact lens wearer) has opted for daily disposable contacts after her reusable lenses regularly sat unused for weeks.

Scientists have successfully applied antimicrobial coatings to biomedical devices such as artificial hips and other objects that are implanted in the body, so a logical next step is to apply this to contact lenses. Currently, there are several options commercially available, and animal models offer promising evidence that antimicrobial treatment for contact lenses can decrease risk of eye infection. It's unclear, though, how these coatings will affect the eye microbiota as a whole.

Simply Sebum

Rub your finger along the crease of your nose: feels oily and greasy, right? Despite popular misconception, this layer of oil is normal. It's a substance called "sebum," which the body secretes out of hair follicles to keep the skin moist and supple, especially on the face. If sebum becomes trapped in a hair follicle it can lead to a buildup of the acne-causing *C. acnes*. Often the bane of teenage years (when you produce more sebum), acne can unfortunately flare up again around menopause for women. Whether we are fifteen or fifty years old, the root cause is the same: changing hormone levels. As relative testosterone levels rise, the skin's sebaceous glands can go into overdrive and produce excess sebum. But whereas things eventually level out once puberty ends, in older women the problem is exacerbated by slower cell regeneration and prolonged buildup of *C. acnes*. Frustrating acne blemishes can pop up near the chin, jawline, and sometimes, upper neck. Unlike the superficial zits teens get on their T-zones, these blemishes are often more like cysts, smaller and more tender, deep below the skin—hence their being more painful and difficult to remove.

Thankfully, this pimply condition diminishes once a woman settles into postmenopausal hormone levels. In the meantime, skin should be treated kindly: Do not strip it with a strong astringent if the skin is not oily. Probiotic applications that supplement the skin's microbiota with a beneficial microorganism might offer promising treatments for older women's acne. One study found that *S. epidermidis* is important to keep *C. acnes* in check. Succinic acid, a fatty acid fermentation product of *S. epidermidis*, inhibited *C. acnes* growth. *S. epidermidis* is not commercially available as a probiotic, and researchers are still developing succinic acid as an organic peroxide acne treatment, particularly for those allergic to benzoyl peroxide. Other antimicrobials such as topical benzoyl peroxide and oral tetracyclines (oral antibiotics) will suppress *C. acnes*. In a recent clever twist, researchers genetically engineered a strain of *C. acnes* to produce a molecule that decreases sebum production. Their hope is that the bacterium that causes acne might actually be used to prevent or treat it!

While oily skin can become troublesome in late middle age, even more common in later life is the opposite problem: The reduction of sebum production, which requires additional lubrication of the skin to protect against pathogens. Sebaceous glands produce less oil as we age. Men experience a minimal decrease after around age eighty, but women gradually start producing less oil after thirty (and even less after menopause). This leads to dry and cracked skin, particularly around the drier skin sites of the knees and elbows. Dryness may be exacerbated by dysbiosis (a microbial imbalance), which further disrupts the skin. One way to combat this tendency and thus protect normal microbes is to bathe less often and only in moderate temperature water. Frequent hot baths can remove moisturizing lipids and oils from the skin and may disrupt the helpful microbes and their defenses against pathogens. We'll see later that particular microbial applications, such as the probiotic *Lactobacillus plantarum*, offer promising options to moisten and nourish dry skin.

Ironing Out the Wrinkles

How would you characterize aging skin? Translucency, age spots, and wrinkles probably come to mind. Although microbes turn out to be key players in these signs of age, they can be used to our benefit to improve overall skin appearance. In a riff on personalized medicine, a research group extracted *S. epidermidis* from twenty-one women aged thirty-nine years on average. The scientists grew each person's individual strain in the lab, and then asked the women to add it–or a placebo–to a mixture, and then apply the mixture to their face before bed twice a week for four weeks. In the double-blind study (neither the participants nor the scientists knew which group any one participant belonged to), they found that this treatment increased skin lipid content, decreased water evaporation, and markedly improved skin moisture retention while maintaining healthy acidic skin conditions. This suggests that we may soon be able to cultivate our own skin microbes for immediate and future facial rejuvenation. If so, we could biobank our youthful skin microbes to apply them later in life when wrinkles and dry skin are more of an issue. An intriguingly novel approach to personalized skin care!

There is also some evidence that specific probiotics can be used to target and improve skin appearance. In a separate randomized double-blind, placebo-controlled trial, 110 volunteers aged forty-one to fifty-nine were fed ten billion *Lactobacillus plantarum*, a harmless probiotic, daily for twelve weeks. The investigators found significant increases in skin water content in the face and hands; this hydration boosted the skin so that it appeared healthier with fewer wrinkles. The probiotic significantly decreased skin-wrinkle depth, improved skin gloss, and enhanced skin elasticity and epidermal thickening. The researchers labeled the probiotic a "nutricosmetic agent" for its beneficial effects. *Lactobacillus plantarum* is widely available in commercial probiotic supplements and in fermented foods such as sauerkraut, kimchi, pickles, and brined olives.

BOTOX: FROM POISON TO POSH

One of the most unusual ways to control wrinkles is the unconventional use of a deadly bacterial toxin (Toxin A) from *Clostridium botulinum*, which lives deep within soil where there is no oxygen. As you might guess from the name, it produces the deadliest known toxin on the planet, one that causes an often-fatal type of food poisoning called "botulism." This organism and its toxin are also famous as a potential bioterrorism agent, since incredibly small quantities of the toxin are so deadly.

Botulism toxin works by blocking neurotransmitter release, and thus paralyzing nerves. Its first real medical use was when very small quantities were injected into muscles that control the eyes, in order to provide a remedy for people who were cross-eyed, and to treat uncontrolled muscle spasms in the face. However, its real infamy came when it was discovered that it could minimize wrinkles. Jean and Alastair Carruthers are a Canadian husband and wife team: an ophthalmologist and dermatologist, respectively. In 1987, Jean injected this toxin into the facial muscles of patients to control eyelid twitching and eye spasms. One day, a patient asked why she wasn't injecting her forehead, and Jean replied that her forehead wasn't spasming. The patient replied that when Jean had injected her forehead in the past, her wrinkles had gone away. Naturally, this came up at dinner with Jean's dermatologist husband, and they decided to try it the next day on their receptionist who complained of forehead wrinkles. The results were spectacular, and Botox was born.

There was remarkable skepticism initially: The concept of injecting the world's most notoriously lethal toxin into a patient for cosmetic purposes was a tough sell. To counter this, Jean injected herself and jokingly says she hasn't frowned since. After conducting controlled studies, Europeans began to use it, and North Americans soon followed suit. Botox is now America's (and Australia's) number one cosmetic procedure, with seven million people receiving injections and four billion dollars in sales per year—making it the mainstay of most dermatology practices. However, it is not without its problems: Among the risks, repeated use causes skin sagging and drooping.

We can also potentially use our microbes to address the root cause of most wrinkles and skin aging: sun damage. In a double-blind study of fifty-four people, scientists discovered that feeding participants a particular probiotic, *Lactobacillus johnsonii*, for eight weeks actually decreased sunburn. The fun part is how they studied it: Researchers irradiated one buttock and used the other side as a non-suntanned control. Several trials indicated that probiotics decrease inflammation (which is associated with sunburns, as the skin is damaged), and researchers for this trial suggested that the oral probiotic minimized sunburn by dampening the inflammation and damage associated with UV exposure. The probiotics induced changes in the skin's immune system, which may have boosted its ability to prevent sunburn and promote skin healing.

Scientists hope that bioengineering of the microbiota will produce a new generation of more effective sunscreens and anti-wrinkle mechanisms. Harvard Medical School researchers have determined how cyanobacteria—an aquatic and photosynthetic bacterium often referred to as blue-green algae—protects itself from UV rays. The bacteria produce protective UV-absorbing molecules: mycosporine, mycosporine-like amino acids (MAAs), and scytonemin. Companies already use MAAs to make bio-sunscreens and anti-wrinkle creams, such as Helioguard 365 and Helionori. There is much biotechnological and commercial potential here as we better understand the natural "sunscreen" compounds produced by microbes, as well as specific biological compounds that absorb UV light—although it might be a tough sell to coat oneself in blue-green algae! Keep an eye out for bio-sunscreens that offer protection against premature aging and sun damage by looking for ingredients like *Porphyra umbilicalis* (rcd algac) cxtract.

It's All on Your Head

For men, and some women, a telltale sign of age is the infamous receding hairline—or worse, a comb-over. While it's easy enough to see with the naked eye whether this process is taking hold of your scalp, we can also now tell whether someone is bald just by analyzing a swab of their scalp for microbes. Bald scalp microbes contain more yeast and mites, and less bacteria. However, microbes may be able to help you keep your hair radiant—and on your head—even as you age. There are no data yet for humans, but when probiotic *Lactobacillus reuteri* was fed to mice during the second half of their lives, researchers observed an increase in sebum production, shiny fur, and (as the authors put it) a general "glow of health" within seven days. Preliminary data show that this probiotic may work by decreasing inflammation through an increase in an anti-inflammatory cytokine (IL-10). The aged male mice eating the probiotic had thicker, more lustrous fur, while the female mice displayed shinier hair. There may be something here we can learn from our furry friends. The probiotic *Lactobacillus reuteri* is readily available in current commercial hair products. The daily dose needs to be large: in the range of one billion to one hundred billion colony-forming units (or CFUs, live bacterial cells). *Lactobacillus reuteri*, like most probiotics, can be taken with food, but not with hot beverages (which would cook the bacteria).

We can even potentially take advantage of microbes to treat dandruff, a dermatologic condition that can get worse in older scalps as the skin's structure and function decline. Scientists found that adults with dandruff have higher levels of a yeast-like fungus *Malassezia restricta*, *Staphylococcus* species, and lower counts of *C. acnes*. The Malassezia fungus lives on the scalps of most adults, and it irritates the scalps for some by causing increased growth of skin cells. These extra skin cells die and fall off in pieces, those white and flaky specks visible on scalps and shoulders. It is not proven, but researchers suggest that a microbiota imbalance may have a role in dandruff production. In one randomized, double-blind, placebo-controlled trial, participants with moderate to severe dandruff took the oral probiotic *Lactobacillus paracasei* or a placebo. Of those who took the probiotic, 72 percent experienced significantly less dandruff in four to five weeks, compared to 34 percent in the placebo group, in the same amount of time. It also had secondary benefits, including reduced scalp erythema (redness or rash), itching, greasiness, and scalp Malassezia yeast counts. *Lactobacillus paracasei* is commonly added to probiotic supplements. There are countless websites promoting probiotics to massage into dandruff-infested scalps, and (so far) a formula with live *Lactobacillus paracasei* cultures and at least forty billion colony-forming units (CFUs) is an intriguing option.

MYTH: Sweat stinks.

FACT: Sweat is essentially odorless: The source of any smell is caused by our microbes.

Sweat It Out

A healthy skin microbiome can make us feel attractive in many ways—fewer wrinkles, plumper skin, better hair—but it has one major drawback: It is the culprit behind body odor. Sweat secretions from the body are generally odorless until microbes (mainly *Corynebacterium* and *Staphylococcus epidermidis*) get hold of these secretions and break down the proteins and lipids into smaller molecules, called "volatile organic fatty acids" and "thioalcohols." These by-products smell but evaporate quickly, hence the body odor that wafts from our armpits.

Sweating is less of a problem in later life as the number and activity of sweat glands decreases (along with changes in the microbiome). However, at any age, the stench of sweat and damp stains can leave you in a pit of embarrassment. We generally control body odor through two products: antiperspirants, which block sweating and decrease body odor; and deodorants, which don't affect the amount you sweat but decrease body odor. Around 90 percent of Americans (60 to 70 percent of Australians) use one of these products, resulting in a multibillion-dollar industry. Antiperspirants contain aluminum salts that dissolve upon application and temporarily block secretion by plugging the sweat glands. They are usually dissolved in ethanol so that they dry faster upon application. Both ethanol and aluminum salts are antibacterial, as are other antimicrobial additives (e.g., triclosan) that help kill the bacteria involved in producing body odor.

One small study examined the effects of deodorants and antiperspirants on the microbiota. Researchers took nine healthy subjects and asked them not to use either product for one month—the time it takes for the underarm skin to be replaced. The scientists found distinct microbial communities depending on whether a participant used these products. The microbial richness was higher when using these agents, especially the antiperspirants. Ironically, antiperspirants led to an increase in *Corynebacterium*, which is associated with producing body odor.

In the future, we can expect to see more effective products that specifically target odor-producing microbes. A few probiotic deodorants are currently available, though these are mostly organic mixtures with unspecified "shelf-stable probiotics" (i.e., live probiotics that are naturally stable at room temperature and do not require refrigeration). DIY recipes combining natural butters and oils with emptied capsules of powdered probiotics abound on the internet. These products likely do not work, as they contain a random assortment of probiotics in varying amounts, not ones specifically involved with the bacteria that cause body odor. As science advances, we can expect to see pharmacy shelves stocked with more precise probiotic deodorants that target specific microbes.

PROBING TOPICAL PROBIOTICS

Despite the volume of topical skin probiotics available, the research on probiotics taken orally is much more promising. One particular challenge is that many topical probiotic products contain preservatives, which are antibacterial. To get around this, most products instead make an extract from a probiotic, rather than storing the live bacterium in it. Despite being promised as a probiotic product (probiotics are live bacterial products), they contain only a probiotic bacterial extract, which is not, by definition, a probiotic. Some companies are working on getting around this by storing a probiotic (*Lactobacillus*) in protective capsules that release the bacterium only when it is applied to the skin. Take a careful look at the "probiotic ingredients" before purchasing anything.

You may have more impact eating fermented foods and oral probiotics to promote your skin health. In one study, taking *Lactobacillus brevis* SBC8803 orally enhanced the barrier of the skin to keep out foreign invaders and helped the skin stay hydrated. Another study showed that orally ingested *Lactobacillus paracasei* NCC2461 also enhanced skin barrier function. An advantage of taking probiotics orally is that it keeps the skin microbiome diverse, whereas a topical probiotic can dominate the skin microbiome, which ironically can be detrimental to the skin biodiversity.

The Future Is Bright

Though it is still early, remarkable strides are being taken to understand the effects of the microbiome on the skin and scalp as we age. Personalized probiotics made from an individual's beneficial microbes show significant promise to both prevent infections and promote skin health. We can imagine a revolutionized approach to skincare in the near future, where we analyze our aging skin and add back specific beneficial microbes. When it comes to personalized medicine, we may even be able to culture and apply our very own "nutricosmetic" microbes to boost skin health and appearance. Similarly, we may take certain microbes from the skin of younger people and apply them in later life as an anti-aging strategy. Biobanking your own personal skin microbes for thirty years may sound futuristic, but we can imagine rejuvenating skincare cocktails that incorporate youthful microbes extracted from younger populations.

Emerging research further suggests that hair growth could be influenced by identifying microbial compounds. Soon we may target balding through microbial interventions that promote the health of hair cells. We may even be able to boost the health and longevity of pigment-producing hair cells to gain more autonomy over whether we "go gray."

Scientific advances will filter microbe-friendly skin regimes into our everyday lives. Deodorants of the future may include a precise mixture of microbes that displace those causing body odor. We know that antibiotics wreak havoc on our skin's microbes, especially topical applications. Mixtures of beneficial skin microbiota could become available to apply after antibiotic treatments to help recolonize the skin microbiota in a healthy way. Given the high usage of antibiotics in older populations and a resulting microbe depletion, this is a particularly important therapy to pursue. With evolving knowledge of the vast differences between people's skin microbiota, we can expect probiotic skincare therapies tailored to individuals. We can also imagine a personalized diet that diminishes typical signs of skin aging by modulating the gut microbiota. We have already seen that certain oral probiotics can affect skin health. Diet is a terrific way to modulate microbiota through the gut-skin axis. Microbes are essential to revolutionize skincare and provide a much-needed fresh approach to achieving youthful, healthy, radiant skin.

KEY TIPS

Moisturize: Regular moisturizing may help maintain a healthy skin microbiome, since just like us, our skin microbes need moisture to thrive.

Steer clear of smoking and air pollution: Smoking and air pollution both alter and damage the skin microbiome. They contain nanoparticles that can become embedded in the skin (in addition to being inhaled into your lungs). If you can't avoid exposure to smoke or air pollution, wash with soap and water afterward to help get the harmful nanoparticles off your skin.

Eat your way to radiant skin: A diet rich in fruits, vegetables, beans, fermented foods, and whole grains (all sources of prebiotic fibers) can support a healthier skin microbiome. While studies have linked gut and skin health, the opposite is also true: Gastrointestinal issues (and systemic inflammation) are often accompanied by skin problems. Certain probiotics, including *Lactobacillus plantarum*, show significant promise for decreasing skin wrinkles and promoting general skin health. Consider incorporating *Lactobacillus plantarum* into your diet through a probiotic supplement and fermented foods.

Consider oral probiotics for eczema: Several clinical trials have shown that orally taking lactobacilli (*Lactobacillus fermentum, Lactobacillus salivarius*) as well as *Bifidobacterium* are protective against eczema (atopic dermatitis). There are no good clinical data yet for topical probiotics and eczema.

Avoid antibiotic ointments: Antibiotics—whether applied topically or even taken orally—can significantly disrupt the skin microbiome. If a wound does not show any signs of infection, keep your skin injury clean, use an appropriate non-adhesive dressing to keep it moist, and keep covered with sterile bandaging.

Avoid antibacterial soaps: Washing your hands with regular soap and running water remains one of the best ways to prevent illness and spread of infection.

Take care with contacts: Reduce risk of bacterial eye infections by washing your hands with soap and water before handling contact lenses. Clean contacts and storage cases thoroughly with fresh disinfecting solution, never water. Leave the empty case open to air dry and replace it at least every three months. If you are an occasional user, do not give bacteria the chance to grow in your static lens case. Never wear lenses stored for more than thirty days without re-disinfecting.

Practice sun safety: The easiest and least expensive way to keep skin healthy and youthful is to stay out of the sun. Emerging bio-sunscreens, such as Helioguard 365 and Helionori, use cyanobacteria UVA filters to naturally protect against the sun; they may be a better alternative to traditional sunscreens, which negatively disrupt the skin microbiota. After any extended sun exposure, consider taking the probiotic *Lactobacillus johnsonii* to help decrease inflammation and sunburn.

Take a pro-hair probiotic: An oral probiotic that might help to avoid hair thinning is *Lactobacillus reuteri*, especially strain ATCC PTA 6475. There are strong animal (mice and rat) data that this probiotic enhances hair growth, as well as many other beneficial effects such as increasing testosterone and vitamin D and B12 levels, and decreasing inflammation. One such source is BioGaia, which sells this strain with one hundred million per dose (the predicted needed dose based on animal studies). It probably won't regenerate hair loss but shows promise for improving the conditions to keep hair for longer.

6

Healthy Smile, Healthy You: The Oral Microbiome

In 1683, while using a microscope he'd invented, Antonie van Leeuwenhoek made the seminal observation that there were more "animalcules" (i.e., bacteria) in his mouth than on all the people living in his home country of the Netherlands. It was humanity's first glimpse of microbes, and the stunning realization that our mouths are inhabited by living organisms. As with so many innovative scientific discoveries, at first nobody believed the "crazy Dutchman," as he was called. It took decades of letters to the Royal Society in London describing microbes in great detail to convince the world. As others peered through van Leeuwenhoek's microscopes, his amazing findings were confirmed, and the field of microbiology was born.

The oral cavity—everything in your mouth from lips to teeth, gums, hard palate, and tongue—normally teems with millions of microbes. It comprises your second largest microbiome in total numbers after the gut, containing over seven hundred species. You swallow billions of bacteria in your saliva every day. The environment of the mouth flourishes with bacteria, given that we constantly provide fluids, nutrients, and a nice warm temperature. Fighting for their own survival just as we do, resident microbes cling to the tongue, inside the cheeks, teeth, and gums in order to resist being flushed away when we swallow. Relative to the few hundred years of microbiology, the fact that there is a whole thriving bacterial community in our oral cavity is a new realization. We spoke to Dr. Richard Ellen, a retired professor from the faculty of dentistry at the University of Toronto. Ellen is a recognized authority on oral microbial ecology. He told us: "No one ever used the term 'microbiome' back in the 1970s when

I started my career." After earning his dental degree, he became a research fellow at Harvard University and Forsyth Dental Center, where he met an inspiring microbial ecologist named Dr. Ronald Gibbons.

Gibbons was interested in how bacteria adhere to surfaces in the mouth and whether similar principles governed the distribution of bacteria that cause disease elsewhere in the body. He sent Ellen off to the library to learn more about the potential for bacterial adhesion in strep throat. Thus began a fruitful collaboration that caught the attention of medical microbiologists. Ellen later applied his expertise to study microbial ecology in periodontology, the specialty of dentistry that studies the supporting structures of teeth such as the gums, as well as diseases and conditions that affect them. In the lab next door to Gibbons, another microbiologist, Dr. Sigmund Socransky, was using the most advanced methods at the time to document the bacterial populations that colonized different oral surfaces. The process involved "picking individual bacterial colonies that grew on nutrient media, then using laborious biochemical tests to identify only those that could grow under lab conditions," Dr. Ellen explained. "This helped us understand a good number of the microorganisms that lived on the tongue, cheek, teeth, and in saliva, but it grossly underestimated their diversity because most of the resident bacteria were not cultivated by these methods." The field has advanced remarkably since then. Dr. Ellen reflected: "I feel ancient, since I started research on these topics when the confident identification of a core but limited cluster of the bacteria in oral samples was just emerging. Today's rapid DNA sequencing and analysis of the oral microbiome seems a bit like interstellar travel to me!"

Scientists and dentists now know that hundreds of oral microbial species generally live interspersed among many different neighbors rather than as a clonal population (think of a city bustling with multitudes of diverse people and buildings). These complex oral communities are fairly stable during an adult's life, but some major changes can occur in older people. Diminished oral microbial communities in older patients give pathogens an invitation to colonize and thrive. This affects not only our teeth and gums, but our entire body.

The mouth reflects overall health at any stage of life and represents the critical first contact point between our alimentary canal (also known as the gastrointestinal tract, which we've already discussed, along which food passes from mouth to anus), the immune system, and the outside world. There is a 45 percent overlap in species between the oral microbiome and the gut. If we envision the gastrointestinal tract as a river, the mouth is the source; the headwaters from which everything flows downstream. In fact, the majority of all systemic diseases (those involving many organs or the whole body such as cardiovascular disease, type 2 diabetes, and dementia) produce oral signs and symptoms.

There is a surprising correlation between the body's microbiota and dementia, as related to oral hygiene. A large twin study showed that early tooth loss (before thirty-five years of age) correlates with higher levels of dementia. The most interesting statistic is that individuals who do not brush their teeth daily have a 22 to 65 percent greater risk of developing dementia than those who brush their teeth three times a day!

How could fastidiously brushing one's teeth possibly affect dementia? As one ages, saliva production slows, which enhances low-grade inflammation in the mouth because saliva is antibacterial; it also reduces one's ability to wash away and swallow oral microbes. Presumably this, and likelihood of gum disease, allows increased numbers of microbes and their inflammatory products to seep into the body's circulation, triggering additional inflammation. Studies show that when antibodies to oral microbes are circulating in increased numbers–an indirect indication that these microbes are entering into the body and seen by the immune system–this is directly related to an increased risk for Alzheimer's disease.

Ultimately, oral health is much more important than just an attractive smile. Your mouth is a window into the condition of your entire body and can serve as a critical vantage point to detect and defend against health problems.

Brush, Floss, Repeat

The oral microbiota live in miniature microbial cities called "biofilms." The "skyscrapers" of these cities are built from molecules called "extracellular polysaccharides" (EPS), which form sticky structures in and around the microbes and protect them from their harsh environment. Biofilms can exist pretty much anywhere, but the most common site in the body is the mouth, in the form of dental plaque. Which microbes inhabit the biofilm is important, and it depends on who adheres first. The early colonizers shape which microbes colonize later–i.e., which "neighbors" get to move in, and this sets the composition of the oral "neighborhood," for better or worse. The most common first colonizers, *Streptococcus* species, help other beneficial microbes subsequently move in. As others colonize and the neighborhood expands, around one hundred microbial species are found intertwined in the plaque. Microbes usually layer three hundred to five hundred cells deep–a microbial skyscraper indeed!

We've all experienced, to some degree, what plaque buildup feels like: the white or dark-colored flakes that dental hygienists scrape off our teeth are calculus (tartar)–old biofilm material from bacteria that has calcified into adherent masses. Unfortunately, plaque is constantly building from the moment you finish having your teeth cleaned, and it accumulates in hard-to-clean spots in the months between visits. Meanwhile, as plaque builds up on and under our gums, direct contact between biofilm and gum tissue causes irritation. The gums inflame (our body's 911 response), and this inflammation summons macrophages and neutrophils: cells designed to damage and kill microbes. However, in many people, prolonged and repeated bouts of inflammation can cause collateral damage to the underlying tissue, and later periodontitis–a destructive form of gum disease that includes loose teeth, receding gums, and bad breath. The microbes shift toward more pathogenic ones as the disease advances, which further damages the soft tissues and underlying bone structure. This allows inflammatory microbial products to seep into the body and increase harmful systemic inflammation.

Surprisingly, two of the most common infectious diseases worldwide are not among the usual suspects that cause devastating pandemics like COVID-19, AIDS, malaria, or tuberculosis; rather they are periodontitis (gum disease) and dental caries (cavities). Nearly all humans have had at least one cavity, and up to half of us experience some form of gum disease. However, unlike the above well-known infectious diseases, oral diseases are caused by a mixture of microbes rather than one particular pathogen. How are they infectious? Periodontal diseases are contagious because they can spread between people through saliva. While the chances of catching periodontal disease-causing bacteria by drinking from the same cup, sharing utensils, or kissing are low, it's not impossible. People with periodontitis have distinctly different microbes. *Porphyromonas gingivalis* and *Treponema denticola* are often among the microbial culprits behind this disease. Germ-free lab animals do not suffer from periodontitis, which makes sense, given that they do not have any microbes.

SHOULD YOU TAPE YOUR MOUTH SHUT?

Do you ever wake up with your mouth completely dry—and perhaps a disgruntled partner who struggled to sleep through your snoring? The internet abounds with claims that taping your mouth shut while sleeping improves your mouth's microbiome because mouth breathing exposes the oral microbiome to a lot of airflow and is linked with an increase in pathogens associated with cavities. Although there have not been any large studies yet proving this, some dentists are now suggesting that if you sleep with your mouth open to consider mouth taping: putting a piece of special porous tape over your lips when you sleep to enhance your oral microbiome. It also is reported to enhance your sleep quality (the primary reason dentists recommend taping to patients), although again large studies have not published yet about its efficacy.

Older adults are more susceptible to gum disease: The CDC reports that nearly half of adults aged thirty years and older have some form of periodontal disease (one-third in Australia), increasing to 70.1 percent (70 percent in Australia) of those over the age of sixty-five. Ultimately, eight out of ten people will experience this. However, it is not a "normal" part of aging: good hygiene and a healthy oral microbiota can prevent this disease. You know the drill: thorough brushing, interdental cleaning (aka flossing), and regular trips to the dentist. Looking to the future, you may also be able to use probiotics to help "good" microbes colonize the gums and keep pathogens away (but there are no good studies yet definitively showing that oral probiotics work). Lactobacilli and Bifidobacteria are the two genera most commonly found in these probiotics. A normal part of the oral microbiota, they are generally regarded as safe and can be consumed through oral probiotics and food products. Dairy sources of probiotics include yogurt, kefir, cultured cottage cheese, and buttermilk; nondairy sources include fermented vegetables such as sauerkraut and kombucha tea. Use caution, however, as lactobacilli and Bifidobacteria can be harmful to people who frequently consume fermentable carbohydrates. These include sugary foods (e.g., cookies, cakes, soft drinks, candy) and less obvious foods such as bread, crackers, bananas, and breakfast cereals. Lactobacilli and Bifidobacteria use the sugars from these foods to produce acids. In technical terms, they are incredibly acidogenic and aciduric members (tolerant of a highly acidic environment) of the deep plaque that causes dental caries. This means that, through acid production, they can make plaque worse.

Oral probiotics are not commonly used at present in the dental profession, due to lack of compelling clinical trials. They may eventually represent a novel therapeutic strategy to help promote oral and systemic health. Localized treatments with a culture of *Lactobacillus acidophilus* have significantly helped those suffering from periodontal diseases (e.g., gingivitis and periodontitis) to recover. Studies show that the probiotic *Lactobacillus* strains *L. reuteri*, *L. brevis* CD2, *L. casei* Shirota, *L. salivarius* WB21, as well as *Bacillus subtilis* can improve gingival (gum) health and reduce the number of periodontal pathogens. Probiotic gum (see "Chewing Your Way to Dental Health" on page 129) also represents an easy method to improve gum health and decrease periodontal disease, although it has not been proven clinically. Probiotic gum not only provides an oral probiotic, but the act of gum chewing would also benefit many older people who suffer from reduced salivary flow rates. As with periodontitis, microbes are at the heart of dental cavities.

When the biofilm builds up on the enamel of our teeth, bacteria associated with cavities (such as *Streptococcus mutans*) colonize and shift tooth microbiota. The microbial diversity decreases, and a few pesky microbes like *S. mutans* and various lactobacilli increase significantly in numbers (*S. mutans* may multiply from about 2 percent of the microbes to over 30 percent). These microbes hang out on tooth surfaces happily munching on the sugars and other carbohydrates that we feed them every day. In return, they produce acids (lactic, formic, acetic, and propionic), which the microbes can withstand but our teeth cannot. Cavities form when the acids dissolve our enamel and decay the underlying dentin layer. This leads to all-too-familiar symptoms of toothache, sensitivity, and mild-to-sharp pain when biting or consuming something sweet, hot, or cold.

We too often overlook the role of microbes in treating teeth cavities, and instead blame the sweets we all love. But germ-free animals on a high-sugar diet do not even get cavities! In addition to well-known dental and dietary habits (i.e., brush, floss, cut back on sugar), an ecologically balanced and diverse oral microbiome might help diminish cavities. Several studies show that consuming probiotics containing lactobacilli or Bifidobacteria can reduce the number of troublesome *S. mutans* in saliva. *Streptococcus salivarius* M18, commonly found in oral care probiotics, destroys harmful *S. mutans* bacteria and helps neutralize acidity in the mouth. Boosting microbial defenses can combat the root cause of cavities.

We all know that regular brushing is important to oral health. However, it seems that not all toothpastes are equal: Those that affect the microbiome population may enhance health benefits. In a recent double-blind, randomized study, 111 healthy adults brushed their teeth twice a day with fluoridated toothpaste for four weeks, after which those participants were divided into two groups: one that continued to use the regular fluoridated toothpaste, while the other began using Zendium, a fluoridated toothpaste that contains three enzymes that generate antimicrobial products, as well as three antibacterial proteins. After using either toothpaste twice daily for fourteen weeks, the participants' oral microbes were analyzed. The results were extremely encouraging: the supplemented toothpaste promoted a positive microbial community shift toward more beneficial microbes (twelve microbial taxa, including *Neisseria*), and a decrease in those associated with periodontal disease (ten taxa, including *Treponema*). The toothpaste seemed to boost the mouth's natural defenses by relying on natural proteins and enzymes that are similar to those found in saliva. Zendium is available in most of Europe and the Middle East, and you can buy it from Amazon and other online retailers in North America.

Jessica tried it out and noticed that it was a bit different from traditional toothpastes because it does not contain the foaming agent sodium lauryl sulfate. Although there wasn't that clean-feeling froth, it tasted good and left her mouth feeling clean. As scientific advances in molecular techniques boost our ability to understand the oral microbiome at the species level, we can expect to see even more specific microbe-friendly toothpastes in the future. Given that oral health largely depends on the balance between health-promoting and disease-associated bacteria in the mouth, we can increasingly tip the scale in our favor by applying supplemented oral products.

HOW OFTEN SHOULD YOU CHANGE YOUR TOOTHBRUSH?

The average person should swap in a new toothbrush every three to four months. This is recommended to ensure that bristles remain effective and bacteria accumulation on the toothbrush is minimal. Should you change your toothbrush after being sick (e.g., with a cold, flu, or COVID-19)? We couldn't find any strong scientific evidence on this. While the virus may survive on your toothbrush for a short period of time, as long as they're your own germs you don't have to worry; you won't make yourself sick again.

Chewing Your Way to Dental Health

Given that periodontitis (gum disease), caries (cavities), bad breath, and other oral issues are all caused by troublesome microbes taking up residence in the mouth, can we rid ourselves of these problems by displacing the bad bacteria with "good" microbes? Oral probiotics may be able to help with this, but again, these have not been proven clinically. One microbe now being used as a probiotic is *Streptococcus salivarius* K12. This beneficial microbe produces bacteriocins (toxins) that kill other microbes associated with both periodontitis and halitosis (bad breath). It was declared safe for people in a randomized clinical trial where ten billion microbes were ingested every day for twenty-eight days. More expansive clinical trials are underway to prove its efficacy, but in small trials, it reduced bad breath and decreased throat infections (e.g., strep throat and tonsillitis).

In a clever twist, *S. salivarius* is marketed as a probiotic gum called "BLIS K12." You can order this chewing gum in two flavors (spearmint-peppermint or raspberry-pomegranate). It has no sugars or artificial sweeteners and contains five hundred million probiotic bacteria per piece. Jessica was curious about the product and ordered a spearmint-peppermint pack online. At first, she tried one piece per day and chewed it for five to ten minutes after brushing her teeth before bed (as suggested). The gum tasted good, though it lost its minty taste rather quickly. The main snag is that at $13.50 for a pack of eight pieces, it was rather pricey to purchase on her grad student budget.

Given its expense, Jessica would consider chewing it on a case-by-case basis, such as on the way home from dental appointments to help recolonize beneficial oral microbes on her freshly cleaned teeth. It might also be helpful when taking antibiotics–which are intended to attack the body's microbes. For older adults, the chewing gum represents a potentially easy way to deliver probiotics throughout the entire mouth while boosting saliva flow.

Other types of probiotic chewing gum available contain *L. reuteri* ATCC 55730 and ATCC PTA 5289, and may decrease levels of pro-inflammatory cytokines, therefore contributing to better oral and systemic health.

Spit and Polish

Saliva plays a vital role in maintaining oral health as it lubricates your mouth, helps you taste and digest your food, and contains defensive compounds that help control excessive buildup of microbial plaque. It's also teeming with helpful microbes: roughly five hundred million bacteria per teaspoon. Good saliva flow thus delivers moisture and nutrients to your microbes, and buffers as well as flushes away acid produced by cavity-causing microbes on the teeth. We each have a unique microbiome within our saliva that remains fairly stable over time. But as we age, our saliva can dry up: hyposalivation (less saliva) and xerostomia (dry mouth) are present in one third of older adults and in 40 percent of those over the age of eighty. A dry mouth makes chewing, eating, swallowing, talking, and even whistling–clearly the most essential activity on this list!–more difficult. Without saliva's defensive properties and nutrient delivery, the good and protective microbes can't thrive, which makes us more vulnerable to pathogenic infections.

There is no significant decline in salivary flow for healthy, unmedicated older adults, so dry mouth is not an inevitable nuisance in later life. Many patients and even doctors do not know that over four hundred frequently prescribed common medications cause dry mouth. Risk increases when taking four or more medications per day. Perhaps a probiotic gum could help boost oral microbes and stimulate saliva: Studies show that *Lactobacillus* species *L. reuteri* DSM 17938 and ATCC PTA 5289, *L. rhamnosus* GG (ATCC 53103), and *L. rhamnosus* LC705, as well as *Propionibacterium freudenreichii* ssp. shermanii JS all have promise in diminishing the risk of hyposalivation and the feeling of xerostomia by replenishing one's supply of microbe-rich saliva.

Microbe-Breath

Can't you just use mouthwash to kill all the bad oral microbes? Antonie van Leeuwenhoek tried the original mouthwash experiment centuries ago. He knew that both alcohol and vinegar could kill the "animalcules" he scraped out of his mouth. So, he did what any good scientist would do: Using himself for an experiment, he tried gargling with alcohol and vinegar and then examined the microbes in his mouth. It didn't work: The microbes were unaffected, likely because they are encased in a strong shield of protective biofilm casing. His experiment holds true today: Common over-the-counter mouthwashes generally are only partially effective (and tongue scraping doesn't work either; don't bother). While they are great for rinsing away food particles missed by brushing and flossing, limiting plaque above the gumline, and freshening odor, they do not rid our mouths of cavity causing microbes or those deep *below* the gumline.

Dr. Ellen explained that commercial mouthwash was initially marketed to "kill the germs that cause bad breath," which fell under cosmetic concerns. Mouthwashes did not need to be approved by the FDA because the companies did not assert specific "health" claims. As researchers and clinicians began to learn about dental plaque and its relationship with gingivitis, clinical models for mouth rinses began to emerge.

The first antimicrobial mouthwash that proved to prevent plaque-induced gingivitis was chlorhexidine, which later became a prescription drug in North America and is available over the counter in Australia. "It tastes terrible, but it works," Dr. Ellen explained. "It prevents the accumulation of plaque. In those without brushing skills, such as elderly patients who cannot manipulate the instruments needed to clean their teeth, it can help reduce plaque and lower risk for gingivitis. It is not a good idea, however, to be on it continuously. And rinsing with chlorhexidine does not reach below the gums to affect destructive forms of gum disease."

What about over-the-counter antimicrobial mouthwashes? These products indiscriminately kill both good and bad microbes, as does chlorhexidine. They also do not necessarily prevent periodontal disease. Dr. Ellen cautioned that consumers need to read the disclaimers in small print on the bottom of the bottle to learn about the product's limitations. While generally harmless, long-term use may result in some negative side effects including teeth stains and antimicrobial drug resistance.

Routine gargling with chlorhexidine (still the gold standard for mouthwash) decreases dental pathogens (including *Porphyromonas gingivalis*, *Treponema denticola*, and *Tannerella forsythia*). So, it appears that frequent gargling with chlorhexidine may help decrease oral pathogens, although additional and longer-term studies on mouthwash and type 2 diabetes are needed.

Keep an eye out for probiotic mouthwashes–they are an emerging and perhaps more effective oral hygiene treatment than traditional models. Published results of preliminary studies show that probiotic mouthwash containing three different oral streptococci reduced plaque and *S. mutans* associated with cavities. There are many options commercially available: Talk to your dentist before changing your oral hygiene routine. Ultimately, Dr. Ellen advised, today's mouthwashes cannot replace manual cleaning: "Mouthwash is topical, temporary, and does not reach critical areas if someone has periodontal pockets, in between teeth, or in fissures." It is just one component of oral hygiene, and secondary to keeping your teeth clean through brushing, interdental cleaning (flossing), and routine professional visits.

AN ONION A DAY KEEPS EVERYONE AWAY

We all have mornings when we need to brush our teeth before greeting any fellow humans. If you have a dry mouth while sleeping, this can cause bad "morning breath." Halitosis (chronic bad breath) occurs in about 25 percent of people and significantly affects quality of life. Microbes living in deep crypts or valleys of the tongue cause bad breath. These microbes make around 150 different volatile molecules—meaning that they evaporate into air—that stink, including sulfur compounds such as hydrogen sulfide (rotten egg odor) and others that smell like rotten cabbage, decomposing seaweed, fish, and garlic. Yuck! No single microbe is responsible for bad breath; it is a mixture of microbes living together on the tongue.

Older adults particularly suffer from bad breath due to hyposalivation (less saliva to wash away these malodorous microbes and their compounds). Furthermore, poorly fitted dentures allow pockets of bacteria to grow in the spaces which, like grooves in the tongue, can lead to microbial production of smelly molecules.

Traditional methods to control bad breath include teeth brushing, dental flossing, tongue scraping, using mouthwash, and drinking ample water. All of these have limited success. Recent clinical studies suggest that replacing the smelly bacteria with good species may be a more effective way of controlling bad breath. Specific probiotic strains that can alter halitosis include *E. coli* Nissle 1917, *S. salivarius* K12, and *Weissella confusa* isolates. Remember that the probiotic gum BLIS K12 contains five hundred million *S. salivarius* K12 bacteria, making it an easy method for fresh breath support. E. coli Nissle 1917 can be found in oral supplements, but those should be used only with extreme caution: One study found that if both the microbiota and immune response are defective, there can be potentially severe adverse effects. *Weissella confusa* has also been suggested as a probiotic, but it can cause sepsis and other serious infections in humans and animals.

These two examples remind us of the need to approach probiotics with caution and a close eye on the scientific literature. The Food and Drug Administration (FDA) regulates probiotics as a food, not as medication. This means that probiotic supplement companies, unlike drug companies, do not have to scientifically demonstrate that their products are safe or effective. The products are not rigorously "approved" to prevent or treat specific conditions, which leads to abundant misinformation and false claims. In Australia, the regulation depends on the probiotic product's intended use and marketing claims. Before you begin to use a new probiotic, research all the specific strains in the product (see chapter 16 on how to read up on medically tested probiotics).

Smoker's Mouth

Smoking has profound effects on the oral microbiota as they are directly exposed to highly concentrated doses of smoke. In biofilms of the subgingival area (under the gums), smoking favors the early colonization of pathogens that cause periodontal disease. Smoking also prevents normal microbes from colonizing early enough to take up the space of unwanted pathogens inside the mouth. Given their unhealthier oral microbiome and the direct negative effects of tobacco smoke on the tissue itself, smokers' mouths do not heal as well when their owners seek treatment for periodontal disease. An estimated 42 percent of periodontitis in the United States is attributed to smoking, and, despite all the known dangers, there are forty-nine million American adult smokers and over one billion smokers worldwide.

Oral microbial communities are less stable in smokers. A lack of healthy and diverse microbes contributes to pathogen colonization in the nasopharyngeal area (head and neck). This leads to additional upper respiratory problems (e.g., ear and throat infections), especially in older adults more susceptible to infection, and causes a buildup of bacteria, which travels from the throat to the middle ear. To add insult to injury, additional gum disease in smokers means that they are much more likely to have bad breath due to their pathogenic microbes.

The damage caused by smoking accumulates, meaning that the longer you smoke, the greater the risk for these ailments. Studies show that using tablets containing *L. salivarius* WB21 can improve gingival health in high-risk smokers and reduce the number of periodontal pathogens in plaque. *L. salivarius* is found in live-culture dairy products as well as probiotic supplements. Beneficial microbes in oral probiotics may help strengthen the barrier against invading pathogens that cause periodontal disease and upper respiratory infections. Of course, quitting smoking represents the best defense and brings immediate health benefits at any age–even in later life. The effects of smoking on the oral microbiome can be seen for years, but after quitting, it does eventually return to a healthier state. For the sake of your microbes and personal health, if you smoke, take advantage of counseling and of smoking cessation medications such as nicotine in gums and patches.

Over the past few years, vaping (smoking e-cigarettes) has been touted as a "healthier" alternative to smoking, especially among younger generations. E-cigarettes are thought to produce fewer toxic chemicals than traditional cigarettes, although they still contain nicotine and other toxic products such as lead. In a recent study, the oral microbiomes of smokers, e-cigarette users, and non-smokers were compared over six months. The smokers showed the expected microbial dysbiosis associated with smoking. However, those that vaped had an intermediate microbiome somewhere between that of smokers and non-smokers, tending more toward the smokers' microbiome, including species associated with gum disease (*Fusobacterium* and Bacteroidales species), as well as increased inflammatory markers. This early evidence suggests that vaping does have a detrimental effect on the oral microbiome, but not as strongly as tobacco smoking.

MYTH: Brushing your teeth immediately after smoking can make up for some of the harmful effects on your teeth and gums.

FACT: Smoking kills beneficial microbes in your mouth that protect against dental disease and bad breath. The destructive microbes settle right back in the mouth immediately after brushing.

Exciting Times Ahead

This is a thrilling time for oral health as we begin to realize the major role of oral microbes. If you are really keen to understand the details of your oral microbiome, there are commercial tests available to analyze it (like you can find for your gut microbiome, as we discussed in chapter 2). These tests usually require a saliva sample and cost about $250–300. They will give you a detailed analysis of your oral microbiome, as well as suggestions to follow to enhance your oral health. One example is the Viome Oral Health Intelligence test: Following your individual analysis, they claim to provide you with a list of food supplements, vitamins, minerals, herbs, pro- and prebiotics, and other suggestions that you can use to improve your oral health. While a fun experiment (assuming you want to know what your oral microbes are!), keep in mind that oral microbiome testing recommendations include many things that have not been clinically proven.

We're increasingly confident that recolonization of the mouth with healthy microbes to establish strong microbial communities can play a major role in the future, in both the dentist's office and personal hygiene. Commercial products such as probiotic gum and supplemented toothpaste are on the rise to boost the oral microbes. We expect that probiotic mouthwashes will help reduce the number of pathogenic bacteria associated with bad breath, dental cavities, and periodontitis.

With the awareness that gum health is critical for lifelong and full body vitality, the medical community will exercise increased vigilance toward the microbes involved in gum disease. Since the mouth is much easier to access than other body sites, we are likely to profile older adults' microbes in order to identify specific risks and recommend targeted interventions. We will also be able to expand personalized treatment to alter the microbes and boost helpful bacteria through diet, prebiotics, and probiotics. Now that is something to chew on!

KEY TIPS

Brush multiple times a day: Early tooth loss is linked to higher levels of dementia. Brushing your teeth regularly—ideally three times a day—may decrease your risk for dementia and Alzheimer's.

Floss diligently: Regular brushing and flossing are still the mainstays for good oral and dental health. If you have gum diseases, water flossers may be a gentle alternative way to remove plaque and promote oral health. These devices use a pulsating stream of water to clean between the teeth and along the gums.

Address the root causes of dry mouth: Talk to your dentist and doctor if you are experiencing dry mouth. Medications are often the culprit, and other drugs may be substituted or dosages changed. If medications cannot be avoided, it is advised to drink plenty of water, chew sugarless gum (consider a probiotic variety), and avoid tobacco and alcohol. Consider trying a probiotic (e.g., *L. reuteri* and *L. rhamnosus*) after taking antibiotics.

Eat a high-fiber, low-sugar diet: High-fiber, low-sugar, low-processed-food diets such as the Mediterranean Diet are an excellent way to promote oral health. Differences in oral health are noticeable within three weeks of changing a diet, with the oral microbiome stabilizing within six to eight weeks. Happy and healthy mouth microbes will help seed the gut microbiome with beneficial microbes, thereby enhancing gut health as well.

Consider oral probiotics: Promising oral health products often include lactobacilli and Bifidobacteria. You can incorporate these "mouthy microbes" into your diet through dairy products and fermented vegetables (e.g., cultured yogurt, kefir, sauerkraut), or consider taking a supplement that includes specific strains. Supplemented chewing gums and toothpastes may also help with bad breath and improve oral health. Using these enhanced products on a regular basis, particularly following antibiotic treatment and after any dental visits, may help recolonize healthy microbes for immune support. However, at present, we lack enough thorough studies showing that oral probiotics really work. Keep this in mind when you consider how best to spend your time, energy, and dollars.

7

Love Bugs: The Heart and the Microbiome

Your heart is a strong muscle roughly the size of the palm of your hand. Like the engine of a car, it's what keeps your body running. It has two main pumps: The first uses arteries to send oxygenated blood away from the heart to the rest of the body. The second uses veins to bring blood back to the heart and send it to the lungs to get more oxygen. The cardiovascular system spans your entire body: your heart, veins, arteries, and blood. Cardiovascular disease (CVD) happens when the engine and its pipes get blocked up. Plaque builds up in the arteries, which becomes a condition called "atherosclerosis." If pieces of plaque dislodge or too much of it accumulates, it can clog an artery and cut off critical blood supply to the body. If the blockage occurs in an artery that feeds the heart itself, it is a heart attack (a myocardial infarction in medical-speak); if it occurs in an artery to the brain, it is a stroke. Blood clots and clogged arteries can also occur in legs (deep vein thrombosis) and lungs (pulmonary embolism).

One person dies from CVD every thirty-three seconds in the United States; one every twelve minutes in Australia. This disease is the leading cause of death worldwide. Every year, roughly one in three deaths globally (over twenty million) is caused by a heart-engine that sputters out and stops pumping as it should (85 percent of these CVD deaths are heart attacks and strokes). Although CVD is traditionally attributed to unhealthy diet and lifestyle, we now know there is a strong microbial component to the disease.

Age is by far the largest risk factor for CVD, although obesity, diabetes, dietary patterns, and a sedentary lifestyle are also prominent risk factors. Changes in the heart and blood vessels as you age increase the threat. The arteries become harder and less flexible, like a bike chain rusting over time, which is why blood pressure goes up with age. Blood vessels can become stiffer, and the heart wall can thicken to assist with blood flow–i.e., more muscle to pump. The valves, which are like one-way doors that open and close to control blood flow, can also become thicker and stiffer. This leads to leaks or more resistance to pumping blood. Eighty-two percent of people who die of CVD are over the age of sixty-five.

There's also a gender element to this rise, as older women are three to five times more likely to develop CVD than men. Cholesterol levels keep increasing in women until around sixty-five years of age (cholesterol buildup in the arteries is one of the things that inhibit the "engine" from pumping), whereas in men, the levels plateau between age forty-five and fifty-five. Some believe this is related to hormones: Estrogen protects the heart, but estrogen levels decline following menopause (see chapter 10 for more about menopause and microbes).

Microbes and CVD Prevention

As with many things we've already examined, when it comes to microbes and disease, how you live now affects your degree of risk later in life–it's never too late to have your eye on a heart-healthy lifestyle. Everyday decisions–like choosing a burger versus a salad for lunch or sticking to your new exercise program versus letting your gym membership slide–lead to effects on blood vessels that accumulate over time. (Think of all the burgers you've enjoyed over the years!) You're lucky if your parents gave you good genes, but when it comes to CVD, most people are in control of their own luck.

It is estimated that nearly 90 percent of CVD is preventable, with only the remaining 10 percent due to family history and genetics. These preventable aspects include high blood pressure, which according to a 2016 study accounts for 13 percent of cardiovascular deaths; smoking, accounting for 9 percent (although if you quit smoking by age thirty this risk disappears later in life); obesity, accounting for 5 percent; poor diet; and excessive alcohol consumption. As challenging as it may seem, there is plenty you can do to prevent or delay CVD caused by these factors. Physical inactivity, which is defined as fewer than five moderate thirty-minute workouts per week, is thought to be the fourth leading factor for mortality worldwide, yet the majority of the American and Australian populations fail to meet this standard. Diets that are high in saturated fats, sugars, salt, and processed meats increase risk of CVD considerably, while diets such as the Dietary Approaches to Stop Hypertension (DASH) diet, incorporating plenty of fruits, vegetables, fiber, and nuts, significantly lower the risk.

Given the major impact diet and exercise play in CVD, it's no surprise that the body's microbiota are involved in the disease's development and prevention. In patients with CVD, we see changes in the main types of intestinal microbiota: increases in the Firmicutes and decreases in the Bacteroides. Some studies even suggest that we can use microbial composition to predict CVD, including one recent human study that showed that increased levels in *Oscillibacter* correlated with lower levels of cholesterol and higher HDL (high-density lipoprotein). But there is currently no "microbes test" for CVD. These changes in the microbiome are similar to changes seen in the microbiota associated with obesity (as discussed in chapter 2), suggesting a shift toward a more problematic "inflammatory" microbiota composition. As we've seen, the body defends itself with inflammation if any bacteria or bacterial surface molecule, especially lipopolysaccharide (LPS), seep into the body. This defense–our body's response to infections–causes destruction of tissue, including damage to blood vessels and the heart. Low-grade inflammation is not healthy for the cardiovascular system.

CVD does not just affect the heart. Many people are unaware of how this condition extends throughout the body, including how the health of the mouth is related to CVD. We saw in chapter 6 that the oral cavity is full of microbes, and that cavities and gum disease involve critical microbial pathogens. As gum disease worsens, pockets of pus develop around the teeth, along with inflammation of blood vessels in the gum tissue. Scientists believe these gum changes enable periodontal pathogens to enter into the body's circulation through blood traveling via veins and arteries, where the pathogens encounter blood vessels and trigger more inflammation. This causes tissue damage, including the tissues of the cardiovascular system. Dental pathogens have been found in the heart valves of CVD patients. This is why if you have CVD, dentists may prescribe antibiotics prior to dental procedures to try to prevent microbes from directly entering the bloodstream during the oral surgery—although antibiotics will have additional, often unintended effects on the microbiota. Given that older adults are more at risk for periodontal disease and tooth loss, they are also more at risk for heart disease. Use this as additional motivation to keep brushing and flossing, and schedule regular cleanings with your dentist.

THE BIG FAT SURPRISE

There is a rethink underway regarding the role of saturated fat in CVD. Dr. Ancel Keys, a powerful scientific figure in the 1950s to 1970s, initially championed the concept that high saturated fat intake leads to high cholesterol and heart disease. He persuasively advocated for the American Heart Association and the broader scientific community to stress the need to decrease fat intake and make it public enemy number one. We all very much "took it to heart": Dietary fat intake in the US dropped by 11 percent from the 1970s to the 2000s, and grocery stores still stock many low-fat and non-fat foods.

But we had to eat something, preferably something that tastes good! So instead, we increased our carbohydrate consumption—this includes adding sugar—by at least 25 percent. We now know that added sugar and refined carbohydrates also increase risk for CVD. Saturated fat is just one piece of the puzzle, and butter, meat, and cheese in moderation are part of a healthy diet. If you want the sordid details, check out *The Big Fat Surprise* by Nina Teicholz.

Here are the American Heart Association's current facts on fat, which are in line with what the National Heart Foundation of Australia says.

LOVE IT: Unsaturated fats lower rates of CVD. Sources of healthy fats containing good HDL cholesterol, such as olive oil, beans and legumes, whole grains, fatty fish, and nuts act like a vacuum for the arteries. They remove bad LDL (low-density lipoprotein) cholesterol and plaque buildup and reduce risk of heart disease.

LIMIT IT: Saturated fats are no longer forbidden but should be consumed in moderation. They occur naturally in many foods, including meat (e.g., fatty beef, lamb, pork, poultry with skin) and dairy products (e.g., cream, butter, cheese). It is recommended to aim for no more than 5 to 6 percent of daily calories from saturated fats.

LOSE IT: Artificial trans fat, hydrogenated oils, and tropical oils, such as palm kernel oil, increase risk of CVD and raise bad cholesterol levels. Try to save commercially fried foods and baked goods for rare occasions.

Heart Chemistry, or the Science Behind CVD

Now, let's get to the "meat of the matter" regarding microbes and CVD. We know that meat eaters, especially red meat consumers, have a higher CVD risk than vegetarians. In studies, germ-free–i.e., microbe-free–animals have a very low CVD risk, even if these animals are fed diets that increase the risk of CVD in animals with a normal microbiota. Why is this? Meat and egg yolks are rich in two structurally related compounds, L-carnitine and choline, and these compounds make up about 2 percent of the Western diet. Through a series of reactions, the gut microbes convert these compounds into a molecule waste by-product called "trimethylamine" (TMA). TMA is then oxidized by liver enzymes to trimethylamine N-oxide (TMAO), which facilitates CVD.

This suggests that if we took the microbes out of the equation, TMAO wouldn't be formed (nothing would make the microbe by-product of digestion, TMA). By extension, the occurrence of CVD would decrease. Remarkably, this process has evidence in real life: Germ-free animals don't make TMAO, and in model systems, they develop less CVD since they can't make TMA in the first place. But once they are colonized with microbes, they start producing TMA, then TMAO, and then get heart disease. In a study of four thousand people, high levels of TMAO equated directly to increased risk of high thrombotic events, including stroke and heart attack, and TMAO levels could be used to predict the degree of risk. So, the higher the TMAO levels, the higher the mortality in heart attacks.

MYTH: Red meat alone causes heart disease.

FACT: Red meat does not cause CVD by itself: It's how our microbes break down the red meat and create harmful by-products that leads to heart disease.

We interviewed Dr. Stanley Hazen, whose groundbreaking research has shown that TMA is a microbial product and TMAO is a major contributor to heart disease and stroke. A clinician and researcher in cardiovascular medicine at the Cleveland Clinic, Dr. Hazen explained that he "stumbled upon a connection to the gut microbiome" in the context of his work on heart disease and stroke. Working from a chemical background, Dr. Hazen's lab made their discovery around 2007 while searching large populations of patients for chemical signatures in plasma. They found a higher concentration of an unknown compound in patients with heart disease. After seeking out the rare and expensive tools needed to identify this compound, they discovered it to be TMAO, which was a known product of TMA, and yet when Dr. Hazen began researching TMA separately, he could locate descriptions of it found only in putrefaction–i.e., bacteria growing on rotting things. He figured that if there were enough bacteria to make it possible to see TMAO in plasma, then it must be coming from the body's microbial stronghold: the gut.

Dr. Hazen's team was shocked when he told them that they were switching gears and turning their focus to the gut. But their surprise soon turned to enthusiasm as the researchers realized that everything we eat is filtered through the intestinal tract, where its microbes digest and help us absorb our food. Dr. Hazen told us: "We like to think of ourselves as clean and sterile beings, but we aren't. We evolved with microbes through all of our eternity: from *Homo sapiens* onward. It started to make total sense." Dr. Hazen explained that in his clinical work, he knew that genetic risk factors for heart disease capture only 10 to 15 percent of patient risk. The vast majority of risk is environmental. "Our gut microbes are the filter of our biggest environmental exposure: what we eat," Dr. Hazen clarified. "When two people eat the same diet, we can see one develop heart disease and the other not. A big chunk of this reason is the microbes." This was the enormous missing piece to understanding human physiology and disease risk.

Dr. Hazen's group took initial animal studies further by demonstrating similar effects in humans. He fed people eight-ounce steaks and then measured their TMAO levels, which increased soon after digesting this meat. He then put these people on antibiotics, which suppressed their TMAO production because the key microbes that make TMA were killed off. After he stopped the course of antibiotics, the microbes and TMAO production increased to previous levels. But his coolest experiment involved getting a vegan of over five years to eat a steak! Though he promised there was no coercion involved for the sake of science:

> In our early studies, it was important to provide some food when giving study participants a capsule. For those who agreed, we

served them a steak. In one test, someone ate a filet mignon prepared on a George Foreman grill in my office—not too untypical during this time. But this person's blood and urine sample stood out like a sore thumb. When we did a follow-up to check for any genetic diseases, this person told us they had only eaten steak three times, ever—I had no idea this particular person was a vegan! This was a game-changing moment that shifted our gears toward considering differences between vegans, vegetarians, and omnivores.

As one would predict, the post-steak TMAO levels of the vegan were much lower than those of regular meat eaters—because the vegan had fewer microbes that could make precursor TMA to begin with. Outside of Dr. Hazen's discovery, further studies have also shown that there are higher levels of TMAO in omnivores than in vegans and vegetarians—which confirms the connection between certain animal products such as red meat and this microbial menace of the heart.

Red meat is not the only source of these compounds: Choline, lecithin, and carnitine supplements can also give rise to the body's production of TMAO. Drinking multiple cans of certain energy drinks, which can include supplemental carnitine, may be equivalent to eating multiple steaks' worth of carnitine a day. Research has shown that feeding mice diets rich in carnitine or choline can cause a tenfold increase in TMAO, as well as an increase in the microbes that form TMA, which then leads to more TMAO.

With growing interest in microbes and CVD, researchers discovered that TMAO is what leads to the "clogged pipe" of atherosclerosis by suppressing reverse cholesterol transport from peripheral tissues back to the liver. It also affects platelet activity, which can lead to more clotting of blood vessels (thrombosis) and inflammation, which correspondingly contributes to vascular damage. Collectively these conditions obstruct blood flow and cause heart disease.

Compelling evidence from fecal-transfer experiments further demonstrates that gut microbes are involved in CVD. When fecal matter from a mouse line that makes high levels of TMAO was transferred to a breed of mice with low TMAO levels, the recipients' TMAO levels went up, as did the microbes with the enzyme that makes TMA. By simply swapping feces (and microbes), it would be possible to alter the likelihood of CVD!

Recent data in human studies have confirmed that high levels of TMAO correlate with major adverse cardiac events. One study showed that, in people with stable coronary heart disease, high levels of TMAO were correlated with a fourfold increase in mortality. Several studies also show that measuring levels of TMA and TMAO are indicative of predicting CVD risk, much like current cholesterol and lipid measurements.

As we have seen, short-chain fatty acids (SCFAs) such as butyrate are key microbial products made from dietary fiber that have significant anti-inflammatory effects. Recent studies indicate that increased dietary fiber intake (think Mediterranean or DASH diets) results in decreased CVD risk and lower blood pressure (decreased hypertension). A common theme throughout this book—decreasing inflammation via SCFAs—is a key benefit to health and longevity.

Although we don't have all the details yet, it seems that microbes have a major impact on CVD through the production of TMA/TMAO and SCFAs. The fact that microbes are involved in CVD would have been an unthinkable concept a decade ago, but now scientists are hard at work to see exactly how microbes are involved in heart attacks and strokes. The goal is to be able to use this information to address the biggest cause of death in the world.

Drugging the Bugs

How can we use these discoveries to decrease our risk of CVD? One might think that targeting the human liver enzymes that convert TMA into TMAO with inhibitors might reduce CVD. But when we try this, we raise the level of the precursor TMA, which smells like rotting fish. Not a good side effect for a drug! Several studies that genetically "knocked down" the liver enzyme resulted in mice that stink like rotten fish—but they were protected from CVD. Targeting liver enzymes as such is difficult pharmacologically in humans—all the compounds are toxic, in addition to the unattractive smell. For these reasons, scientists have been unable to target the key liver enzyme in TMAO formation.

Perhaps we could go after the microbes directly? Hazen's group has done this in animals. They identified a naturally occurring compound: 3,3-dimethyl-1-butanol, or DMB, found in grape seeds, red wine, and cold-pressed extra virgin olive oils (think of the Mediterranean diet). This compound inhibits the bacterial enzyme (called a "lyase") that initially forms TMA from choline and L-carnitine. Amazingly, when scientists fed the inhibitor DMB to mice, they observed decreased TMAO production and atherosclerosis. DMB didn't kill the microbes–which is good because that would put pressure on them to evolve and increase their resistance (much like how resistance to antibiotics develops). Although this inhibitor has been tested only in mice and the team is looking for even better inhibitors, the results certainly suggest that drugging the bugs may soon become a viable strategy to decrease risk of CVD.

Cardiologists and physicians are beginning to incorporate some of these findings into patient care. TMAO testing is now available, and some are using TMAO as a clinical diagnostic tool to recognize previously unidentified individuals who are at risk for CVD, and those who may be overlooked by traditional tests, such as markers for cholesterol. Dr. Hazen advised that someone with a high TMAO level should take a progressive approach to CVD prevention through weight reduction, improvements to diet (such as cutting down on animal products), and watching traditional markers of blood pressure and cholesterol. As always, Dr. Hazen cautioned, there is a need to tread carefully regarding modifying TMA or TMAO levels, given the lack of reliable proof of efficacy and long-term safety. "TMAO is just the tip of the iceberg. Dozens and dozens of other connections between gut microbes and cardio-metabolic processes exist. It's going to get a lot more complicated before it gets simpler." Dr. Hazen expressed his belief in rigorous scientific trials to ensure that we do no harm.

Hypertension

Hypertension refers to increased blood pressure, which causes stress on the heart (making it harder to pump blood). According to the WHO, a staggering 1.28 billion adults have hypertension (defined as a systolic blood pressure greater than 140 mmHg, and diastolic pressure greater than 90 mmHg), and nearly half of all adults in the USA, and roughly one-third of adults in Australia. The problem with hypertension is that there are no obvious symptoms (nothing hurts, things seem normal) and you think you are fine until you have CVD. This is why doctors regularly test your blood pressure to try to catch it early. Hypertension can be controlled initially by diet (including reduced salt intake), exercise, losing weight, and not smoking. However, if that doesn't decrease your blood pressure enough, there are drugs that are commonly used to control it.

In the past few years, evidence is accumulating that the microbiome is involved in affecting this silent killer disease. Initially, like so many other diseases we have seen, studies showed that people with hypertension have a dysbiotic microbiome. This wasn't surprising, as the risk factors include poor diet, obesity, lack of exercise, and smoking. This was also studied in animal models among rats and mice. Fecal transfer into germ-free mice from hypertensive people caused an increase in blood pressure in these animals, which is currently the best causation data we have about microbes and hypertension.

Further studies are now starting to show that the microbiome could affect blood pressure by impacting blood vessel function. As we discussed above, one of these mechanisms includes SCFA production which decreases inflammation, a major cause of damage to blood vessels. A recent double-blind clinical trial showed that by taking high-amylose starch (a fermentable fiber), blood pressure dropped by 6 mmHg and human participants saw a significant increase in SCFAs. High-salt diets have also been shown to cause dysbiosis and inflammation, including depletion of lactobacilli, in both mice and humans. A study that added back *Lactobacillus* for eight weeks dropped blood pressure. TMAO is also associated with hypertension, mainly through affecting blood vessel vasoconstriction and stiffening of the arteries. As expected, studies are now starting to appear using the microbiome to predict hypertension risk, although they have not reached the clinical stage yet.

NO WHINING ABOUT RED WINE

Alcohol overuse is perhaps the second-best known risk factor in CVD after meat, but its consumption is a double-edged sword when it comes to the heart. There is no doubt that high levels of alcohol consumption increase the risk of heart attack. In a study, people who had heart attacks were asked if they had a drink within the hour before the attack; those who had consumed hard liquor drinks (e.g., gin, vodka, whiskey) had increased their risk more than if they had consumed beer or wine, but the risk with beer or wine was still greater than for those who did not have an alcoholic beverage. Binge drinking is defined by the National Institute on Alcohol Abuse and Alcoholism "as a pattern of drinking alcohol that brings blood alcohol concentration [levels] to 0.08 g/dL"—typically occurring after four drinks for women and five drinks for men, in about two hours. Binge drinkers are 72 percent more likely to have a heart attack than those who consume alcohol moderately—defined as those who consume up to one drink per day for women, and up to two per day for men. Even infrequent binge drinkers can have increased gut permeability and higher levels of inflammatory LPS and bacterial DNA. This indicates microbes in their blood serum following the binge could contribute to general inflammation.

The good news is that a glass of red wine a day is protective for CVD, similar to its health-promoting work in the gut, as discussed in chapter 2. (We think it's the best part of the MIND, Mediterranean, and DASH diets!) Although we previously thought it was the antioxidants in red wine that helped protect our arteries from inflammation damage and CVD, no such mechanism had been found. Instead, it's microbes that are causing us to rethink how red wine might be beneficial.

Red wine, grape seeds, and olive oil all contain a compound called "DMB" (see page 146), which inhibits the microbial enzyme that converts meat products into TMA. This ultimately decreases TMAO levels and atherosclerosis in animals. The benefits of resveratrol, a polyphenolic compound found in the skin of grapes and other berries (and in red wine), may be similar. Researchers found that resveratrol causes a reduction in TMAO levels in mice—but it also causes a restructuring of all the intestinal microbiota, most importantly the decrease of the microbes that produce TMA. Although it is early days for trials on humans, it is suggested that red wine polyphenols (such as resveratrol) favorably change the microbiota over a month.

All this definitely calls for a glass of red wine and a toast to our microbes!

Sweating the Microbes

Exercise plays a key role in protection against CVD, and new data suggest this may occur in part through changes to the microbiota. When mice were fed normal or high-fat diets, both lean and fat mice that then "exercised" (on a running wheel in their cage) did not have the arterial damage seen in those that didn't exercise (no wheel in the cage). There were also more beneficial shifts in the mice's microbiome following exercise, including increases in *Faecalibacterium prausnitzii*, which protects against obesity and IBD, since it decreases inflammation. Researchers found that exercise also improved the integrity of the gut (meaning less leakage of LPS and resulting inflammation), and, regardless of diet, it was uniquely beneficial to the microbiome. Of particular relevance here is another key factor: Even exercise in older animals reduced inflammatory markers and increased intestinal health.

Further interesting studies like this suggest how microbes affect endurance as well (we may be on the cusp of a bug-doping trend; see chapter 11). Earlier studies (with different animal welfare ethics standards) found that when mice were made to swim to exhaustion, the mice colonized with microbes fared much better than germ-free mice. Animals colonized with microbes also had increased muscle mass and increased antioxidant activity, which helps protect against intense exercise-induced oxidative damage (read: sore muscles).

What does this mean for us? Given that most of the population is considered inactive, these studies suggest that boosting our activity may decrease CVD incidence. A study from Ireland sheds light on similar effects in humans. The research group studied a professional Irish rugby team during their pre-season camp and compared them to normal people. They found that the athletes had a much higher diversity in their microbes–which is generally good for health. Controls with low BMI and the athletes also had higher levels of *Akkermansia*, a beneficial bacterium that increases SFCAs; this is in contrast to low levels of this microbe found in those with obesity and metabolic diseases. Other studies show that exercise is associated with increased SCFA production, and the type and intensity of exercise (e.g., running, cycling, high-impact interval training) may have distinct effects on microbiome composition. Combining various exercises (e.g., aerobic exercise and resistance training) was better than a single form of exercise, increasing microbiome diversity, and decreasing inflammation. They also found that more exercise was better for improving microbial diversity, both in length of session (ninety minutes was optimal), and number of sessions/week (two to five times/week was needed for sustained changes in diversity). And beyond eight weeks, the longer you stuck with it, the better the effect on the microbiome. Unfortunately, the changes were reversed within three weeks of being sedentary. For serious runners, a pre-race taper (the phase of reduced training load before an important competition) was not associated with changes in the microbiome, and for those who have exercised for many years, significant changes were not seen during sedentary periods. What these studies seem to point to is that exercise, like diet, does directly and beneficially influence the microbiota, which in turn are beneficial for us.

Healthy Hearts: A Look Ahead

Given the exciting developments described in this chapter, CVD prevention could undergo a major revolution in the next few years. We are now learning how microbes are beneficially affected by lifestyle (e.g., exercise) and diet (e.g., red wine). The most promising leads involve targeting microbial enzymes to prevent disease with new drugs that will stand a much better chance of minimal side effects, since the pathway they are targeting is found only in microbes, rather than in humans. One possibility is designing probiotics or prebiotics to outcompete these unwanted organisms and their genes. Moreover, preventive analysis of an individual's microbiome can deliver an indication of the level of microbes present that contribute to CVD. This could provide us with specific diet modifications to target and decrease these microbes before a heart attack or stroke occurs–we can already analyze the microbes' presence, but the exact dietary changes needed to correct them are less clear. Specific microbial interventions promise new ways to target the world's number one killer in the future.

KEY TIPS

Aim for at least thirty minutes of moderate activity most days: Regular exercise is essential to the health of your heart and your microbes. Aim for a mix of aerobic (cardio) and strength-based activities. The most important point is to keep it up for the long term. So, choose activities you enjoy, and know that it doesn't have to all be done at once. Ten-minute blocks of exercise can be just as beneficial as longer blocks (if not more so, since you are sitting less continuously the rest of the day).

Increase the fiber and antioxidants in your diet: Incorporate plenty of fruits, vegetables, whole grains, and nuts into your diet. Cold-pressed extra virgin olive oils and foods rich in antioxidants (e.g., dark chocolate, green tea) and good HDL cholesterol (e.g., nuts, avocados) in moderation can also protect the heart.

Avoid high-fat and high-sugar diets: Meat, egg yolks, and high-fat dairy products contain high levels of choline, phosphatidyl choline, and carnitine, precursors to TMA and TMAO. Similarly, avoid carnitine-supplemented energy drinks.

Drink in moderation: Red wine can inhibit TMAO production and help protect the arteries. The CDC defines moderate drinking as one drink or less per day for women, and two drinks or less per day for men.

Follow the Mediterranean and/or DASH diets: There is extensive clinical evidence and studies showing that these diets significantly decrease CVD and hypertension risk and modify the microbiome to a more beneficial composition.

Pause the probiotics: There are currently no studies in humans that show that probiotics decrease CVD risk (although there are a few studies using *Lactobacillus* strains that show decreased markers associated with CVD). Several mouse studies have shown positive results, but the data for probiotics in humans are still preliminary.

Take care of your teeth: Regular brushing, flossing, and dental checkups can help keep away heart disease. As noted in chapter 6, don't rush when you brush to get all those deep crevices where microbes can settle down!

8

Take a Deep Breath: The Lung Microbiome

Take a really deep breath. Hold it. Now breathe out. What happened? Even though you had some conscious muscle control of your breathing just now, it's unlikely that you regularly consider the precise mechanics of this autonomic process. It goes like this: As you inhaled, your diaphragm muscle–located just under the lungs, at the bottom of the rib cage–contracted and pushed itself downward. This increased the space in your chest cavity for your lungs to expand and fill with air, a movement aided by the intercostal muscles between your ribs. Your expanded lungs then sucked in air from outside the body through the mouth and nose. Air traveled down your windpipe and into your lungs, passing through your bronchial tubes into the alveoli (tiny air sacs). You also sucked in microbes from the surrounding air. The oxygen then traveled through the thin walls of the alveoli into the surrounding capillaries (blood vessels) to diffuse throughout your entire body. At the same time, carbon dioxide moved from the capillaries into the alveoli. Exhaling relaxed your diaphragm and intercostal muscles, which reduced the space of your chest cavity and forced carbon dioxide and moisture out of your lungs and windpipe.

This entire process happens effortlessly somewhere between seventeen thousand and thirty thousand times per day–that's twelve to twenty times per minute on average, when at rest. Without it, we would die. While we can live without food for many days and water for a few days, we can only live without air for a few scant minutes. Every day we breathe in about eight thousand liters of air. The maximum amount of air your lungs can hold at once is about six liters (three large soda bottles).

We tend to think of the lungs as an inverted Y structure with two lobes at the end of the central windpipe. If we look very closely, however, we see that it is an intricate structure with thousands of tiny alveoli branches to increase the surface area of our lungs to exchange oxygen and carbon dioxide. If we flattened out all these tiny airways, the surface area would be thirty times that of our skin!

Aging Lungs

What happens to our lungs as we age? First of all, maximum lung function (the maximal force you can generate when breathing in or out) naturally decreases with age. After the age of thirty, the rate of airflow through the airways slowly declines, as well as the amount of oxygen diffusing from the alveoli into the blood. Later on, other structural changes start to play a role in lung capacity. The rib cage can become thinner and change shape due to shrinking muscles, thereby altering the bones' ability to respond to the expansion and contraction of the lungs and diaphragm with breathing. With nowhere to expand into, the diaphragm weakens, which in turn decreases the capacity to inhale and exhale to our fullest. The muscles and tissues keeping the airways open can lose elasticity, and the alveoli can lose their shape and become slack. The part of the brain controlling breathing may no longer send as strong a signal to the lungs in old age (due to age-related decline), and nerves in airways that trigger coughing may become less sensitive to foreign particles. The immune system can also weaken, meaning that the body is less able to fight off lung infections (e.g., pneumonia and bronchitis) and other diseases. As a result of these changes, older adults are more at risk for shortness of breath, low oxygen levels, and abnormal breathing patterns such as sleep apnea.

Despite these declines, older people should be able to maintain enough lung function for everyday activities. In our youth, we have "extra" lung function: This is why healthy, younger individuals can tolerate the surgical removal of an entire lung and still breathe reasonably well. In healthy individuals, even these age-related changes seldom lead to serious decline. In fact, poor heart health and obesity are more often the culprits for breathing problems than changes to the lungs and their surroundings. Exercise is thus essential to both overall fitness and breathing. Studies have shown that exercise and aerobic training can improve lung capacity, even in very old populations. Aerobic workouts can improve lung capacity by 5 to 15 percent as exercise "works out" two of your most important organs: the lungs and heart. Not smoking is the number one way to minimize the effect of aging on the lungs. More than any other demographic, older adults need to be aware of the need to stand up, move around, and breathe deeply and regularly–especially during illness or after surgery. Lying in bed or sitting for long periods of time, at any age, allows mucus to build up in the lungs, putting them more at risk for infection.

Exploring the Lung Microbiome

Every time you breathe in, more than just vital oxygen is entering your body. The air around us teems with millions of microbes, mixing with some of the microbes in your mouth that ultimately make their way through your windpipe and downward. We have a strong defense system against unwanted microbes, including the lungs' surface, which is coated in mucus, a slimy substance designed to trap microbes. Cells of the lung push that mucus upward into the mouth, where you swallow and digest it. This is called "mucociliary action." Think of the last time you had a cold and coughed up slimy mucus–that was your body's way of expelling unwanted bacteria and cellular debris. In addition, there are special cells called "alveolar macrophages" that patrol the lower airways of our lungs looking for harmful microbes to engulf and destroy (we covered macrophages in chapter 3).

MYTH: The lungs are sterile and devoid of microbes.

FACT: Our lungs are exposed to upward of a million bacteria each day and most likely have their very own, essential, microbiome.

But breathing involves much more than just the lungs. There are two main parts of the respiratory tract: Your nose, pharynx, and larynx constitute the upper respiratory tract; and the trachea, bronchi, and lungs compose the lower respiratory tract. All our classic science textbooks say that the lower airway is sterile, and thus no home to microbes. To learn about the history of this paradigm, we interviewed Dr. James Hogg, Professor Emeritus of Pathology at the University of British Columbia and longtime lung researcher at St. Paul's Hospital in Vancouver, Canada. "That sort of thinking is all gone," he confirmed. "The lung is not sterile! That light went on recently–certainly after interest in the microbiome came along." When asked why the sterile lung idea was so prevalent, Dr. Hogg explained that researchers, in part, contributed to this misconception. It is part of a well-established, widely used technique to wash the airway during a normal bronchoscopy–a test that allows doctors and scientists to examine the airway and lungs. Bronchial washing is when clinicians spray saline solution over the surface, particularly areas that can't be seen, to then collect cells washed off of the surface to examine under a microscope. The problem is that these washings are subject to frequent contamination from the oral cavity as the tube is pushed down the airway, resulting in what everyone always thought was contamination from the mouth.

For a variety of reasons, scientists also couldn't grow microbes from the lungs to study through traditional laboratory methods such as agar plates–Petri dishes that contain agar, which acts as the solid growth medium–along with nutrients to culture and grow microorganisms. But with the advent of culture-independent techniques–i.e., DNA sequencing–at last we were able to detect microbial signatures deep inside the lungs. As with many discoveries, this claim did not arrive without controversy. Some scientists continued to assert that the microbial signatures were contaminants from the upper respiratory tract due to washing techniques. Dr. Hogg stated that oral contamination remains a highly contentious argument and complication. To avoid such contamination, he prefers to freeze the lungs from cadavers before studying them. Better sampling techniques and differing compositions from other oral sites over the past few years have dispelled most of the controversy; however, the process is far from perfect. Dr. Hogg joked that pathologists have become veritable tissue hounds, constantly scouring hospitals and clinical trials for diverse lung samples in an attempt to enhance our understanding of the respiratory system.

Appreciation for the lung microbiome is starting to spread among clinicians and researchers, but much more hard science needs to be done. "A lot of people are talking the talk, but not walking the walk," says Dr. Hogg. We are still not able to culture these microbes, so there remains some hesitation to fully accept the "lung microbiome" concept. The existence of microbial DNA doesn't prove the existence of live microbes. The predicted numbers of microbes are incredibly small in comparison to those of other body sites: one thousand times fewer than in the mouth, and one million to one billion times fewer than in the gut. If you follow the math, this works out to approximately two thousand bacteria per square centimeter in the lungs (which may sound like a lot but is very little in microbial terms). Despite this low biomass, the lower lung microbiome, unlike most other microbiomes in the body, is characterized by dynamic fluxes in microbes, rather than a constant composition (making it all the harder to characterize). Generally, there are species in the Firmicutes (including *Streptococcus* spp. and *Veillonella* spp.), Bacteroidetes (including *Prevotella* spp.), and Proteobacteria phyla, with up to 140 bacterial families found in the adult lung. The constant clearing of microbes by the mucociliary action, inhalation of new microbes, and other factors such as inflammation all play a role in making the lung microbiome dynamic, now described as "transient but not resident." These lower microbes include varieties of aerobes, microbes that tolerate oxygen, as one would expect in the lungs; aerotolerant microbes, which do not utilize oxygen but can protect themselves from reactive oxygen molecules; and anaerobes–because they can't grow in oxygen, they are buried deep in the tissues and other protected areas devoid of oxygen. Among the few things we know lower microbes do for us is prevent the pathogens we breathe in from colonizing by producing antibacterial products that can kill them off. They also help to shape the immune response of the airway mucosa, thereby helping to control infections and other health risks we encounter throughout daily life.

What exactly are these microbes protecting us from? Given that lungs are constantly exposed to particles from the air, the lung microbiota respond to everything we inhale. One key exposure is air pollution, which causes oxidative stress and inflammation in the lungs and alters the lung microbiome. Microbiota seem responsive to pollutants. For example, they may break down inhaled pollutants or modulate how the lung immune system responds to them. People exposed to smoke from both forest fires and tobacco have higher rates of pneumonia caused by *Streptococcus pneumoniae* (also called the "pneumococcus").

STAY SAFE FROM HAZARDOUS AIR QUALITY

AQI: This is an acronym that many of us are increasingly familiar with as we check on the air quality index (AQI) in our local areas on hazy days. With increased wildfire smoke and urban smog, it is important to protect yourself (and your lung microbes!) from air pollutants. If outdoor air quality is low, stay indoors with windows and doors closed. Avoid prolonged or heavy exertion outdoors and wear a face mask if you must be outside. Buildings filter many of the smaller pollutant particulates out of the air, and air conditioning units can be set to "recirculate" to prevent bringing in air from outdoors, thereby reducing your and your microbes' exposure to harmful pollutants.

So, what we can definitively say is that there are microbes in small numbers in the lungs, and that they are a dynamic population! This claim, vague as it may seem, nonetheless represents a major rethinking of the lung microbiome, with significant implications for medical research and personal health.

THE GUT-LUNG AXIS

Much like the gut-brain axis, there also appears to be a gut-lung axis largely mediated through the immune system. Research in Brett's laboratory has shown that certain gut microbes encountered early in life can have a major impact on a person's chance of developing asthma as they age. This has been confirmed in several other studies, and it seems that the early life microbiome affects how the immune system develops, pushing it toward one that is more or less susceptible to later asthma. In addition to these early life gut microbes affecting the lungs via the immune system, there are new reports of oral probiotics, including certain lactobacilli, suggesting that the microbes you ingest can modulate lung inflammation via the gut-lung axis. For example: *Lactobacillus reuteri* and *Lactobacillus plantarum* can decrease allergic airway inflammation, while *Lactobacillus casei* can have positive effects in treating bacterial and viral pneumonia in mice. In other words, microbes that affect inflammation in the gut also affect inflammation in the lungs. It also works the other way as well: Alterations in the lungs affect gut microbes. For example, when lung inflammation was triggered in mice by adding LPS to the lungs, it caused a significant change in intestinal microbes. The concept that the lung and gut are linked also suggests that keeping your gut microbiome healthy (and other microbiomes throughout your body) may also enhance lung health.

Antibiotic medications we ingest also alter the lung microbiome, as do anti-inflammatories and steroids. Given our still-limited knowledge of the lung microbiome, it is too early to say whether these changes are detrimental. However, it's safe to assume that any upset to normal microbial composition anywhere in the body is associated with detrimental effects—at some point or another. It's likely just a matter of time before we know more about why avoiding antibiotics could improve our lung function, among other things. We also know that lung microbiota are altered in lung diseases such as Chronic Obstructive Pulmonary Disease (COPD), asthma, and cystic fibrosis—as is the gut microbiome. While we don't know whether these changes cause the disease or are a result of changing lung environment during disease, we are using this information to find new ways to promote lung health as we age and advise on which activities might exacerbate current conditions and therefore should be avoided.

Smoking

A collection of studies shows that smoking causes differences in the oral and upper airway microbiomes but does not cause changes in the lower airway microbes. As we saw in chapter 6, smokers have fewer normal, helpful oral microbes to begin with, and more pathogenic ones. This may be related to smokers' higher rates of pneumococcal pneumonia and susceptibility to respiratory infections. The hypothesis is that smoking disrupts the normal microbiota so that it is not as protective against harmful pathogens. Smoking also dampens the immune system and destroys our body's defenses in the respiratory tract. This likely leads to increased infection. The good news for smokers is that if you stop smoking, the microbiota revert to their healthier composition.

More puzzling to scientists are the changes that occur in the more distant gut microbiota due to smoking. Smokers have a reduced ratio of Firmicutes to Bacteroidetes in their gut (which is usually not healthy—see chapter 2 for more on these key gut bacteria), and reduced numbers of anti-inflammatory Bifidobacteria. Smokers also have more pathogenic bacteria in their guts. We do not yet understand exactly why smoking affects intestinal microbes. Scientists hypothesize that it may be because changes in the environment and host (the person affected) impact the immune system and thereby influence microbes in the gut. That smoking is a known risk factor for Crohn's disease speaks to this microbial connection. However, smoking is perplexingly protective against another inflammatory intestinal disease, ulcerative colitis, and for some reason, Parkinson's disease. We have no idea why–but, again, none of this evidence supports taking up smoking as an exercise in preventative medicine.

Chronic Obstructive Pulmonary Disease

COPD refers to a group of chronic lung diseases, including emphysema and chronic bronchitis, that make it difficult to breathe. Though heart disease, cancer, and stroke often receive more attention in the media and medical literature, COPD is a widespread and deadly killer, and the third leading cause of death worldwide. In 2020, 480 million people were estimated to have COPD. It causes over 3.5 million deaths per year, with about 90 percent in those under seventy years of age occurring in lower and middle-income countries. More than fifteen million Americans have been diagnosed with COPD, and many more do not know they have it. It can cause serious long-term disability, even death, and currently there is no cure.

MYTH: Only smokers develop COPD.

FACT: While smoking tobacco is the leading cause of COPD, there are many other risk factors that contribute to development of the disease.

Causes of COPD include everyday exposure to air pollution, secondhand smoke, and dust; exposure to fumes from forest fires and polluting open cooking fires; and exposure to workplace chemicals. Smokers are especially at risk for COPD, with about 20 percent of smokers getting the disease, and 70 percent of COPD patients in high-income countries being smokers. When a cigarette burns, it creates more than seven thousand chemicals, and the inhaled toxins weaken and damage the lungs in the same way that other external pollutants can. Smoking has a linear relationship with COPD: The longer you smoke, the greater your risk.

COPD is often not diagnosed until very advanced stages because people do not know the early warning signs. Symptoms include shortness of breath progressing to a chronic cough and heavy mucus production. Frequent respiratory infections, blueness of the lips or fingernails (cyanosis), fatigue, and wheezing are other early warning signs. It is important not to wait for symptoms to become severe, because early detection of COPD is essential to successful treatment. You can't reverse the damage to lung tissue, but you can treat the symptoms and manage the disease. There are several treatment options, including medications, surgery, and other therapies that can improve quality of life. Symptoms wax and wane in cycles, with most damage to the lungs caused during flare-ups. Respiratory viral infections can cause these exacerbations, making the flu shot and the pneumococcal vaccine extra important for COPD patients.

Many studies document major changes in the lung microbiota of COPD patients, especially during COPD exacerbations. As these cycles worsen, the lung defenses weaken, inflammation and damage increases, and dysbiotic changes in the microbiota increase while bacterial diversity decreases. This disturbed microbial imbalance is harmful in general and can make lung inflammation even worse. Scientists have shown that changes in the lung microbiota occur early in COPD, including increases in Proteobacteria and known respiratory pathogens that help drive inflammatory damage. This hints, but does not prove, that the microbiota are involved in this disease. Another clue is that bacterial pathogens, such as those that cause pneumonia, are isolated at a higher frequency in COPD patients. While there is ample evidence the COPD lung microbiome is different than the normal lung microbiome, we still do not know whether this is driving COPD, or a by-product of the changes in the lungs.

There is agreement that the COPD microbiome is more inflammatory and helps drive inflammation. Some studies show that treatment with antibiotics for seven to ten days during exacerbations decreases COPD. However, this remains controversial, because little effect was seen in mild or moderate disease states. We may be able to use this information to help identify COPD in its early stages. One study found that researchers could identify COPD by looking for ten microbial strains in the lungs. Given that millions of Americans, and several hundred thousand Australians, unknowingly have the disease, this method of identification could become a useful tool for early diagnosis and help rule out other lung diseases.

Probiotic Potential

Since probiotics can decrease inflammation, could they help with lung infections and inflammatory diseases such as COPD? Maybe in humans, and definitely in mice. Test tube studies indicate that *Lactobacillus rhamnosus* and *Bifidobacterium breve* can reduce inflammatory responses in isolated macrophages–a type of white blood cell that engulfs and digests harmful particles, especially at sites of infection. *Lactobacillus casei* can improve the function of specialized natural killer cells isolated from smokers. In addition, some probiotics (*L. rhamnosus*) decrease lung inflammation in mouse models of COPD that were induced by cigarette smoke.

Given the strong gut-lung axis, oral probiotics that enhance the immune system have been shown to decrease pneumonia and other lung infections in mice. At present, only a few studies have tried delivering probiotics directly into the lungs (an interesting concept), and these were all in mice, including trying to protect against viral influenza infections. In humans, a recent study in Ireland showed that a blend of herbs and a *Lactobacillus* probiotic given orally for a month was well tolerated in both healthy and asthmatic patients, and improved lung function in the asthmatics. This finding lays the groundwork for a larger future controlled clinical trial. In conclusion, oral probiotics that enhance the immune system should also decrease lung infections and other lung diseases via the gut-lung axis, but the clinical trials haven't been performed yet. Keep an eye out for future studies that link the lung microbiota to the progression, exacerbation, and treatment of COPD in humans.

The Angel of Death

Pneumonia is a common lung infection caused by bacteria, a virus, or fungi–most commonly the bacterium *S. pneumoniae*, a normal inhabitant of the oral microbiota that, under the right conditions (such as weakened lungs) can cause this disease. If invading germs get through the upper respiratory tract's defenses, they colonize the lower respiratory tract to cause significant damage and inflammation in the lower lungs. This leads to fluid and debris accumulation, and pneumonia in one or both lungs. The infection and its symptoms vary from mild to severe. Chances of faster recovery are greatest in the young, if the infection is caught early and hasn't spread, and in those with healthy immune systems if they are not suffering from other illnesses. Most healthy people recover in one to three weeks, but it can be life-threatening, particularly for infants, young children, older adults, and those with chronic health problems.

MYTH: Everybody who is a carrier of the bacterium *S. pneumoniae* (a common bacterial cause of pneumonia) will get sick from it.

FACT: It is quite common for people, especially children, to carry the bacteria in their throats without getting pneumonia.

Pneumonia causes millions of deaths worldwide each year. It is disproportionally hardest on older people. Historically (before antibiotics), it was called "the old man's friend" and "the angel of death" because it caused a swift and relatively painless death for already weakened and fragile bodies. Lung defenses are especially vulnerable if weakened by infection, a waning immune system–which occurs as one ages–and/or smoking.

Pneumonia affects lungs in two ways: lobar pneumonia, which may be present in only one part (lobe) of the lung; or bronchial pneumonia, which may be widespread with patches throughout both lungs. It causes a cough (often with mucus), fever, shaking, chills, and shortness of breath. These initial symptoms can be confused with a common cold or the flu. However, unlike a cold–which left untreated will generally run its course in one to three weeks as the body's immune system restores health–pneumonia often requires treatment for full recovery. Most cases can be eased by staying hydrated to help loosen lung secretions and bring up phlegm. Also useful are extended rest, over-the-counter medications to control the fever, and if the condition becomes serious, prescription antibiotics. Do not take cough medicine without first talking to your doctor, as coughing is one method the body uses to get rid of the excess mucus and debris and might be helping you get better. In the past, penicillin worked extremely well in treating bacterial pneumonia, but the rise of antibiotic resistance now often requires new antibiotics. In severe cases, people are hospitalized to receive fluids, oxygen therapy, and stronger antibiotics.

You can reduce your risk of pneumonia by taking a few simple steps.

1. Get your annual flu shot (see "Should I Get a Flu Vaccine?" on page 164), as the flu makes you more susceptible to pneumonia due to lung damage. The CDC recommends different types of vaccines depending on age (i.e., children under two and adults over the age of sixty-five) and for those with certain medical conditions who are at higher risk of bacterial pneumonia (pneumococcal), and recommendations also differ in Australia. Talk to your health care provider to determine which vaccine is best for you.
2. Make it a habit to wash your hands frequently during cold and flu season (viral airborne infections are often spread via coughing, sneezing, and even breathing, which we can pick up from contaminated surfaces and transfer with our hands).
3. Avoid smoking, as we know that tobacco damages the lungs' ability to fight off infection.

External bacteria are behind pneumonia, but do the microbes within our lungs also affect the disease? Recent studies suggest that they may have a larger role than we previously thought. The current hypothesis is that an imbalance in the oral microbiota (dysbiosis) predisposes us to an overgrowth of pathogens, especially the pneumococcus. This leads to subsequent diseases in the lower respiratory tract. Studies have shown that the upper respiratory tract microbiota is vastly different in those with pneumonia compared to those who don't have the disease. Researchers in one study were able to predict pneumonia by analyzing five specific microbial species found in the upper respiratory tract–with 95 percent

MYTH: Pneumonia happens only in cold-weather seasons.

FACT: Though we've all heard the warning "put on your coat or you'll catch a cold," air temperature in fact has little impact on the ability of microbes to cause infection. The origin of this myth likely stems from the fact that we gather indoors together more frequently during winter months, so microbes can spread more effectively from person to person.

specificity and 84 percent sensitivity. This suggests that the oral microbiota play a major role in lung protection and, ultimately, in seeding lower lungs with pathogens.

SHOULD I GET A FLU VACCINE?

Yes!

(The same goes for COVID-19 vaccines and boosters, which also protect against a potentially nasty respiratory virus; you can read more about COVID-19 vaccines in chapter 15.)

The influenza virus causes the flu, a viral infection that affects the nose, throat, bronchi, and occasionally lungs. Most of us have suffered from the flu at some point: fever, aching muscles, headache, sore throat, cough, chills, and fatigue. Jessica got the flu a couple of years ago and literally couldn't get out of bed for a few days, she was so sick. It was a good reminder that influenza should be taken seriously as it can be deadly. Older adults are particularly susceptible to the flu: 80 to 90 percent of flu-related deaths are in people over the age of sixty-five. This is because the immune system typically weakens with age, and the flu can worsen other health problems such as heart disease, lung disease, and asthma. The flu weakens respiratory defenses, which often leads to secondary bacterial pneumonia—a disease that can be life threatening. As such, in addition to the traditional flu vaccine, there is a federally approved high-dose vaccine for those over the age of sixty-five. It contains four times the regular dosage and provides a stronger immune response and antibody protection.

We are still at an early stage in assessing how we can use this knowledge to protect people against pneumonia; however, scientists are getting pretty skilled at saving mice. When treated with broad spectrum antibiotics in one study, mice were more susceptible to pneumonia caused by *S. pneumoniae* (probably because their oral microbiota were disrupted). But when scientists then did a fecal transfer from healthy mice, this effect was reversed! The infected mice recovered from pneumonia. The reasons why this worked are still unclear—perhaps because they recolonized the gut microbiota, or maybe even the oral microbiota (since they did the fecal transfer orally). Either way, this is an exciting finding because it suggests that certain probiotic-like microbial strains might be used in the future to prevent and treat pneumonia.

We generally get our flu vaccine in the fall to prepare for winter, when people spend more time indoors, making it peak infection season. The influenza virus transmits as an aerosol directly between people—more easily accomplished in close quarters than outdoors. You cannot get the flu from the vaccine. It is made with the killed—i.e., inactivated—virus; the worst it can do is produce a slight reaction of redness, soreness, and swelling. Recent data suggest that it's the microbiota that may play a role in our body's response to flu vaccine. Microbial products stimulate the host immune response, which then increases the vaccine response, at least in mice. So, wear it as a badge of honor if you get a slight reaction to the vaccine! It may signify that your immune system really recognized the vaccine, which could lead to better protection.

You may have heard that in some years the flu vaccine does not work as efficiently as other years. This is because the influenza virus is a chameleon: It constantly changes its surface to camouflage itself from our immune system and to try to outsmart our defenses. But we formulate vaccines specifically to protect against these ever-changing components, primarily called H and N antigens (think of the H1N1 swine flu). Every February, the World Health Organization (WHO) looks to the southern hemisphere to see which flu strains are prevalent there and makes their best estimate of which strains will appear in the fall in the northern hemisphere. This leaves six frantic months for vaccine companies to ramp up production of that year's vaccine. Some years, they get it just right, and the vaccine provides great protection; other years (like when Jessica got sick despite having her annual flu shot), the virus changes during those six months and different strains arise, thereby making the vaccine less effective. This process is closely watched by the WHO to begin the process all over again to formulate flu vaccines in time for the southern hemisphere's winter flu season. In either case of effective or less effective flu vaccine years, it is recommended to get yearly vaccines for residual protection from the primary strain. Vaccines even provide cross protection from other strains that arise that year or in later years. Even if a vaccine is not fully protective, one usually has a milder form of flu.

Still not convinced? Consider this: There are hints (in mice) that the vaccine may help stave off dementia and other inflammatory diseases (such as cardiovascular disease and type 2 diabetes), by decreasing inflammation damage associated with respiratory infections. When young mice are vaccinated, they are healthier and have fewer chronic diseases as they age. This suggests that one should be vaccinated early and often—yet around 60 percent of Canadian and American adults, and about 68 percent of Australian adults, do not get the flu vaccine. Everyone over the age of six months should get their annual vaccination; the rare exception being those with severe, life-threatening allergies to the vaccine.

Looking Forward

Recent recognition of the lung microbiome and its dynamic nature, as well as its relationship to the oral and gut microbiota, opens up a whole new way of looking at lung diseases. However, longitudinal (over a prolonged period) clinical intervention and mechanistic studies in humans are lacking due to the unfamiliarity of the field. We still don't know the role of the lung microbiome in diseases–whether it is causing or is an effect of the disease. New generations of probiotics may soon be developed to reduce risk for respiratory conditions such as pneumonia. The other central player in lung diseases, inflammation, also affects the microbiota. Encouraging early studies suggest that some *Lactobacillus* probiotics have an impact on reducing lung inflammation. We may also be able to diagnose diseases such as COPD and pneumonia in the future by analyzing a person's microbiome and looking for key species. This means less of a need for chest X-rays, alongside faster interventions resulting from our ability to identify respiratory diseases at an earlier stage than we were previously able to.

KEY TIPS

Know the warning signs: Early symptoms of pneumonia and COPD can often seem like a regular cold or age-related change. Seek immediate medical attention if symptoms persist. Early detection is essential to effective treatment.

Live smoke-free: Minimize exposure to smoke and harmful pollutants as much as possible. If you smoke, the best way to improve your respiratory health and boost your lung microbiota is to quit.

Consider probiotics: Taking lactobacilli products can help manage allergic lung disease. It may even help with COPD symptoms to reduce inflammation.

Get your annual flu shot: Due to increased risk of bacterial pneumonia, if you're over the age of seventy in Australia, also get the one-dose pneumococcal vaccine (if applicable) to protect against illnesses such as meningitis and pneumonia. Indigenous Australians over fifty should begin with the single dose.

Mind your gut health: Boost your gut microbiota to help keep your lungs healthy via the gut-lung axis. This includes lifestyle strategies like diet (eating plenty of fiber and prebiotic/probiotic foods) and exercise.

9

Belly Bugs: The Stomach Microbiome

Eating is a fairly simple process. Food goes in your mouth, you chew it into smaller pieces, and swallow. The food then enters the stomach. But have you ever thought about what happens next: how you actually digest your food so that what you eat benefits your body? The stomach can hold roughly one liter of food. It is extremely acidic (a pH level of 2) due to the hydrochloric acid needed to further break down food into its components. Digestion in the stomach is aided by proteins called "proteases" and other digestive enzymes that chop up larger molecules such as proteins and complex carbohydrates. But digestion doesn't stop there: Following this acid bath, food is pushed farther down into the small intestine, where most of the action occurs. Enzymes disassemble fats, proteins, and carbohydrates into their components so that the micronutrient building blocks the body needs can be absorbed and passed into the bloodstream, which sends the nutrients to other areas of the body. In the large intestine, trillions of microbes devour what we can't–mainly fiber and other prebiotic carbohydrates. The intestinal microbiota synthesize a variety of vitamins for us, including vitamin B12 and vitamin K.

Because of the stomach's low pH, we long assumed that no microbes could live there–that it was a sterile environment similar to the lungs (another view that is changing, as we just saw in the previous chapter). It had been thought that to protect the body from infections, this high acidity purposefully killed most microbes that were swallowed during eating. However, this line of thought changed in 1982 with the groundbreaking discovery of the spiral-shaped bacterium *Helicobacter pylori*, which lives in the stomach. As we shall see, *H. pylori* has rewritten the book on gastric health, disease, and treatments. Through recent DNA sequencing technologies, we are beginning to realize that there is indeed a small stomach microbiome entirely distinct from that in the gut. There are anywhere from one thousand to ten thousand microbes per milliliter in the stomach, mainly farther down the stomach (in the gastric antrum) where the pH is slightly higher. This may sound like a lot, but remember, in the large intestine there are billions of microbes per milliliter. These stomach microbes are acquired from ingested food, the mouth, lungs (swallowing mucus), and from the upper intestinal tract (which is directly connected to the stomach). The most prominent microbes detected in the stomach are the usual suspects: Proteobacteria (including the pathogen *H. pylori*), Firmicutes, Bacteroidetes, Actinobacteria, and Fusobacteria, with several other minor lineages. Like most microbial populations in the body, they vary extensively from person to person. For bodies colonized with *H. pylori* (which is over half the world's population), this organism is the dominant bacterium in the stomach. It also influences the other microbes by altering stomach inflammation, which then changes the environment of the stomach and the resident microbiota. While we can say with certainty that there are microbes in the stomach, their exact functions are still being explored.

MYTH: Spicy foods cause ulcers.

FACT: Hot sauce lovers, rejoice! We now know that the microbe *H. pylori* causes most ulcers. Spicy foods may aggravate symptoms in some people, but they won't literally eat a hole through your stomach, unlike *H. pylori*. Ulcers are caused by inflammation in the stomach lining triggered by *H. pylori*: When stomach acid seeps through the protective mucus barrier, a lesion grows and further damages the tissue lining the stomach.

Ulcers and Microbes

When Brett was growing up, his father had ulcers (sores that develops on the lining of the esophagus, stomach, or small intestine) that were supposedly caused by too much worry and stress. Everyone nodded in agreement with this diagnosis and instructed him to find ways to relax and avoid spicy food. At the time, the only way to treat the symptoms of ulcers was to take antacids such as Pepto-Bismol. Brett still remembers the big pink bottles filled with chalky liquid that his father drank daily to alleviate symptoms and presumably decrease the damage being done to his stomach. The active ingredient, bismuth subsalicylate, coats irritated tissues in the esophagus and stomach lining to help protect them from stomach acid.

We spoke to Dr. Martin Blaser, a distinguished professor in Rutgers University's Medicine and Pathology Department and a world expert on *H. pylori*. He is a physician by training whose evolving research interests in microbiology over the past forty years have focused on bacteria of the human microbiome, including *Helicobacter* species. Dr. Blaser repeatedly noticed that people with certain diseases had lower rates of *Helicobacter*, which "led to the idea that *Helicobacter* wasn't so bad at all. Its effect is mixed, with both costs and benefits for its human hosts." As a medical doctor, he knew that there was a link between acid reflux and asthma. As a microbiologist, he saw that if *Helicobacter* decreased, asthma increased. By integrating medical practice and microbiology research, he became open to the idea that *H. pylori* was protective against asthma.

Most clinicians operate under the outdated mindset that if a patient with stomach ulcers has *Helicobacter*, you destroy the microbes. Dr. Blaser's findings were a huge shift—one that has taken over twenty-five years to convince various audiences of its efficacy. But as was the case with the truth about *H. pylori* and ulcers, the tide is changing. As he told us, "Now when I speak to microbiologists about potential protective elements of *H. pylori*, they respond: 'Of course, that makes perfect sense.' However, in the clinical community, doctors are still searching for and destroying *H. pylori*. If a patient's symptoms are at all related to *H. pylori* and gastrointestinal issues, their doctor tries to destroy the microbe. This is a huge extrapolation based on limited data." He likened *H. pylori* to the canary in the coal mine: It's a disappearing organism, and without its protective and effective efforts, we may suffer the consequences.

A NOBEL EFFORT

The story of how *H. pylori* was discovered is a classic underdog story that stood science on its head. As previously discussed, the stomach was long thought to be a sterile, even hostile, acidic environment. However, as far back as 1875, forgotten German papers described spiral bacteria seen in the stomach, although no one could grow them. Italians also saw them in 1893, and Polish researchers reported them in 1899. In the 1950s, researchers conducting an extensive American study of stomach biopsies failed to see any of these microbes, further cementing the concept that the stomach was germ-free. Then, just a few years later, in 1979, Dr. Robin Warren—a gastroenterologist in Australia—observed these spiral shaped microbes and convinced a medical fellow working with him, Dr. Barry Marshall, to go after them. They were convinced that these spirals were associated with ulcers; they needed, somehow, to grow these "unculturables" to know more.

In a story remarkably similar to Alexander Fleming's discovery of penicillin, Marshall accidentally left some plates on his laboratory bench top for five days over the long Easter weekend. When he came back, what do you think he found? Microbes: the same he'd seen in every patient who had ulcers and gastritis (stomach inflammation). Marshall and his team were thus convinced that ulcers were not caused by stress and spicy foods, but by this microbe. Although confirmed within months by several microbiologists, their initial paper in 1982 was met with skepticism in the scientific community. So, to prove the role of *H. pylori* in ulcers, Marshall made the ultimate sacrifice for science—he performed an experiment on himself.

He first proved that he did not have any *Helicobacter* in his stomach by way of an endoscopy. He then scraped two Petri dishes that contained a growing strain of *H. pylori* isolated from a patient. Wisely, he first checked to make sure that this strain was sensitive to antibiotics so he could treat himself. Marshall assumed that it would take years before he saw anything, but instead, after five days he became sick with nausea and vomiting. Again, using an endoscopy, he found that he had gastritis (possibly an acute, self-limited infection—i.e., it goes away on its own), and was colonized with *H. pylori*. He treated himself with antibiotics and recovered fully. This caught the world's attention. The scientific community gradually accepted his finding that a microbe could cause gastritis—and now all doctors know that gastritis, ulcers, and most gastric cancers are caused by this microbe. Doctors Marshall and Warren were awarded the 2005 Nobel Prize in Physiology or Medicine for their discoveries.

H. pylori colonizes over half the world's population and is considered the most common human pathogen on the planet. Having coevolved with humans for the last sixty thousand to one hundred thousand years (see "Ötzi the Iceman" in the following box), it is usually acquired early in life, often from our mothers. The microbe is corkscrew-shaped with a special tail (a flagellum) that allows it to burrow deep into the mucus of the stomach, where the pH is much more reasonable for a long-term stay (about 6 to 7). *H. pylori* has an enzyme, urease, that breaks down urea into ammonia, a chemical base that neutralizes the stomach acid even further. To top it off, the microbe has a specialized syringe-like system that allows it to pump virulence factors directly into stomach cells to reprogram them to suit the microbe's purpose. Clearly *H. pylori* used those one hundred thousand or so years of coevolution with humans wisely!

ÖTZI THE ICEMAN: FROZEN IN TIME

In 1991, German hikers found a human body encased in ice in the Alps. After it was chipped out of the glacier, the body was taken to an Austrian lab where they determined he had died 5,300 years ago (between 3359 and 3105 BCE). He was named Ötzi, after the nearby Ötztal Valley. Since his discovery, much has been learned about this individual. Scientists sequenced his genome and found that he is closely related to people living in Corsica and Sardinia today. Ötzi had sixty-one tattoos, making him the oldest tattooed mummy. He had whipworm (an intestinal parasite), was lactose intolerant, had cardiovascular disease, poor knees from extensive walking, and was involved in copper smelting. We also know a fair bit about Ötzi's last day alive: his final meal was red deer and bread, and he was killed by an arrow to the back or a crushed skull—either way he met a violent end. Luckily for us, he was rapidly covered by snow and promptly freeze-dried by the environment, which prevented destruction of his body by predators and decomposition. Ötzi even has the distinction of having his own institute, the South Tyrol Museum of Archaeology, located in Bolzano, Italy, where they continue to study him.

After several years, researchers realized that his stomach hadn't disintegrated as assumed but was hidden within the body. What's more, scientists could get microbial genetic material from the stomach. Using this precious material, they were able to sequence the entire genome of an old *H. pylori* strain! It more resembles an Asian strain than the European strains we see in that area these days. This has provided clues about how *H. pylori* evolved in humans. The current European strain originated from an African strain, which must have arrived after Ötzi met his sudden death over five thousand years ago.

H. pylori gets a bad rap these days, since we pay a great deal of attention to the 10 percent of people who harbor it and get peptic ulcers–although ulcers are not an inevitable outcome. When this connection is present, there is the worry that prolonged ulcer formation and genetic mutations can cause cancer. Only 1 to 2 percent of those colonized with the strain get gastric cancer; however, *H. pylori* has the distinction of being the only bacterium that is a Class A carcinogen–that puts it in the same cancer-causing category as cigarettes–because it causes 80 percent of gastric cancers (the third leading cause of cancer deaths worldwide). A big risk for stomach cancer is age. The longer *H. pylori* lives in the body, the greater the chance it will cause cancer due to cell turnover and mutations. Most people diagnosed with this cancer are in their late sixties through their eighties.

So, if *H. pylori* causes all these problems, why not just get rid of it, as people were doing for years? Because, as Dr. Blaser cautioned, the organism has so many benefits that the drawbacks may be a small evolutionary price we have to pay. Epidemiological studies suggest that having *H. pylori* protects against asthma, obesity, allergies, various infections, and inflammatory bowel diseases.

This protection has, in many ways, allowed our species to survive; he explained, "Humans and *Helicobacter* are very clearly a story of co-evolution. This co-evolution has late-life costs to people, which are gastric cancer to a major degree, and ulcer disease to a lesser degree. However, a critical question remains as to early-life benefits from *H. pylori*. It likely provides benefits from fighting off infection. We have lots of evidence that a healthy microbiome is important, of which *H. pylori* is an essential part. It's something that has lived in many of our species for at least two hundred thousand years. Now *H. pylori* is present in fewer than 5 percent of children that were measured in the United States, Germany, and Scandinavia. This is a huge ecological change in just a few generations. One that's frightening. We are monkeying with our heritage." Dr. Blaser emphasized that we have to better understand who is truly at risk for gastric cancer instead of indiscriminately killing off the organism that might cause it. Those who are at a high risk of gastric cancer should clearly get rid of *H. pylori* if colonized, but those with low risk should consider prioritizing its protective effects. Given its protective boost against asthma, we may increasingly question how to return *H. pylori* to future generations.

The second reason to not get rid of *H. pylori* is its incredible persistence in the body. There is no vaccine to block it—it's resistant to up to seven different antibiotics—and there are no good therapies to completely remove it. Current *H. pylori* eradication therapies use two different antibiotics and a proton pump inhibitor (PPI) to decrease stomach acidity. Tens of millions of people worldwide take PPIs, making them among the most profitable drug classes in the world. The current thought is that PPIs are safe and can't hurt, but this approach may need revising. PPIs quite clearly have a strong impact on the stomach microbiota by increasing the stomach pH; just one of their effects is increasing infections of *Clostridium difficile* and pneumonia. Plus, they are overprescribed and not as effective as we'd hope: Over 70 percent of prescriptions may be inappropriate, and even their hammer-like effect eradicates only 50 to 70 percent of *H. pylori*.

Third, there is emerging evidence that the microbiota may also play a role in gastric cancer rates separately from *H. pylori*. Models using mice show that altered microbiota cause different disease levels when infected with *H. pylori*. In Colombia, people living in the coastal regions have a much lower rate of gastric cancer than those living at high altitudes. They also have different diets: The coastal communities eat more fruits, vegetables, and seafood, while the higher altitude populations eat more potatoes and fava beans. A recent study compared the gastric microbiota of people from two Colombian towns—one at a high altitude in the Andes, the other a coastal village. Twenty participants from each village were matched by age and sex. Those who lived in the high-altitude village had a twenty-five-times higher risk of gastric cancer than those living in the coastal village. Not surprisingly, people from the same village had more microbiota similar to each other than to people from the other village. The researchers also found significant differences in the microbiota between the two populations. Two microbial groups (*Leptotrichia wadei* and a *Veillonella* species) were noticeably more abundant in the high-altitude population, and other microbial groups were much more prolific in the coastal village participants. These differences make sense given that the two villages had dramatically different diets. However, both populations had shockingly similar *H. pylori* levels. This remains puzzling because they had different diets and levels of gastric cancer. Did the diets affect the ability of *H. pylori* to cause cancer? Were there differences in the *H. pylori*? Could other microbes be involved? Other recent studies have shown that particular microbiota compositions are associated with gastric cancer. As expected, these microbes are more inflammatory and have toxins associated with tissue damage. While this doesn't prove that microbiota other than *H. pylori* are involved in gastric cancer, it provides compelling reasons for researchers in stomach health and disease to further investigate the role of these and other microbes, as well as diets and foods. It also hints at a potential future way to detect stomach cancer via the microbiome, as early detection of this cancer is extremely difficult.

TESTING, TESTING

There are four methods to test for an *H. pylori* infection.

Breath test: You swallow a harmless pill, liquid, or pudding that contains urea (a waste product the body produces as it breaks down proteins). If *H. pylori* are present, the bacteria will convert the urea into carbon dioxide. A device can then detect the carbon dioxide when you exhale. This test can identify nearly all people who have *H. pylori*. It can also be used to check if the microbe has been fully eradicated.

Stool test: A stool test can detect traces of *H. pylori* in the feces. More specifically, the laboratory analyzes your stool for antigens (foreign proteins) associated with *H. pylori* infection. This test can diagnose an infection and confirm that it is cured after treatment.

Blood test: Analyzing a blood sample can detect evidence of an active *H. pylori* infection or a former one. However, breath and stool tests are better at detecting active *H. pylori* infections because a blood test can be positive for years, even if the infection is cured.

Biopsy: A tissue sample is taken from your stomach lining during an endoscopy. You'll be sedated for this test as the doctor threads a long flexible tube equipped with a tiny camera (endoscope) down your throat and esophagus into the stomach and the top part of the small intestine. The samples are then analyzed for *H. pylori* infection. Generally, this test isn't recommended solely to diagnose *H. pylori* infection because it is more invasive than a breath or stool test. It is often done for other reasons, including diagnosing an ulcer, treating bleeding, or making sure there is no cancer.

Probiotics versus PPIs

Given the difficulties in safe and effective elimination of *H. pylori*, there are increasing efforts to use probiotics to help rid the body of this organism. Live microbes taken orally could outcompete *H. pylori* for space and dampen inflammation associated with *H. pylori* colonization. The usual probiotic suspects, *Lactobacillus*, *Bifidobacterium*, and *Saccharomyces boulardii* (a yeast), have been tested, not only because they're common but because they can handle the low pH levels found in the stomach. So far, these studies show a partial improvement in gastric symptoms but not a complete eradication of *H. pylori* (*Lactobacillus reuteri* was the best at decreasing inflammation). When these probiotics were used in combination with the standard triple therapy of two antibiotics and a PPI, the probiotics were more effective at eradication than therapy alone. There were also fewer side effects (diarrhea and abdominal pain), which made it easier for patients to stay on the therapy. An interesting study compared a combination of a probiotic yogurt and a PPI with a treatment of two antibiotics and a PPI. They yielded similar results, but the yogurt/PPI group had fewer side effects. Overall, the addition of a probiotic to the triple therapy may make it a more effective and pleasant treatment for ulcers, but probiotics are unable to completely eradicate *H. pylori* on their own.

There is no doubt that *H. pylori* is central to both stomach health and disease. However, it is likely that other stomach microbes have an impact, by either affecting *H. pylori* colonization or the inflammation associated with it. It is also likely that more and better probiotics will be found to alter *H. pylori* colonization and gastric inflammation, especially given the increase in antibiotic resistance currently seen in *H. pylori*. For example, strains of *Weizmannia coagulans* isolated from human stomach lining (i.e., normal stomach inhabitants) show promise as potential probiotics for decreasing *H. pylori*. As science advances, we will gain a better understanding of what the "normal" stomach microbiome composition is, and whether it affects gastric issues. It is likely that microbes will be increasingly used to counter *H. pylori* and gastric issues.

KEY TIPS

See a doctor about concerning stomach symptoms: Check with your doctor if you suffer persistently and/or severely from any stomach symptoms, including poor appetite; abdomen discomfort, fullness after eating a small meal, swelling, or fluid build-up; unintentional weight loss; abdominal pain or discomfort; heartburn or indigestion; nausea or vomiting; and anemia. Unfortunately, early-stage stomach cancer rarely causes symptoms; having these symptoms may be a sign of more advanced-stage illness.

Consider *H. pylori* **carefully:** If you have stomach issues and are colonized with *H. pylori*, have a frank discussion with your physician about whether to try to eradicate the organism.

Try probiotics for *H. pylori* **treatment:** If you are on a PPI treatment, taking probiotics containing *Lactobacillus* and/or consuming a probiotic yogurt could potentially increase the therapy's effectiveness and decrease side effects. Probiotics, in combination with PPIs, are more effective at eliminating *H. pylori* than antibiotics alone.

10

Microbes Down Under: The Urogenital Tract Microbiome

As an avid triathlete-turned-runner, Jessica is constantly seeking scientific information on training, nutrition, and recovery. Her constant frustration, however, is that the science is often based on college-aged males. In fact, until the 1980s, it was generally assumed that physiological responses to exercise did not vary between the sexes. Yet we cannot simply "shrink it and pink it," given the very fundamental physical and hormonal differences between males and females, when it comes to exercise and the microbiome.

So far, this book has been fairly sex-neutral, and for the most part, the microbiome can be discussed as a constant across men and women. This chapter focuses mainly, but not exclusively, on hormonal and microbial processes that most individuals with uteruses and vaginas experience. We have used the term "women" throughout for simplicity, although we recognize that these processes are not experienced by all women, and are not exclusive to people who identify as women. In general, there are fundamental physiological and hormonal differences between males and females that are reflected in their unique microbiomes. The vaginal microbiome changes throughout a woman's lifetime, especially as she ages. This chapter discusses specific microbial signatures of the vagina, changes that can occur during menopause, the role of the gut microbiome in moderating estrogen levels, and why pee is yellow (yes, due to the microbiome). It also dives into emerging understanding of the urinary tract microbiome and even covers the microbiome of semen.

Habits of a Healthy Vagina

Females are not the same as males in a strictly biological sense. The vagina—the elastic, muscular part of the female genital tract that extends from the vulva to the cervix—is unique to women and critical to sexual intercourse, childbirth, and the menstrual flows it channels. It is interrelated to other organs in the female pelvis, including the urinary bladder and the bowel, which lie in close proximity. The vagina harbors a remarkably characteristic microbiome that forms a mutually beneficial relationship with the rest of the body and has a major impact on both health and disease. Like the gut, the vaginal microbiome can form a complex ecosystem of more than two hundred bacterial species, although it is usually much simpler than that, with just a few lactobacilli. Its composition is affected by numerous factors, including environmental and behavioral factors, pregnancy, sexual activity, and stage of life—prepuberty, adolescence, reproductive years, and menopause.

Because it is relatively easy to access, the vaginal microbiome has been cultured for many years. Traditionally, it was thought to be dominated by four *Lactobacillus* species (*L. crispatus*, *L. iners*, *L. paragasseri*, and *L. mulieris*), which produce lactic acid and give the vagina an acidic pH (3.5 to 4.5), providing strong protection against pathogenic microbes. Lactobacilli also produce other antimicrobial products (bacteriocins) that specifically lyse (disintegrate) and kill other bacteria, again protecting the vagina from pathogens. Interestingly, humans are the only animals that have *Lactobacillus*-rich vaginal microbiomes with a low pH, including even other non-human primates. Thus, there are no animal models to study the human vaginal microbiome.

We significantly advanced our understanding of the vaginal microbiome when culture-independent sequencing methods came of age, allowing us to pick up microbes that weren't as easily cultured as *Lactobacillus*. Scientists identified five general types of vaginal microbiomes in normal healthy women, each with a unique microbial signature. Four are mainly *Lactobacillus*-dominant, and the fifth is characterized by other (non-*Lactobacillus*) microbes. Studies finding that healthy women can have a non-lactobacilli microbiome and a vaginal pH greater than 4.5 has really challenged the conventional wisdom about what was previously thought to be needed for vaginal health, and continues to do so to this day.

Vaginas vary significantly from woman to woman. Periods also range widely: While the average menstrual cycle is twenty-eight days long, it can last anywhere from twenty-one to thirty-five days in adults. Menses cause significant changes in the vagina, which are reflected by transient changes in the vaginal microbiome. In general, during menstruation the lactobacilli decrease and there is an increase in other microbes that can be associated with vaginal infections. Sexual intercourse also disrupts the vaginal microbiome, decreasing the lactobacilli and their protective effects. This can lead to a more dysbiotic composition, which is one of many factors explaining why some women can get urinary tract infectious (UTIs) following intercourse—with less of the protective, acidic environment, more harmful microbes can enter the body. In some women, bacteria can also enter the bladder during intercourse.

MYTH: The vagina naturally smells bad.

FACT: It's normal for the vagina to have a slight odor. This can vary depending upon menstrual cycle, sexual activities, and sweat. Distinct causes of abnormal odors include bacterial vaginosis, which occurs when the delicate balance between "good" and "bad" vaginal bacteria is upset and causes an overgrowth of anaerobic bacteria (cannot live in oxygen). It is different from yeast infections, which are caused by a fungus (candida). A yeast infection generally itches; has a thick, white discharge; and doesn't smell. Bacterial vaginosis, in comparison, has a thin white, gray, or green discharge; a burning sensation when you pee; and a fishy smell. A doctor may prescribe a course of antibiotics for bacterial vaginosis, while antifungal medications are generally used to treat yeast infections.

Like the rest of the body, the vagina and vulva change significantly with time, as of course does the vaginal microbiome. Prior to puberty, females have a polymicrobial community rich in Gram-negative anaerobic bacteria and low in lactobacilli and *Gardnerella vaginalis*. Following puberty and incumbent hormonal changes, women develop one of five vaginal microbiomes. Postmenopausal women have lower levels of estrogen, which reverts the microbiome to one that resembles a pre-puberty composition.

Maintenance of the normal vaginal microbiome is important in preventing disease. Bacterial vaginosis (BV) is the most common vaginal infection in reproductive-age women. It affects approximately 30 percent of women in the US and in some countries over half of women (about one in eight in Australia), and results in millions of health care visits. The risk of BV is increased by changes to the vaginal environment, including menstrual blood, a new sexual partner, and vaginal douching. In the United States, an estimated 20 to 40 percent of women aged fifteen to forty-four years old douche. The Australian data is limited but it's possibly around 10 percent. Most of the time, BV does not cause serious health problems, but it can lead to infertility, genital tract and pregnancy complications, pelvic inflammatory disease, and increased susceptibility to sexually transmitted diseases. BV is often accompanied by vaginal discharge and odor (see page 179).

Not surprisingly, BV is associated with dysbiosis of the vaginal microbiome. It features a decrease in the lactobacilli and an overgrowth of a polymicrobial community consisting of strict or facultative anaerobes (microorganisms that either cannot survive in oxygen or can adapt to grow in oxygen-free environments). Although about one quarter of women have microbes similar to this kind of microbiome and are normally healthy, we just don't understand why at this time. Women with BV tend to have thick biofilms (large clusters of adherent microbes) growing on the vaginal surface. However, there does not appear to be a single microbial causative agent. This leads to the theory that BV is linked to changes in the overall vaginal community–which, as we have seen, seems to be a recurring theme when discussing dysbiotic microbiota. Biofilms are infamously resistant to antibiotics, as antibiotics have trouble penetrating the microbial layers. Treatment of BV with antibiotics such as metronidazole is often unsuccessful, resulting in recurrence rates of about 30 percent after three months, and 60 percent after six months. The two classes of antibiotics used for treatment are the same that were recommended in 1982, making new therapeutics and approaches sorely needed.

Further, antibiotics can disrupt the vaginal microbiome and increase its pH, resulting in further risk of BV or yeast infections. There is a promising product coming to market to treat BV that is not an antibiotic. pHyph is made by the Swedish company GEDEA Biotech AB and is a natural substance (Glucono-delta lactone) delivered directly to the vagina. It helps restore the acidic pH of the vagina and promote growth of lactobacilli, which helps protect against BV and fungal infections. Its cure rate for BV is similar to that of antibiotics, yet its recurrent infection rates are less. The clinical trial data look excellent (90 percent cure rates), and the product is undergoing final testing in the US. Hopefully this will be a non-antibiotic treatment option for vaginal infections in a couple of years. In Australia, pHyph isn't yet fully approved.

In chapter 2, we discussed fecal transfers or fecal microbiome transplants (FMTs), which were the first deliberate transfer of microbiomes from one individual to another. Recently, vaginal microbiome transplants (VMTs) are being tested as a potential treatment for recurrent BV. In a small trial, transplanting vaginal fluid from a healthy donor led to successfully treating two of the five participants for recurrent BV. Like FMTs, there are problems in that the donor must be extensively screened for potential sexually transmitted pathogens and semen contamination, among other things. Recent unpublished work on a much larger scale also showed promising results. It is difficult to scale up as a widespread treatment for BV since donors require extensive screening. However, like FMTs, it suggests that we can identify the microbes involved, and then move to a live biotherapeutic product (LBP)–a mixture of live microbes applied to the vagina to treat BV. Because the vaginal microbiome is much simpler than the gut's, this approach should be feasible.

MYTH: Douching–spraying the inside of your vagina with a mixture of water and vinegar or any of a multitude of other "cleansers"–is an effective way to clean your vagina.

FACT: You do not need to douche to clean your vagina. The body naturally flushes out and cleans the vagina, whereas douching disrupts its normal flora and pH. Most doctors recommend that women do not douche, as studies have not found any health benefits. Douching is linked to health problems including bacterial vaginosis, pelvic inflammatory disease, pregnancy complications, sexually transmitted infections, and vaginal irritation–all likely affected by the microbial disruptions it causes.

Full Stop: Microbes and Periods

There are two major instances in a woman's life that involve profound bodily changes linked to reproduction: when menstruation begins and when it stops. These are the bookends of a woman's ability to bear children. Women are born with a finite number of eggs, which are stored in the ovaries. The ovaries also make the hormones estrogen and progesterone, which modulate menstruation and ovulation. At puberty, the ovaries begin releasing those eggs once a month, and if no embryo is conceived, the lining of the uterus is shed during menstruation. (The word "menstruation" comes from the Latin *mensis*, meaning "month.") When a woman's full store of eggs has been released, menstruation stops. This point is referred to as menopause (think: "menstruation" + "pause") and usually occurs around age forty-eight to fifty-five in the United States (fifty-one on average), and forty-five to fifty-five years, with an average of fifty-one, in Australia, after a woman has gone without a period for twelve consecutive months. The years following the point of menopause are often referred to as "postmenopause."

Menopause is a normal phase of life. It is a part of aging, not a disease. Experiences of menopause are more and more common given the increasing life expectancy of women worldwide, with women on average spending three decades in postmenopause. Menopause is associated with lower levels of reproductive hormones, given the reduced functioning of the ovaries, especially estrogen. Overall lower reproductive hormones are associated with increased risk for osteoporosis, bone fractures, and loss of muscle (sarcopenia; discussed in chapter 11). Low estrogen can result in body temperature swings (hot flashes and sweating), psychological changes (mood shifts, irritability, and depression), insomnia, vaginal dryness, and bladder control problems. Lower androgen levels (sex hormones) can contribute to reduced sex drive. There is great variation in how women experience menopause, and not all women undergo all of these symptoms. For those who encounter severe symptoms that affect quality of life, hormone replacement therapy (HRT) is designed to help. HRT is basically a way to supplement estrogen. Hormone replacement can bring risks, however, so talk to your doctor if you are considering treatment.

The human gut microbiome is increasingly thought of as an endocrine organ: one that produces (or affects) hormones, which impact body function. Although the ovaries are the primary producer of estrogen prior to menopause, later in life, other cells of the body can still produce estrogen.

This includes cells in the gut. Germ-free rats secrete very low levels of estrogen compared to microbially colonized rats–levels so low that they do not have menstruation cycles and have trouble reproducing. When the germ-free rats were recolonized with microbes, their estrogen levels increased, and reproduction and menstruation cycles were restored. The gut microbiome clearly affected estrogen levels.

Postmenopausal women have significantly greater risk of metabolic diseases such as obesity and type 2 diabetes then premenopausal women, and this may be tied to ovaries and their production of hormones. Researchers removed the ovaries of mice, thereby disabling their production of estrogen and other hormones. They found that their gut microbiomes became dysbiotic, their intestines became more permeable, and they had increased inflammation, all of which are associated with metabolic diseases. During menopause, the ovaries stop producing estrogen and other related hormones, which likely contributes to the increase in metabolic diseases among postmenopausal women.

Throughout life, female bodies strive for balance in estrogen levels. Too little estrogen can cause headaches, hot flashes, night sweats, vaginal dryness, and other menopausal symptoms described previously that can affect quality of life. On the flip side, having too much estrogen can also wreak havoc with irregular periods, bloating, weight gain, headaches, anxiety, decreased sex drive, and increased symptoms of premenstrual syndrome. We want to keep hormonal levels balanced, like an equally weighted seesaw, to avoid these health symptoms. Because gut microbes have specific enzymes (beta-glucuronidases) that can cleave precursors of estrogen, called "phytoestrogens," the gut microbiome may play a role in regulating estrogen. This presents a novel avenue to potentially help moderate estrogen levels in menopausal women, including through diet.

Phytoestrogens are found in some plants: isoflavones in soy products (milk, bean curd, sprouts) and lignans (a compound abundant in seeds, particularly flax, berries, fruits, vegetables, and whole grains). The gut microbiome deconjugates (breaks down and metabolizes) these estrogen precursors to produce active forms of estrogen that can then be absorbed by the body. Once in the body, they can act like weak hormones and may reduce the risk of some diseases associated with low estrogen, such as osteoporosis.

Studies show that strict vegetarians have increased conjugated estrogens in their feces. This indicates that the microbial enzymes in their gut that normally deconjugate these compounds to release active estrogen in the body are not present, or not active to the same extent, compared to omnivores. Studies of women on a Western diet (high fat, low fiber) compared to vegetarian women showed that vegetarians had 15 to 20 percent less estrogen in their circulation and triple the conjugated estrogens in their feces. In a study of sixty menopausal women, researchers found that women with diverse microbiomes had less estrogen and more breakdown products than women who had a less diverse microbiome. We don't yet know exactly why this is, but it is certainly a topic for further studies.

The concept that the gut microbiome might alter estrogen levels is an exciting one. Perhaps we can design HRT to work even better by incorporating a microbial approach to modulate estrogen levels during menopause. This could decrease risk for menopausal conditions including obesity, glucose intolerance, and metabolic diseases. Stay tuned for additional scientific research focused on the relationship between estrogen levels and microbial enzymes.

Menopausal Microbes

Given the significant changes in the vaginal environment during menopause, it is not surprising to see more direct changes in menopausal and postmenopausal vaginal microbiomes–though, unlike premenopausal vaginal microbiomes where there are monthly shifts in the community, the postmenopausal vaginal microbiome seems remarkably stable. During menopause (the point when periods stop), the microbiome is still dominated by lactobacilli (although to a lesser degree in total numbers), including *L. crispatus*, and *L. iners*, as well as *Gardnerella vaginalis*, and *Prevotella*; and a lower abundance of *Candida*, *Mobiluncus*, *Staphylococcus*, *Bifidobacterium*, and *Gemella*. The lactobacilli can degrade glycogen (a sugar) into organic acids, especially lactic acid, which keeps the vagina acidic. In postmenopause, there is an overall decrease in lactobacilli and replacement with other microbes, therefore less lactic acid production. This then increases the vaginal pH, which some believe may help to explain an increase in risk for UTIs and gynecological infections among older women.

Estrogen keeps the vaginal surface healthy by triggering the depositing of glycogen on the vaginal mucosal surface. Like plants in need of regular fertilizer, these vaginal microbes need glycogens for sustenance. Lack of estrogen causes the genitourinary syndrome of menopause (GSM)—also termed vulvovaginal atrophy, vaginal atrophy, and atrophic vaginitis. This leads to a thinning of the vaginal wall, which means less glycogen deposition and fewer beneficial resident microbes. Symptoms of GSM include dryness, itching, burning, urgency to pass urine and/or urinary leakage, lack of lubrication and bleeding during intercourse, vaginal discharge, susceptibility to sexually transmitted infections, and inflammation of the vagina. Many postmenopausal women experience these symptoms, with vaginal dryness being the biggest complaint.

In a Swedish study that compared twenty premenopausal women to twenty postmenopausal women, the premenopausal women had far more diversity in the subspecies of lactobacilli. Another study confirmed the correlation between glycogen levels and *Lactobacillus* species: Postmenopausal women have decreased glycogen and lactobacilli. There are strong correlations between vaginal health and lactobacilli—and inverse correlations with *Gardnerella* and *Atopobium*, two biofilm-forming species also seen with BV. Generally, but not always, GSM is associated with lower levels of lactobacilli. One study of postmenopausal women divided them into groups based on vaginal dryness. In the group that had no to mild vaginal dryness, the women were rich in *Lactobacillus* species and had low bacterial diversity, both positive markers of vaginal health. In the group that had more severe vaginal dryness, the women were colonized with fewer lactobacilli, and had more bacterial diversity, including *Prevotella*, *Porphyromonas*, *Peptoniphilus*, and *Bacillus*. Individuals with more severe signs of GSM tend to have higher vaginal microbiota diversity that is not dominated by lactobacilli. In a sense, vaginal health is promoted through a dysbiotic microbial population—contrary to nearly every other finding in this book. Somehow, we need to restore high lactobacilli levels while decreasing the bacterial diversity for postmenopausal vaginal health.

If lack of estrogen causes these issues, wouldn't adding it back do the trick? Estrogen levels and healthy microbes do seem to go hand in hand. In one study, 44 percent of postmenopausal women not on HRT lacked lactobacilli compared to only 6.9 percent of postmenopausal women on HRT. All routes of estrogen administration (oral, injected, topical, or vaginal) can improve vaginal health and microbiota. Lactobacilli species normally seen before menopause seem to return to similar numbers, to the benefit of vaginal health. In a study of women treated with estrogen for three months, 20 percent of controls compared to 80 percent of women on estrogen reported improvements to vaginal dryness and irritation. The group also saw increases in lactobacilli and lowered vaginal pH. There were no changes in sexual complaints based upon placebo or estrogen. This suggests that low-dose estrogen therapy may work well for those with GSM to bring the lactobacilli back and decrease diversity and vaginal pH.

Yet there are also perfectly healthy women who have a high vaginal pH of 6.6, extremely little lactobacilli, and high microbial diversity. Like the gut, every vagina is unique: What a healthy microbiome looks like in one woman can differ markedly from other healthy women, which means that broad generalizations are not universally applicable. It's also worth keeping in mind that high doses of estrogen in postmenopausal women can increase risk for endometrial and breast cancer. The potential dangers of HRT are higher for certain groups of women, including those already at risk for breast cancer, coronary artery disease, stroke, or active liver disease. Estrogen supplementation can be given as low-dose vaginal supplements in the form of cream, tablets, or estrogen-eluting rings (vaginal inserts).

Given the importance of the vaginal microbiome, there is significant promise and early progress using microbes (especially lactobacilli) as probiotic treatments, although no conclusive evidence. These can be delivered orally or vaginally. Vaginal probiotics presumably work in several ways: reconstituting the normal microbiome, decreasing the pH, outcompeting microbial pathogens, and enhancing the vaginal epithelial barrier and mucosal immunity. There are several reports of both oral and vaginal delivery of *Lactobacillus* in postmenopausal women suggesting that probiotics, compared to controls, may improve vaginal symptoms and health. A trial that tested the effect of vaginal delivery of low-dose estriol (estrogen) and *Lactobacillus acidophilus* in postmenopausal women found that it improved vulvovaginal symptoms compared to controls. The concept of delivering both estrogen and a healthy normal flora microbe, *Lactobacillus*, is particularly appealing given that both of these tend to decrease postmenopause. However, as noted earlier, there are health risks to HRT, including heart disease, stroke, blood clots, and breast cancer. The bottom line on vaginal probiotics (both oral and suppository) is that they hold promise, but there is not enough evidence to deem them safe and effective. Similarly, probiotics do not influence infertility.

VAGINAL GUMMIES

Yes, these products exist. One example is a line of oral vaginal probiotic gummies with the tongue-in-cheek name of Lemme Purr, advertising balanced pH, healthy odor, yeast balance, flora support, and immune health. They consist of pineapple extract, vitamin C, and a "clinically studied" probiotic strain *Bacillus coagulans*.

Are vaginas supposed to smell like fruit and flowers? Not according to experts. Scientific data suggest that these gummies do not work. Pineapple extract will be broken down in the gut into small molecules and cannot contribute to vaginal smell directly. There is no evidence that vitamin C significantly affects the vaginal microbiome, and we already consume a fair bit of it in our diets. The probiotic *B. coagulans* has not been associated with improving the vaginal microbiome. There is no evidence it works against BV, and the clinical studies they used were not performed in a rigorous manner. According to one expert, "they are basically like taking candy."

Vaginal Microbiome Testing

There are now several commercially available vaginal microbiome tests. These work similarly to gut microbiome tests: You take a vaginal swab or tampon to collect the microbes, place it in a preservative tube, and then return it to the company for analysis and wait for them to send a list of the microbes found. Some companies also offer further consulting services to suggest what you might do knowing the results.

There are several reasons you might consider vaginal microbiome testing (besides being a curious microbiologist!): 1) you want to see if you have BV or fungal infections; 2) you are experiencing fertility challenges;

or 3) you are entering menopause. These tests cost about $125 to $150, though tend to be most expensive in Australia, and some companies suggest you do take them a few times a year. Some companies offer additional specific screening for sexually transmitted pathogens.

A critical component to consider when deciding if testing is worth it is what you are going to do with the information. Several companies offer consultations with experts (some are MDs), which might be useful but perhaps limited. These tests can satisfy curiosity, but you probably already know if you have BV or thrush due to clinical symptoms and should likely consult a physician rather than try to self-diagnose and treat. Although there are correlations between the vaginal microbiome and fertility, currently there are no medically approved ways to correct this, as we just don't know enough yet. Finally, you will probably have a good idea if you are entering menopause, and again, knowing that, there is little you can do to alter the vaginal microbiome besides going on hormone replacement therapy. Thus, while these tests are certainly interesting, they may not be worth it given limited evidence-based steps to take with the information.

WHY IS URINE YELLOW?

For the past 125 years, we have known that a molecule called "urobilin" makes urine yellow. We have only recently identified the mechanism that explains this. Certain microbes (Firmicutes) can convert bilirubin (an orange molecule created when old red blood cells are broken down) into urobilinogen, which then further breaks down into yellow urobilin. So it's microbes that make urine yellow! Brett was rather skeptical, so he asked a colleague who studies germ-free sheep. Sure enough, the colleague confirmed that urine from microbe-free sheep is colorless!

The Bladder Fallacy

Scientists traditionally thought that urine and the bladder that holds it prior to urination were sterile. This thinking goes back to the mid-1800s based on the fact that a sealed vial of urine does not turn cloudy. Dr. Lynn Stothers, a professor of urology at the University of British Columbia, a research scientist, and a practicing urologist, explained this history of urology: "The bladder was long thought to be sterile. Somehow the urethra was like the gatekeeper between the vagina and the bladder. But later we found that some people have 'asymptomatic' bacteriuria [i.e., bacteria can be in the urine but there may not be any symptoms]." Much of the research on the vagina was conducted under the impression that there were no organisms in the bladder. If any microbes were detected from the bladder, they were explained away as likely contaminants from the vagina or the result of a UTI. The Human Microbiome Project (data collected from 2008 to 2013) did not sample the bladder for sequencing, as it was considered sterile at that time. This dogma persisted until very recently. Sequence-based analysis has now revealed that there are indeed microbial signatures in the bladder. Dr. Stothers admitted: "This discovery generated a lot of surprise. Clinically, we know that approximately 20 percent of women have bacteria growing in their urine and are asymptomatic. How can that be? It has created clinical confusion that persists to date." Many clinicians, still under the assumption that the bladder and urine should be sterile to be healthy, unnecessarily and inappropriately prescribe antibiotics to rid the body of bacteria that are not causing any symptoms.

Jessica encountered this recently when a post-kidney-stone urology appointment detected fairly low bacteria levels in a urine sample. The urologist prescribed three days of antibiotics. Since Jessica did not have any UTI symptoms and was conscious of the potential impacts of unnecessary antibiotic exposure on herself and her baby in utero, she called the urologist's office asking to discuss reasons for and against taking the antibiotics. They dismissed her concerns and instructed her to "just take the antibiotics." Jessica's midwife team was thankfully more thoughtful and open in their medical approach and agreed that given the low bacterial numbers and lack of symptoms, Jessica could hold off on taking antibiotics unless she began to develop symptoms. The midwife ordered a urine test for the following week, which showed that bacterial numbers had dropped even further, and no antibiotics were necessary to keep Jessica and the baby healthy.

Extended efforts are underway to culture microbes from urine. "We are trying to move into the idea that the bladder is not always a sterile environment," Dr. Stothers explained. "The trouble is, however, that it is difficult to obtain suitable specimens from the bladder. How can we collect urine? It is easiest and most practical for people to pee into a cup and then study the voided urine. To get urine directly from the bladder is much more difficult. We can pass a catheter (a hollow tube) up the urethra or put a needle through the abdomen to aspirate urine from a full bladder, but either way urine is acquired in an invasive manner. This is a barrier to research." A lot of work has been done to compare voided samples to urine obtained directly from the bladder. Under the right conditions (enhanced quantitative urine culture to detect live microorganisms in most urine), scientists have found that there are indeed microbes in the bladder. There are greater than one hundred thousand viable microbes per milliliter of urine, which consists of a variety of microbes, many–including *Lactobacillus* and *Gardnerella*–similar to those in the vagina. This number of microbes has traditionally been used as a threshold for determining bladder infections, but we now realize that even numbers much larger than this do not necessarily represent infections.

Do microbes in the bladder and urine play a role in health and disease? Like so many examples in this book, there are hints that they do, but we don't know much about the mechanisms yet. The urinary microbiome, for example, is different in female overactive bladder patients compared to controls. Those with an overactive bladder have more diverse microbes and fewer lactobacilli–so it is thought, but again not proven, that microbes like lactobacilli are protective against pathogens that can infect the urinary tract. The microbiome of urgency urinary incontinence patients is different still, with more *Gardnerella* and diverse species than continent controls. Dr. Stothers clarified that until we can routinely collect clinical samples that provide a specific profile of organisms in the microbiome, it will be difficult to translate scientific discoveries into medical practices: "We are now just barely dipping our toes into the world of the urinary microbiome. The tipping point into clinical medicine is when we can get urinary microbiomes on a day-to-day basis. At the moment, clinicians can only get a standard urine culture. We need to be able to see reports with the urinary microbiome." To do this, we need to convince clinicians who are still skeptical that a urinary microbiome even exists.

Dr. Stothers was hopeful that advancing knowledge of the urinary microbiome could be harnessed to better identify and treat urinary conditions. "First of all, we can potentially influence our urinary microbiomes through diet. We know that compounds from foods we eat, such as cranberries, end up in our urine. Hopefully we can use things like diet to more precisely alter the urinary microbiome to prevent UTIs." UTIs also involve a variety of microbial pathogens, especially *E. coli*, that infect the kidneys, urethra, or bladder. A healthy vaginal microbiome may serve a protective role by outcompeting pathogens.

Could we use probiotics to increase this protection? There are not strong enough data to make this claim. In a review of nine published studies (735 participants total) that tested the effectiveness of probiotics to prevent UTIs, reviewers concluded that the currently available evidence indicates no significant reduction in risk of recurrent bacterial UTIs.

Dr. Stothers also mentioned important intersections between the vaginal and urinary microbiome, and how these two regions change in women as they age and experience changes in hormonal status. She felt strongly that there is immense potential to advance opportunities to work with our microbes instead of seeking to get rid of them: "I encourage my patients to think of their bodies like a canvas upon which the bacteria live." This is an important symbiotic relationship.

MYTH: Cranberry juice can cure UTIs.

FACT: Prevention of a UTI is different from treating an active symptomatic infection. The body of evidence supports that cranberries prevent—but don't cure—UTIs. Scientists originally thought that the acidity in cranberry juice decreased vaginal pH, which could protect against pathogens. More recent data indicate that components in the juice bind to—and plug up—structures (pili) on the microbial pathogen's surface, therefore blocking its ability to adhere to host cells. Numerous clinical studies have tested the ability of cranberry juice to block (prevent) UTIs. Because some studies suggest that cranberry products may reduce repeated infections in women, some medical professionals may advise the use of cranberry supplementation in the prevention or treatment of a UTI. Dr. Stothers recommended it as "a 'low risk' prevention strategy in patients with recurrent UTIs with potential upside (as opposed to using chronic antibiotics)."

OVERDOSING WOMEN ON ANTIBIOTICS

Antibiotics are frequently prescribed for specific bacterial infections, including respiratory tract infections, bronchitis, and UTIs. A 2016 analysis of eleven studies encompassing antibiotic use in over forty-four million individuals found some highly surprising results. Women are 27 percent more likely to receive an antibiotic prescription in their lifetime than men. Compared to men in the same age groups, women aged sixteen to thirty-four receive 36 percent more prescribed antibiotics, and women aged thirty-five to fifty-four receive 40 percent more. Two types of antibiotics often used for respiratory tract infections—cephalosporins and macrolides—were particularly high in prescriptions to women.

We know that women have unique issues with UTIs, and at first glance, one might assume that this may in part account for gendered differences. However, this doesn't hold true when examined more closely: The types of antibiotics usually used to treat UTIs (quinolones) were not increased in women compared to men. It is well documented that outpatient treatment of respiratory tract infections with antibiotics is overprescribed, with 40 to 50 percent of patients receiving "inappropriate" prescriptions. Women generally visit their physicians more than men and are more likely to see their doctors for a respiratory tract infection than men.

Antibiotics are not the only class of drugs where gendered differences are evident; medication for thyroid therapy and depression are also skewed toward women, and these differences can't be fully explained by medical reasons. Still, antibiotics show the highest disparity in prescription practices among male and female patients, so women should pay particular attention to these prescriptions. Inquire about the medical reasoning to make sure that the prescription is medically necessary. It is traditionally said that "an antibiotic might not work, but it can't hurt." Given all that we know about antibiotics and their effects on the microbiome, this concept needs serious revisiting for members of both sexes.

The Semen Microbiome and Fertility

Until recently, we assumed that semen was microbe-free unless there was an infection. But as we have seen throughout this book, microbes keep surprising us. Within the last few years, we've realized that there is a semen microbiome. By applying standard sequencing methods to semen, researchers compared the sperm microbiome in males experiencing fertility issues (poor sperm motility or viability) compared to males with proven biological paternity (i.e., children). They found a diverse but largely consistent sperm microbiome, although the sperm of those experiencing fertility challenges had differences in microbial diversity, especially with changes in *Pseudomonas* species and an increase in *Lactobacillus iners*, a bacterium common to the vaginal microbiome. This is one of the four lactobacilli often linked to a healthy vaginal microbiome, but it is also associated with female infertility and bacterial vaginosis. This *Lactobacillus* was the strongest difference between the two groups, and it was also associated with lower sperm motility. Although the exact reason this bacterium may contribute to infertility is not known, this organism does produce a lactic acid (L-lactic acid) that is associated with triggering inflammation. This is why it may also contribute to female infertility if inflammation may damage the fallopian tubes. In addition, the production of this acid may also inhibit sperm swimming ability (one hypothesis is that the acidic environment of the vagina caused by lactobacilli helps select for healthy sperm that are able to fertilize the egg).

A recent study showed that the gut microbiome can affect offspring via sperm. It is well established that the health of the mother's microbiome impacts the placenta and newborn, a major reason not to use antibiotics in pregnancy unless needed. In this study, the researchers showed that treating male mice with antibiotics was linked to less fetal weight gain and survival in their offspring. Researchers used in vitro fertilization and other methods to show that this effect was directly transmitted by the sperm to the paternal offspring. If confirmed in humans, it adds another layer of complexity to healthy conception.

Along a similar line, the vaginal microbiome is now thought to play a role in female fertility. In addition to *L. iners* triggering inflammation through L-lactic acid, the presence of non-lactobacilli bacteria is associated with infertility. This result suggests that it may be helpful in the future for women being tested for infertility to analyze their microbiomes. Researchers have also found that the vaginal microbiome at twelve weeks gestation is different between those who conceived without medical intervention versus by in vitro fertilization (IVF). Microbes associated with bacterial vaginosis such as *Gardnerella* and *L. iners* were associated with the IVF group, hinting that there is a correlation between IVF and preterm birth–a higher risk for IVF pregnancies–and may be in part microbial.

These fertility concepts are quite new. They may have significant implications for fertility, although we certainly don't understand them all yet. Who would have thought microbes would have such an intimate role in our bedrooms?

Looking Ahead

The realization that the bladder is not sterile is a major paradigm shift in how we think of urinary tract biology and might be leveraged into novel applications to improve bladder health, including how we treat UTIs. Older adults tend to suffer more from bladder problems as weakening muscles make it harder to fully empty the bladder. When urine stays in the bladder longer, infections are more likely.

Vaginal health is tightly tied to the vagina's resident microbes. The ability to modify or deliver particular vaginal microbes holds much promise for better treatment of vaginal infections, in addition to enhancing menopausal vaginal health. Given that the gut microbiome can modulate estrogen levels postmenopause, in the future, we will hopefully be able to improve symptoms of menopause through dietary practices, including the consumption of particular probiotics, prebiotics, and fermented foods. Because the vagina has a mucosal surface (which ties into the immune system), there is speculation that vaginal microbes might be used in vaccines, or to alter immune responses.

KEY TIPS

Eat with estrogen in mind: You may be able to help moderate your estrogen levels through diet (unbalanced levels can lead to menstrual cycle changes, hot flashes, troubles sleeping, low sex drive, mood swings, and weight gain). The gut microbiome can break down and metabolize soy products, flax seeds, fruits, vegetables, and whole grains to produce active forms of estrogen to be absorbed into the body.

Pause the probiotics: Despite all the hype, there are currently no robust clinical studies to indicate that probiotics taken either orally or vaginally actually work to improve vaginal health.

Don't bother with vaginal microbiome testing: If you want to take a test to satisfy your inner microbiologist, great! However, there are currently limited options to use test findings to modify your microbiome. It is advisable to consult with a physician regarding your medical concerns (and they can order testing if warranted).

Be wary of overprescribed antibiotics: Antibiotics taken for infections can disrupt the vaginal microbiome and increase the pH, resulting in BV or yeast infections. Women are significantly more likely than men to receive antibiotic prescriptions, and are at greater risk for sexist, gender-based medical care. When your doctor prescribes antibiotics, double-check that the prescription is warranted given your health condition and symptoms.

Avoid antibiotics when pregnant or trying for a baby: If you are trying or planning to try for a baby, minimize your antibiotics exposure whenever possible. It is well established that maternal antibiotics affect offspring, including influencing rates of obesity, asthma, and other chronic health issues. To be extra safe, future fathers should also avoid antibiotics. The paternal gut microbiome affects sperm, which in turn, affects fetal weight gain and survival (at least in mice).

Beware of "alternative" treatments for BV and yeast infections: Antibiotics and antifungals are currently the only ways to treat BV and yeast infections (thrush). The internet is full of potential treatments (such as putting garlic cloves in the vagina), but medically, only these antimicrobial compounds have been shown to consistently work. Beware of other methods, especially those which may exacerbate discomfort and infection risk.

Don't douche: The inside of the vagina is completely capable of self-cleaning and ridding itself of unwanted fluids and bacteria. Douching disrupts the vagina's normal microbial communities and pH, which can result in irritation and lead to severe gynecological conditions. Just use water to wash your vulva (soap disrupts the microbial balance) and stay away from harsh or fragranced soaps.

Practice safer sex: Unprotected sex leads to disruptions in the vaginal microbiome, which can increase risk for bacterial vaginosis and thrush. Safe sex also protects against sexually transmitted infections. One of the best ways to protect you and your partner is to use a barrier, such as condoms and/or gloves when you have oral, anal, or vaginal sex. It may also be helpful to pee after sex, particularly for females. Because female urethras are shorter than men's, bacteria can more easily enter and cause a urinary tract infection Peeing after sex may help flush out bacteria.

11

Flex Your Microbes: The Musculoskeletal System

Weakness. Weight loss. Low energy. Agonizingly slow gait. These are the telltale signs of frailty visible among many older people. Contrary to these clichés, however, frailty is a medical condition but not an inevitable result of aging. It can be prevented or delayed with deliberate choices that affect lifestyle, behavior–and your microbiome. Dr. Heather McKay, professor in the Departments of Orthopaedics and Family Practice at the University of British Columbia, is keen to educate people on why these "decline and decay" narratives aren't true. Her research focuses on addressing the needs of our aging population, specifically related to exercise physiology. This stems from her own personal experiences as an elite athlete (she represented Canada as a sprinter on the world stage, including at the Commonwealth Games) and as a mother. When she had children, her experiences showed her it was "really obvious that we set the course of our lives by what we choose to do in young childhood." She set her sights on medical school even though she had young children at home. "But then I realized that I don't care as much about treating people once they're already sick. I want to keep them healthy!" In an abrupt turn away from traditional medical practice focused on acute care and treatment, her work became all about prevention.

The need for this kind of focus has never been greater. Dr. McKay acknowledged that she's partially drawn to aging research because of the increase in the population over sixty-five, a group more numerous "than those under the age of fifteen–a first in North American history, and soon to be the case in Australia. If our health care system is to have any chance of surviving whatsoever in the future, we need to make sure older adults age well–and age actively." Dr. McKay reflected that as bones grow in children, so do bones decline in older adults: "This is a logical extension of my earlier work. Turns out I've been looking at old bones for a really long time! Understanding how everything is connected across the course of life is important to sustain and maintain skeletons wherever possible. Exercise and diet can play a huge role in the health of our bodies at every age." Dr. McKay is fascinated by longevity and thinking through how we can plan for the final thirty years of our lives, which she calls our "third trimester." "I'm convinced that physical activity and mobility are the keys to a longer life," she said, "and, more importantly, a high quality of life."

She qualified that physical activity does not necessarily mean the blanket prescription of sixty minutes of moderate to vigorous physical activity five days per week. This is just "not in the wheelhouse" of the low-mobility older people she works with. Instead, Dr. McKay takes an incremental approach with light physical activity: "Every little bit counts. If you're lying in bed most of the day, try to sit up at [your] bedside. If you're sitting at [your] bedside, walk to the door. If you can get to the door, walk around the block. Do a little more every day, ideally with friends and family around for encouragement and connection." Even things like patio gardening and playing with grandchildren count as ways to make people stronger, prevent bone loss, improve balance and coordination, boost mood and memory, and ease the symptoms of numerous chronic conditions.

Fighting Frailty

In 1900, the average American lived forty-seven years (the average Australian into their fifties). Nowadays, our average life expectancy is nearly seventy-eight years. Adding thirty years to the human lifespan is an amazing success story, but it also brings new challenges, including frailty–a syndrome characterized by weakness, weight loss, and low activity. Its two main physiological contributors are loss of bone mass (osteoporosis) and muscle mass (sarcopenia). In the United States, approximately 15 percent (about 11 percent in Australia) of the older non-nursing home population–aged sixty-five and older–are considered frail, meaning that they score highly on the frailty index by having three or more of the following symptoms: exhaustion, low physical activity, weakness, slowness, and shrinking; another 45 percent are considered pre-frail (one or two symptoms). In those aged ninety and older, frailty rises to 38 percent. It is estimated that by 2050, over one billion people worldwide will be frail.

Frailty is a strong predictor of disability and multiple adverse health outcomes. A Johns Hopkins study found that frailty doubles the risk of surgical complications, extends hospital stays, and increases the odds of moving into nursing homes or assisted living after a surgical procedure by up to twentyfold. Up to half of frail people in the United States (about a quarter in Australia) have reported a fall in the past year, and about one fifth of those who have sought medical treatment for a fall have required overnight hospitalization (around three-quarters in Australia). Frailty is a more accurate predictor of mortality and hospitalization than actual chronological age. In other words, aging well requires minimizing and hopefully preventing frailty.

What can we do to protect ourselves? Per a major theme in this book, diet and exercise do wonders for a person's general health and longevity—and both involve microbes, as we've discussed. One cause of frailty is the age-related loss of muscle mass, so try to be active and moving most days of the week, choosing activities that can improve strength and thereby reduce weakness. You don't necessarily need to hit the gym to achieve this—as Dr. McKay advised, carrying grocery bags, taking the stairs, and lifting and holding grandchildren all count. Another cause of frailty is that as we age, our microbes become less effective at reducing nefarious low-grade age-related inflammaging. With age, the number of microbes making anti-inflammatory molecules such as butyrate decreases, while other more inflammatory microbes increase in number. Both of these microbial shifts increase inflammation. This is why supporting your microbes by maintaining a balanced and nourishing diet, including fruit, vegetables, protein, healthy fats, whole grains, and low-fat dairy products, is so important. We can see that people who faithfully adhered to the Mediterranean diet were 74 percent less likely to become frail.

There is also a general decrease in microbial diversity associated with frailty, in addition to the many other diseases discussed throughout this book. It is still not clear whether these microbial differences are due to external changes in diet and housing that accompany aging (see chapter 14 for more on the role of the environment in later life), or whether they are caused by the aging body's biological changes.

Although causation hasn't been proven, several studies have now examined how the gut microbiome is associated with frailty (microbiomes from other body sites have not yet been examined). In one small study of twenty-three individuals (median age of eighty-six), researchers compared the gut microbiome of ten highly frail individuals to thirteen low-frailty people sharing the same diet and living in the same care home. They found seventeen key gut microbes that showed significant differences between the two groups. Those with high frailty had lower numbers of anaerobic microorganisms lactobacilli, Bacteroidetes, and *Faecalibacterium prausnitzii*. Remember that these microbes produce butyrate, an anti-inflammatory short-chain fatty acid—so having fewer of these helpful microbes leads to more inflammation. These individuals also had higher numbers of *Enterobacteriaceae*, which are associated with increased inflammation.

In a much larger study of a total of 728 female twins in the UK, researchers sequenced the participants' fecal microbiomes to explore this connection with frailty. The average age of participants was sixty-three (ranging from forty-two to eighty-six). Because of the younger ages, many participants still lived in the community and overall frailty scores were lower, yet their results show a similar trend to the smaller study described above. Overall, frailty was associated with a decrease in diversity in the microbiome. Frailty was more strongly correlated with microbial diversity than someone's age, diet, alcohol intake, smoking, or weight. Researchers also found a negative correlation with Clostridiales, especially *F. prausnitzii*, a key butyrate producer. This means that frail participants had lower numbers of anti-inflammatory microbes (and presumably increased inflammaging). They found positive correlations between certain other microbes and frailty, although we don't know at this time if they actually increase frailty.

Another major study on the microbiome and frailty was conducted with 178 individuals of Irish descent aged 64 to 102 years old. They used thirteen younger adults with a mean age of thirty-six as controls. One interesting aspect of this study is that researchers included analyses of the microbiome by diet and residence: eighty-three lived in the community, while sixty resided in long-term residential care. It took a year for those entering long-term care to fully shift from a diverse "community dweller" microbiome to a diminished "long-term care" composition (more on this in chapter 14). Long-term residents had a higher frailty index score, as measured by the five symptoms described earlier–which makes sense as they were in long-term care–and higher levels of circulating inflammatory cytokines, such as TNF alpha. These studies show that we need to keep our microbiomes in mind when it comes to the long-term strength of our bodies.

Brittle Bones

Loss of bone mass is a natural process following its steady increase and strengthening in childhood. There is strong evidence that it is vital for children to do weight-bearing exercises such as jumping and running to build healthy bones that will set them up for life. Jessica remembers her pediatrician mother once instructing her and her brother to go outside before dinner to jump up and down twenty times. At the time, she thought it was just a fun game–but now she sees how her mom was trying to protect her bones!

Dr. McKay's work, and that of others, shows that we gain about 26 percent of our adult bone mass in the two years around puberty. This is as much bone as we lose across fifty years of adult life. Osteoblasts (cells that secrete the protein matrix for bone formation) build bone, while osteoclasts (cells responsible for bone dissolution and absorption) tear it down. Peak bone mass happens between the age of twenty and the mid-thirties, which is the most bone you will ever have. Then as you age, the bone remodeling process changes: Your body continually builds and breaks down bone structure, replacing about 10 percent of your skeleton every year, but the new bones come in at a slower rate. This can lead to osteopenia: the condition of thin bones, usually a precursor to osteoporosis if not treated properly. Osteoporosis results in significantly weakened bones and increased risk for unexpected fractures. Women are four times more likely than men to get osteoporosis (the same in Australia). However, men still make up 20 percent of all cases in the US (about 20 to 30 percent in Australia), meaning more than two million men in the country have osteoporosis (about a quarter of a million in Australia), and another three million have osteopenia (about 3.7 million in Australia). Over the age of fifty, the odds of experiencing a major fracture become one in two for women and one in six for men. Postmenopausal women are twice as likely as men of the same age to suffer a fracture partly due to women's generally lighter frames and smaller, thinner bones, and the hormonal changes that accompany menopause.

What causes osteoporosis? The causes are complex and many. It starts in our youth where–depending on genetics (which accounts for as much as 50 to 80 percent of bone mass), childhood activity patterns, and diet–an individual's bone mass, density, and strength are first established. Throughout adulthood, changes in, or maintenance of, nutrition and lifestyle factors are important. Diets low in calcium and cigarette-smoking can both weaken bones. Also, weight-bearing physical activity through *mechanotransduction*–when cells convert mechanical stimulus into electrochemical activity–has direct effects on bone accrual and loss. Because women have longer lifespans than men, they have more time to incur wear and tear on their bones.

There are hints that microbes are involved in osteoporosis. First, people with inflammatory bowel disease (IBD) are at a much greater risk. Second, we learned in chapter 10 that menopause is characterized by decreased estrogen levels, which contribute to decreased bone mass and density. As estrogen declines, there is an increase in pro-inflammatory hormones such as TNF alpha, produced by T cells, which cause an increase in osteoclasts (the cells that break down bones). Third, we know that microbes are involved in diet, nutrition, and exercise, all of which can affect osteoporosis. The microbial role in all three factors suggests that bacteria might have to do with development of, or predisposition to, the disease.

Scientists are beginning to formally examine how the microbiome plays a role in osteoporosis with germ-free animals. Some studies have shown that a specific breed of germ-free mice (C57BL/6) had higher measures of bone volume than regular mice. When they exposed these germ-free mice to microbes, their bone density decreased to the levels of regular mice. Studies with a different strain of germ-free mice (BALB/c) found the opposite: These mice had weaker bones. Long-term colonization of microbes in certain germ-free mice has resulted in increased bone formation and bone mass. These contrary findings may be explained given different mouse strains, or differences in mouse sex and age.

New studies using conventional (i.e., colonized with microbes) mice show that microbes may play a key role in osteoporosis. Production of SCFAs is important, and feeding mice high-fiber diets increased their bone mass, prevented bone loss, and significantly reduced osteoporosis. SCFAs seem to inhibit breakdown of bone without affecting bone formation. The microbes also affect bones by regulating the immune system. By stimulating the production of anti-inflammatory cytokines (TGF-beta and IL-10), they inhibit the production of osteoclasts and decrease their number, which also results in less osteoporosis. Finally, there is some evidence that the microbiome affects bones by regulating hormones and neurotransmitters such as 5-HT (5-hydroxytryptamine), which regulates bone formation.

The few human studies on the subject found that the microbiome can have a large effect on bone remodeling (the natural processes of osteoblasts and osteoclasts) and bone mass. The largest study so far looked at 181 individuals, predominantly females, with an average age of sixty-four. Researchers found significant differences in the microbiomes of health controls, those with osteopenia, and those with osteoporosis. In a study of ninety-six individuals, those with osteoporosis had higher levels of *Dialister* and *Faecalibacterium*.

Calcium absorption is another factor that plays a role in bone density, and several studies find some evidence that the microbiome is involved. When gut microbiota break down dietary fiber consumed in foods, and produce acids such as SCFAs, the gut pH decreases; the lower pH boosts calcium absorption into the body. These SCFAs, especially butyrate, can also modulate signal pathways in the gut, which can increase calcium absorption and affect bone density.

Some of the best evidence that the microbiome affects bone density comes from research with probiotics and prebiotics. Several mouse studies show that modulation of the gut microbiome by probiotics (mainly lactobacilli) increases bone mass and can prevent estrogen-mediated bone loss. There are also data coming out about humans. In a study of the probiotic *Lactobacillus reuteri*, researchers found that it increased circulating levels of vitamin D, which promotes calcium absorption and bone health. There was also a large study of 417 older patients with broken arms, some of whom researchers gave the probiotic *Lactobacillus casei*. They found that fractures healed faster among those who received the probiotic than those who did not. It has also been shown that women with osteopenia who received a probiotic mix of six microbes for six months showed decreases in the inflammatory cytokine TNF alpha. They had increased markers of bone formation, but researchers didn't see any effect on bone density during this short period of time. Finally, in a study of seventy women (average age seventy-six years) who took *Lactobacillus reuteri* daily for a year, those taking the probiotic had decreased bone loss compared to the controls. So, there are hints that probiotics (especially *Lactobacillus*) might help decrease bone loss, especially in postmenopausal women, but so far, the trials have been fairly small and of limited time, so we await larger-scale clinical trials to further confirm this.

These findings usher in a new area of research generating significant excitement. While conclusive data are yet to come on the many linkages between the microbiome and bone density, measures like taking probiotics, enhancing microbial diversity through dietary sources and, of course, maintaining a calcium-rich diet are all recommended to reduce risk for osteoporosis–and to improve health in general.

Microbes with Your Muscle Milk

Along with osteopenia and osteoporosis, muscle loss (sarcopenia) plays a major role in frailty. The diagnosis refers to generalized muscle loss, which includes both muscle mass and strength. It is associated with physical disability, heightened risk of falling, and ultimately, increased risk of death. Sarcopenia generally accelerates around the age of seventy-five, although it can vary in intensity from ages sixty-five to eighty to increase one's overall frailty. Several factors account for sarcopenia, including a decrease in nerve cells connected to muscles, changes in hormones such as growth hormones and testosterone, and decreases in protein intake and synthesis.

Why do we lose muscle in the first place? Muscle mass peaks later than bone mass, at around the age of thirty. With age, the balance between muscle growth and loss shifts, and more muscle is lost than synthesized, resulting in a decline in both muscle mass and function. Physically inactive people can lose 3 to 5 percent of their muscle mass every decade. That's up to 30 percent of muscle mass loss between the ages of twenty and eighty! The primary treatment for sarcopenia is resistance or weight training to increase muscle strength and endurance. These workouts differ from cardiovascular exercise, although they often overlap. Several studies show significant benefits within two weeks of starting training. Continued exercise helps prevent further muscle loss and can even build some back, but it can't totally prevent it.

The links between sarcopenia and the microbiome are only beginning to emerge. In a mouse model of leukemia–which features muscle atrophy–there was a correlation with changes in the gut microbiome, including reduced *Lactobacillus*. Adding back specific species of lactobacilli reduced the muscle atrophy. Microbiome studies have also been conducted on aging rats (who undergo sarcopenia, like humans). Comparing the gut microbiome to muscle physiology, researchers found specific age-related changes in the microbiome that correlated with the physiological decline of musculoskeletal function. We view this result cautiously because, as we saw in chapter 2, there is a general change in the gut microbiome as one ages. Whether this change is causing musculoskeletal changes or is just correlated with it remains to be determined.

Recent studies analyzing the microbiome find a correlation between microbial composition and sarcopenia. A study of 1,417 participants showed a characteristic microbiome profile associated with sarcopenia compared to controls. They even developed a model to predict sarcopenia based on microbiome composition, and found they could differentiate those with sarcopenia with fairly good accuracy. In another study with sixty controls and twenty-seven individuals with sarcopenia, they found a marked decrease in the butyrate producers in those with sarcopenia. Another study indicates there may be an association through diet. As part of the TwinsUK study, 2,570 women between the ages of eighteen and seventy-nine were asked to follow a Mediterranean diet. They were then scored for their adherence to that diet. Results reflected a direct positive correlation between higher muscle mass and strength with higher adherence to the diet. Interestingly, there was an inverse correlation between meat consumption and muscle strength. In other words, those who ate more meat had less muscle strength (which helps disprove the common myth that you can't build muscle on a plant-based diet). The dietary effect was greater in women over fifty, which is also when there is increased sarcopenia. This is the first study on sarcopenia to look at diet across ages, rather than only in older populations, and it suggests that how we treat our microbiome throughout life can affect our health as we age.

Feel the Burn

There are tantalizing hints from recent human studies that exercise influentially boosts the microbiome–as we touched on in chapter 7–with an overarching theme: Exercise increases microbial diversity because it selects for helpful SCFA producers, which can decrease inflammatory responses and facilitate overall health.

Several studies in rats and mice provided early evidence of the effect of exercise on the gut microbiome. A study of rats placed in cages with running wheels for "voluntary exercise" found that these rats had higher levels of the SCFA butyrate in the colon compared to sedentary animals with no access to a running wheel. These exercisers also had an increase in beneficial butyrate-producing Firmicutes microbes in their intestine. In another mouse study, researchers compared three groups of mice: germ-free, sedentary (no running wheel available) with a normal microbiome, and an exercise group (a running wheel in their cages). As other studies support, the data here showed that exercise increased microbial diversity and butyrate-producing microbes, which translated into decreased inflammation. Researchers then transplanted the microbiota from the exercised and sedentary mice into the germ-free animals; the transplanted microbiota from exercised mice decreased inflammation in a mouse model of inflammatory bowel disease (IBD). Collectively, these studies show that exercise alone may modulate microbial composition and cause changes in the microbiome to decrease gut inflammation.

Only one mouse study that we know of thus far has examined the reverse scenario: how the microbiome affects exercise performance. This study tested endurance during swimming of normal mice, germ-free mice, and germ-free mice colonized with a single bacterium (*Bacteroides fragilis*). It found that mice colonized with normal microbes or even the single bacterium were able to swim for longer times than germ-free animals. This suggests that the microbiome might affect exercise performance. This is probably not surprising, since we know that the microbiome can affect energy metabolism, immune responses, and stress responses–all of which play a role in exercise performance.

Although there are only a few human studies so far, a similar trend appears to hold true. One fascinating study looked at the changes in eighteen lean and fourteen obese sedentary individuals when they began exercising. They started with thirty minutes of moderate exercise (walking) three times a week, and over six weeks, progressed to sixty minutes of vigorous exercise (vigorous jogging or cycling) three times a week. They did not change their diets. Participants then stopped the exercise program, and researchers tracked them for another six weeks in the "washout period." As in the animal studies, researchers saw an increase in microbial diversity and microbes that produce SCFAs for all exercisers, although the changes were more pronounced in the lean individuals. After stopping the exercise program, the microbiome reverted back to its original composition.

In a 2017 study of women, moderate physical exercise was shown to modify the composition of the human microbiome and increase the abundance of health-promoting bacteria such as *Bifidobacterium*, *Akkermansia*, and *F. prausnitzii*. All of these microbes are associated with SCFA production and anti-inflammatory activity. Similarly, an analysis of 1,493 participants in American Gut showed that increasing moderate exercise boosted microbial diversity in the Firmicutes, including the butyrate producer *F. prausnitzii*. Physical exercise is commonly recommended to prevent and treat chronic inflammation in many diseases such as type 2 diabetes, coronary disease, and obesity, all of which are characterized by dysbiotic microbiota. These exercise studies collectively suggest that moderate exercise increases the levels of anti-inflammatory SCFAs by beneficial modulation of the microbiome.

BUG DOPING

Given all that we are learning about the role of the microbiome in exercise, it's possible that we might be able to design the perfect (and presumably legal) microbiome to enhance the performance of elite athletes. There is only one study thus far that has focused on elite athletes' microbiomes: that of Irish rugby players (described in chapter 7). In our eyes, this is a prime area for stealth scientific innovation. Here we describe the ingredients of our hypothetical microbial cocktail.

1. First, we know that elite athletes' training habits differ from most "weekend warriors." They train frequently (often two to three times per day) and repeatedly find creative ways to push themselves to the limits to meet specific goals. Extreme exercise triggers significant inflammation in the body, which includes inflammatory cytokines. Athletes generally recover quickly, and their levels of inflammation drop back rapidly to very low levels. So, to design our perfect bug-doping concoction, we first need to include microbes that produce anti-inflammatories (namely the butyrate producers we discussed previously) to even further enhance this response.
2. Second, we need our microbial elixir to include a mix of microbes that break down lactic acid, which is a by-product of intense exercise. Think of that nauseated feeling you got in elementary school after sprint repeats in gym class, or if you push yourself through grueling high-impact interval training. Lactic acid can limit performance by triggering muscle pain when oxygen cannot reach the muscles as efficiently, and energy breakdown (metabolism) switches to pathways that don't use oxygen (anaerobic metabolism). One can recover upon decreasing exercise intensity or resting, which returns the metabolism to its aerobic state (using oxygen), and the blood circulation washes away the lactic acid. In one study looking at runners training for and running the Boston marathon, researchers found that post-race runners had a major enrichment in a microbe that breaks down lactic acid. Jessica previously ran the Boston marathon and can personally attest to grueling long runs and tough workouts that likely selected for this microbe.
3. Third, we'd need microbes that could efficiently break down food to rapidly generate energy during a race and increase protein uptake to help repair muscles. This is especially important for the ultramarathoners tackling fifty- to one-hundred-plus-mile races. Although scientists have found microbes in these athletes that efficiently and selectively break down carbohydrates and fiber, applying that knowledge broadly will be a bit tricky until optimized personal diets gain more headway.

4. While we are dreaming, we may as well throw in some microbes that affect the brain. Perhaps we can find microbes that dampen pain, which would help us push through soreness and fatigue. As we saw in chapter 4, we can probably dig up some microbes that overcome stress, too, and alleviate symptoms for athletes who suffer from crippling pre-race nerves at the starting gate. And as we have seen in this chapter, let's add some microbes to strengthen our bones and muscles to reduce injury and fractures. Gymnasts might especially benefit from having stronger muscles to ensure a perfect landing every time.
5. Finally, let's tackle jet lag, a major problem for international athletes. We can likely bring in microbes that affect circadian rhythm to regulate body clocks and keep athletes performing at their best in any time zone. We also have to remember that elite athletes are only human, so they still get colds and other communicable diseases—and could be more susceptible while traveling on planes or running themselves ragged with training. Imagine the devastation of getting sick while competing at the Olympics (think of the 2024 Olympics in Paris, where disastrous COVID-19 infections cost some athletes medals)! So, let's throw in some beneficial oral microbes that outcompete respiratory viruses, and for good measure, wash it down with probiotic yogurt. In forty-six female endurance swimmer athletes, probiotic yogurt was linked to a reduction in the number of respiratory infections and some of the symptoms.

For a final touch, this hypothetical world would call for some creative coaching strategies: Take the very best person in your sport—a multi-gold medal Olympian and world champion will do quite nicely—and pay them an exorbitant amount of money for their feces, which they'd just flush away anyway (so what's the loss?), then line up medical fecal transfers for your athletes to receive a dose of microbes from this individual. At present, there is no regulation regarding athletes' microbiomes—so the biggest hurdle might be getting the athletes to cooperate with this unorthodox training technique!

KEY TIPS

Know that no one is "too old" to move: A mix of physical activities that are weight-bearing (these can be short and sharp, like jumping), make your heart beat faster (this can be short and fast, like high-impact training, or long and slow, like walking or running), and increase your strength (weight training) are important at any age. Finding a functional and enjoyable exercise routine is an important way to get regular bursts of activity instead of sporadic sweat sessions at the gym. As Dr. McKay recommends, small bouts of exercise that help you sneak in physical activity have cumulative benefits in strengthening your bones and muscles—and in the process, boosting your microbes as well.

Eat your veggies: Plant-based foods help boost dietary fiber intake, which can increase calcium absorption through the gut microbiota to improve bone health. Choose fiber-rich foods such as beans and legumes, whole grains, brown rice, nuts, baked potatoes with skin, berries, bran cereal, oatmeal, and vegetables—all staple components of the Mediterranean and MIND diets (see chapter 4). You can double down by serving these foods with calcium-rich dairy products, such as bran cereal with milk and baked potatoes with sour cream, to further strengthen your bones and reduce risk for osteoporosis.

12

Microbes Meet Cancer

An editorial published in the influential medical journal *The Lancet Oncology* declared that cancer is no longer the big, scary word it once was. The medical reality of cancer is changing as doctors and scientists come to recognize that many cancers can now be manageable for a very long time–and many more are even curable. However, the word still elicits an understandable rush of dread and visceral fear for most. A cancer diagnosis is terrifying and can exact an immense toll on the physical and mental health of patients and their loved ones. After diagnosis, life expectancy can range from months to decades.

Cancer is not a single monster of a disease. Rather, it describes more than one hundred diseases in which normal cells grow out of control. Healthy cells divide in an organized way so that when they are worn out or damaged, new cells take their place. When cancer develops, however, this orderly process breaks down. The cells divide continuously, forming the growths we know as tumors. Cancer can occur anywhere in the body–the brain, lungs, breast, colon, even in the blood. Some cancers grow and spread fast, while others grow more slowly. They also respond to treatment in different ways. The most common treatments are surgery, chemotherapy, and radiation, which can have significant side effects. But there are promising new ways to treat cancer, such as immunotherapy and precision medicine-based approaches, including sequencing the tumor, which can offer treatment with fewer side effects. The FDA and TGA are continually approving new tests and therapies, providing many new options for cancer treatment. We are also getting better at preventing cancer through methods such as tobacco avoidance, healthy diets, regular physical activity, asbestos removal, and sun protection. Prevention is the ultimate goal, but many factors that cannot be controlled contribute to cancer. On average, annually, twenty million people worldwide learn that they have cancer and 9.7 million people die from the disease. It is the second leading cause of death worldwide (behind cardiovascular diseases). Novel approaches and advances in cancer treatment are needed to reduce the global burden of cancer, and microbes appear poised to take center-stage.

Having studied cancer for over thirty years, Dr. Shoukat Dedhar—distinguished scientist at the British Columbia Cancer Agency and professor in the Department of Biochemistry and Molecular Biology at the University of British Columbia (and a longtime collaborator of Brett's)—has seen the highs and lows of the field's evolution. When he spoke with us, he noted that scientists are beginning to realize that microbes play a much bigger role in both cancer and its treatment than anyone previously thought. Dr. Dedhar became aware of the microbiome when he learned that a microbe, not stress, contributed to stomach ulcers and cancer (a topic we explored extensively in chapter 9). "It was surprising, and yet also unsurprising if you really think on it. We can see the influence of microbes everywhere." His list of such conditions included ulcerative colitis (a chronic inflammatory bowel disease that we came across in chapter 2, induced by microbes that increases one's risk for bowel cancer), colon cancer, viruses involved in liver cancers, and more.

> **MYTH:** Cancer is cellular, so microbes aren't involved.
>
> **FACT:** Microbes are intimately involved in many cancers. They influence the risk for developing cancer, immune responses that affect both cancer and tumor control, disease progression and metastasis, and response to treatment.

Why are we just coming to this knowledge? Evolving technologies enable researchers to better "see" the microbiome and its many interactions with cancers. Dr. Dedhar was particularly interested in observing tumor micro-environments: "Are there bacteria within growing tumors that help them flourish? What role do they play? Perhaps a tumor is more aggressive because of assisting microbes? Nothing is known." Yet that is changing fast. Emerging data suggest the possibility that colon cancers are driven by mutations in certain genes (such as ZEB2), which may promote bacterial infiltration into the tumors. Treatment with antibiotics could inhibit tumor growth. "Now that is an area," Dr. Dedhar said, "that I would like to explore."

Microbial Carcinogens

An estimated 20 percent of all cancers are linked to microbial agents. We saw in chapter 9 how *H. pylori* is linked to stomach cancer; it can inject a bacterial molecule into host cells that activates a cell division pathway, which triggers the cells to divide without stopping. Gall bladder cancer is also associated with *Salmonella typhi* infections. Since the chronic inflammation triggered by microbes causes tissue damage, subsequent mutations that occur during repair can lead to cancer in both the gall bladder and stomach. In mouse models, *Helicobacter hepaticus*, a microbe that causes intestinal tissue inflammation, triggers an increase in mammary tumors in several mice strains. This is probably through activation of the body's immune system and inflammation.

This inflammatory response is one of the key ways that microbes' impact on immune system development and function relates closely to cancers. Our immune system's defenses normally detect and try to control tumors in a process known as immunosurveillance, a kind of alarm system that protects us. If the alarm system is triggered, it calls on the body's response, which in turn, stops any unwanted invaders. If microbes make our immune system less efficient (think of power being intermittently cut to the alarm system), this can increase our rate of developing tumors. As we saw in chapter 3, another tactic our immune system uses to defend the body against invading microbes is inflammation. Activating the alarm, a pro-inflammatory response, can be pre-carcinogenic as it leads to further cell damage and faulty repair. With alarm bells increasingly ringing, an inflammatory state increases cancer risk.

So far, the International Agency for Research on Cancer has designated a total of ten microbes as carcinogenic to humans; this is actually an incredibly small fraction of the estimated trillions of microbes that are found on Earth. Nearly all of these cancer-causing microbes are viruses, including Hepatitis C (liver cancer), human papillomavirus (cervical cancer), Epstein-Barr Virus (the first virus shown to cause a wide variety of cancers), and of course the bacterium *Helicobacter pylori*.

Rapidly evolving knowledge about the microbiome's role in the body at large also suggests further microbial-cancer associations. For example, numerous risk factors for cancer–including obesity, cardiovascular disease, type 2 diabetes, and aging–have established microbial links. There is even a proposed "cancer hygiene hypothesis" based on the more general hygiene hypothesis, in which increases in certain cancers are linked to modern lifestyles that avoid microbes and encourage sterility, as well as to consumption of highly processed food.

We also experience risks and benefits from the many different molecules that microbes produce and secrete into the body, a subset of which can impact cancer. Several gut microbes break down fibrous food substances, for example, and produce the short-chain fatty acids (SCFA) butyrate, propionate, and acetate. These molecules can suppress inflammation, which in turn reduces cancer incidence, but other microbial metabolites can promote carcinogenesis–the production of cancer. This includes bile acids, hydrogen sulfide gas (the rotten egg smell in intestinal gas), and naturally occurring, microbially modified steroid hormones. Learning more about the presence of any of these molecules in the body could be a powerful tool in our war against cancer.

COLEY'S TOXINS

The use of microbes in cancer therapy goes as far back as the late nineteenth century, when American physician William Coley began treating various tumors with a mixture of two heat-killed bacteria: *Streptococcus pyogenes* and *Serratia marcescens*. Called "Coley's Toxins," this cocktail was injected locally into the tumor. This produced significant inflammation, which could assist the body's immune system in controlling tumors. The method was applied from 1893 until the early 1960s in the United States, and up to 1990 in Germany. However, the results of this treatment were mixed, so treatments were stopped. Clinical trials were not conclusive, and the scientific evidence did not support it as a viable cancer treatment.

This experiment didn't die entirely, however, for the Coley's Toxins concept is behind the current treatment for bladder cancer. Bacillus Calmette-Guérin

(BCG) is a strain of *Mycobacterium bovis,* which is closely related to *Mycobacterium tuberculosis.* Because *M. bovis* is related but does not normally cause tuberculosis, it is used extensively as a live-attenuated (a fancy name for a weakened but live microbe) vaccine for tuberculosis. *M. bovis* is the only FDA-approved treatment for bladder cancer, though not the only one approved by the TGA. Live microbes are injected into the bladder following surgery. There, they presumably trigger a strong localized inflammatory response, which helps prevent tumors recurring. The method eradicates the cancer in 70 percent of patients.

The Fear of Lumps

Breast cancer affects one in eight women in the United States (one in seven in Australia) and is the second leading cause of cancer deaths in women after lung cancer, as in Australia.

Men are also affected: Every year nearly three thousand men are diagnosed (about two hundred and twenty men in Australia). Their mortality rate is slightly higher than in women, perhaps because awareness is lower, and they are less likely to assume that a lump is breast cancer. Overall, breast cancer accounts for forty thousand deaths per year in the United States alone (about three thousand three hundred in Australia). Breast self-exams are recommended for both genders to check for any persistent lumps or changes in breast tissue.

Some risk factors for breast cancer can't be changed, including sex, age, and genetics. But lifestyle changes can affect other factors such as being overweight, lack of exercise, unhealthy diet, and smoking cigarettes. As with many diseases, risk of breast cancer increases with age. About two in three invasive breast cancer cases involve women aged fifty-five and older. High estrogen levels are a risk factor, especially for current or former users of hormone replacement therapy (HRT).

Given the link between the gut microbiome and estrogen levels, as discussed in chapter 10, are there connections between the microbiome and breast cancer? Maybe. In a preliminary study, forty-eight postmenopausal women with breast cancer had altered gut microbiomes. They had decreased microbial diversity and altered composition compared to cancer-free controls, in addition to higher estrogen levels. There are also several epidemiological studies showing that consumption of fermented milk products (e.g., kefir, yogurt) is associated with a decrease in breast cancer risk, although it has not been established whether this occurs through the gut microbiome and the enzymes it encodes. We need more scientific studies to determine whether the microbiome has a direct causal effect on breast cancer risk. It may be correlated simply because decreased microbial diversity is associated with obesity, insulin resistance, and other risk factors associated with breast cancer.

Antibiotics, especially ampicillin–which is used to treat different types of bacterial infections, including ear infections, bladder infections, and pneumonia–eradicate gut microbes that produce enzymes that break down and metabolize estrogen. This means lower circulating estrogen levels and higher conjugated estrogens in the feces (as discussed in chapter 10). There is also increasing evidence that dysbiosis associated with extensive antibiotic use (including commonly used tetracycline and sulfonamide) correlates with breast carcinomas (tumors).

Does that mean we should avoid taking antibiotics, except when medically necessary, to protect ourselves against breast cancer? Perhaps. But there are currently no data to indicate that minimizing antibiotic exposure could directly protect against this specific disease. In a large North American study of nearly ten thousand women, increased prior antibiotic use increased the risk of breast cancer. All classes of antibiotics were associated with this increased risk. Other studies have found a slightly higher risk of breast cancer associated with antibiotic use. Antibiotic-induced changes to the microbiome may affect the metabolism of sex hormones such as estrogen, and in turn, the risk of breast cancer. The general consensus is that there is a small increase in risk with antibiotics, but their use is so ubiquitous it is difficult to prove a clear link.

Alcohol consumption also increases the risk of breast cancer, especially in postmenopausal women. Again, the gut microbiome may be involved in this. There are always significant changes in the gut microbiomes of individuals with chronic alcohol abuse, including the appearance of large intestinal microbes in the small intestine, a condition called Small Intestinal Bacterial Overgrowth (SIBO). Excessive bacteria in the small intestine are frequently implicated as the cause of chronic diarrhea and malabsorption, and SIBO patients may also suffer from weight loss, nutritional deficiencies, and osteoporosis. SIBO is found in animal models of alcoholic liver disease. How alcohol-induced microbiome changes relate to estrogen and breast cancer is currently undefined, although several metabolites linked to estrogen production were altered in the animal models. This could influence breast cancer susceptibility if true for humans.

A surprising new finding is that there is a breast tissue microbiome with a diversity similar to that found in the gut. Researchers have observed differences in the breast microbiome of those with breast cancer compared to controls without the disease. Several small studies suggest that the breast microbiome in breast cancer patients, as well as in the control subjects, is different from nearby healthy tissues. In a study of forty women (twenty of whom had breast cancer), scientists observed fewer microbes in tumor tissue and more microbes in healthy breast tissue. Recent work in Brett's lab, in collaboration with Dr. Shoukat Dedhar, has identified a specific strain of *Bacillus* that promotes breast tumor metastasis (spread of a tumor into other parts of the body) in a mouse model of breast cancer. In humans, the presence of this bacterium is associated with an increased mortality rate during breast cancer, hinting that this microbe somehow enhances tumor spread in the body.

Further complicating this emerging field, another study—of seventy women who had breast cancer (normal adjacent tissue was also collected) and healthy controls—provided a different picture. This study found that the microbiomes from cancer biopsies and normal adjacent tissue were not different, but when compared to healthy control breast tissue, *both* were different. In other words, there doesn't seem to be a microbiome profile specific to tumors, but there is a different overall profile for both healthy and cancerous breast tissue from individuals with breast cancer compared to healthy controls. Women with breast cancer had elevated levels of *Enterobacteriaceae* (including *E. coli*) and *Staphylococcus*. Using cultured human cells in the lab, researchers also showed that these microbes increased DNA breaks. This is associated with increased tumor formation, although it remains an incredibly preliminary lab observation.

While there were no differences observed based on menopausal status, one interesting finding is that breast cancer patients' bacteria encoding the enzyme beta-glucuronidase were enriched–which, as we have seen, increases estrogen levels.

A common form of cancer treatment is radiation, but many cancer patients develop severe dermatitis during radiotherapy (termed "radiodermatitis," or inflammation and damage to the skin). In a recent small study of female breast cancer patients, researchers found that women who have an altered skin microbiome on their breasts develop more severe radiodermatitis, while those with normal skin microbes developed only mild or moderate dermatitis. Although still in the early days, the researchers are now looking at breast skin microbiomes before radiotherapy, and at how disinfecting the skin microbiome can lower the amount of inflammation-triggering microbes to reduce the likelihood of radiodermatitis.

To sum up, there are certainly differences in the breast microbiome of women with breast cancer compared to healthy controls, but we are not at the stage yet where we can use the microbiome as a tool to detect, prevent, or treat breast cancer. In the next few years, we anticipate intensive studies in this exciting new area of breast cancer research.

Microbial Cancer Diagnosis

Many studies have shown that there are significant differences in individuals with cancer compared to controls. This has led to the concept that, in theory, we should be able to diagnose cancer based on microbial signatures, or by screening for molecules they produce. In 2020, a landmark paper came out saying that different tumor types could be identified by characterizing microbial molecules in tissue and in blood. Researchers looked at thirty-three types of tumors in over eighteen thousand individuals and used machine-learning algorithms to predict whether individuals had cancer or not, forming the basis of a microbiome-based cancer diagnostic tool. Several studies (and at least one new company) followed up on these results.

However, not everyone agrees with the findings. Another group has claimed that the computational results were not done correctly, and that there were "major data analysis errors." This has led to significant angst in the field, and a follow-up paper in the scientific journal *Cell* by the original group. It highlights the difficulty in doing complex microbial analysis (which requires significant bioinformatic computation), as opposed to a traditional observational experiment. Recently the original paper was retracted. Currently there are many involved in sorting all this out, and time will tell how good a microbe-based diagnostic could be for cancer. At present, there aren't any microbiome-based cancer diagnostics available clinically.

DIET AND CANCER

Health-promoting diets such as the Mediterranean diet are well known for decreasing cancer risk. It now seems they can also enhance recovery from cancer. One recent study showed that a plant-based diet, low in dairy and meat and high in fruits, grains, and nuts (all foods that promote healthy, diverse microbiota), improved sexual and urinary health in men treated for prostate cancer. This included average improvements in sexual function (8 to 11 percent) and urinary health (14 percent), and increased energy and lowered depression (13 percent). The authors also point out that a healthy diet significantly reduces cardiovascular disease risk, which also enhances chances of survival.

Recent work in mice has also suggested vitamin D plays a role in both increasing immune resistance to implanted tumors in mice (i.e., increased tumor resistance) and enhancing checkpoint inhibitor treatment (treatment that blocks proteins, known as checkpoints, that control the immune system, thereby enhancing the immune response against the tumor), which may improve cancer treatment. Previous studies in humans have proposed a link between vitamin D and cancer prevention, but the evidence is not conclusive. You can boost your vitamin D levels through (careful!) sun exposure, certain foods (e.g., flesh of fatty fish such as trout, salmon, tuna, and mackerel; some mushrooms; fortified milks), and dietary supplements.

Antibiotics and Cancer

Part of the argument for the "cancer hygiene hypothesis" described earlier has to do with the role of antibiotics in cancer, since several studies indicate that antibiotic-driven dysbiosis can affect cancer rates over time. For example, a cohort study in Finland observed individuals who took little to no antibiotics (zero to one prescription) in comparison to those who had six or more antibiotic prescriptions. They found that heavy antibiotic users had a 15 percent increase in risk for developing colon cancer during nine years of follow-up. Similarly, a large study of colorectal adenoma (the precursor to colorectal cancer) in female nurses found that long-term antibiotic use beginning in early to middle adulthood was associated with an increased risk of colorectal adenocarcinoma after age sixty. Interestingly, in the past four years, antibiotic use did not increase the incidence, although this makes sense given that colon cancer often takes a decade to develop.

There are also hints that antibiotic exposure may affect other cancers throughout the body. Epidemiological evidence in a large study of over six hundred thousand people indicated that antibiotic exposure may increase rates of lung, prostate, and bladder cancer. These results support exercising caution when deciding whether to use antibiotics. While they are very effective at treating bacterial infections, they may have longer-term consequences of increasing cancer risk. This science linking antibiotic use to cancer is still in its early days and we do not yet fully understand the mechanisms involved, but it certainly smacks of microbial involvement.

Colorectal Cancer

Given the many interactions between intestinal microbes and the gut, it is not surprising that there are linkages between gut microbes and colorectal cancer (CRC). Often referred to as colon cancer, CRC is the second most deadly cancer worldwide. Approximately 1.9 million people worldwide are diagnosed with colon cancer and over 930,000 succumb to the disease annually. About one in twenty-four Americans (one in twenty-one Australians) will be diagnosed with CRC in their lifetime. But especially worrying is that cases are rapidly rising among people under the age of fifty, having nearly doubled between 1995 and 2019 and now comprising 20 percent of CRC cases (about 12 percent in Australia). This is an age group that is rarely screened for this disease. Some experts predict that colon cancer rates among people aged twenty to thirty-four will increase by 90 percent by 2030.

Colon cancer is a silent killer, often without obvious symptoms. Approximately one third of CRC cases are attributed to genetics, or family history.

It is unclear what accounts for the remaining two thirds of cases, but, as we will see, the long-term effects of diet and microbes contribute to the disease. Indeed, colon cancer is preventable and highly treatable–there is over a 90 percent chance of being cured when diagnosed early. CRC can take ten to forty years to develop, partly because genetic mutations in the colon accumulate over time, which can lead to abnormal and cancerous cell division. The resulting overgrowth of intestinal cells forms an adenoma: a polyp, or small growth of tissue, that is typically benign. But in some cases, cancer can start in the adenoma. Colonoscopies are used as a preventive measure to search for and remove larger and suspicious adenomas. Advanced CRC is very deadly, so we emphatically stress the importance of being proactive about getting colonoscopies. Starting at age forty-five–and even earlier for those with a history of family risk–everyone is urged to have a colonoscopy to screen for colon cancer. The sooner the disease is caught, the better your chances for treatment and survival. Those few days of discomfort could save your life.

Besides proactive screenings for polyps, there are many risk factors for CRC you can control, and others you cannot. You won't be able to change your risk when it comes to being older, or having a family history of colorectal polyps, inflammatory bowel disease, and/or the presence of adenomas. This makes it even more critical to focus on the factors we can control, such as being overweight or obese, being physically inactive, smoking, and heavy alcohol use–all of which can be lessened with lifestyle modifications. High-fat diets and those rich in red meat and processed meats increase the risk of CRC, while diets rich in fiber are thought to be protective. This is where our microbes enter the conversation. As we learned in chapter 7, both red meat and processed meats have proteins and other molecules that gut bacteria can modify to produce compounds that are harmful to the gut lining. They trigger mutations in cells that can lead to polyps, and ultimately CRC. Diets rich in saturated fats can also increase the body's bile acid production. While bile acid helps solubilize and break down these fats, it is also a very destructive detergent. Gut microbes strongly affect bile acid metabolism and modify bile acids to form several other compounds, which may contribute to cellular mutations that cause CRC.

Many of the immune-microbial connections discussed earlier play a particular role in the development of CRC. Dysbiosis increases the number of inflammatory microbes, triggering inflammation and subsequent CRC. In animal models, mice lacking innate immune pathways–cell-signaling pathways that are integral to activating the immune system and therefore key to inflammation–are more resistant to CRC.

There is ongoing debate regarding whether particular microbes are responsible for CRC. One microbe receiving a lot of attention is *Fusobacterium nucleatum*, a common oral microbe and minor component of the intestinal microbiota that can also trigger an inflammatory response. By studying the microbial composition of adenomas and colon tissue, scientists found higher numbers of *F. nucleatum* in colonic adenomas (polyps) and colonic tumors when compared to normal colon tissue from the same patient. When germ-free mice susceptible to tumors are inoculated with this microbe, there is an increase in tumors. *F. nucleatum* is invasive, which means it can adhere strongly to host cells and even enter them. Adding to this, the unwanted microbe has a cell surface protein (FadA) that is able to bind to a cell receptor and tell the cell to multiply uncontrollably. More studies have followed, showing that *F. nucleatum* is found in 50 percent of colon tumors. However, it appears that there are two strains of this bacterium, and only one is associated with tumors. The one associated with tumors seems to have more genes that would allow it to survive the perilous journey from the mouth, where it is normally found, to the intestine. We need more studies to better understand these mechanisms and how to manage *F. nucleatum*, which may in fact be a biomarker for CRC, one we can measure to decrease the incidence of tumors or even prevent tumor progression in patients who have an increased risk of CRC.

Microbiome studies in both younger and older CRC patients revealed that there were marked differences in their dysbiotic microbiomes, which are different than those who don't have CRC. Scientists hope that knowing these differences may help us further understand why there is this worryingly large increase in CRC among younger adults.

There are other particular microbes being associated with CRC such as *Akkermansia*, but data in humans are still at an early stage. We need to treat discoveries critically and thoughtfully, and wait for studies that confirm findings before claiming causation. Remember, just because a particular microbe is associated with tumors (or any other disease, for that matter) does not mean it causes them—perhaps the tumor environment merely favors that particular microbe's growth. The other problem with studying CRC is that its tumors are extremely slow growing. The microbe(s) that could have triggered it may well have long ago left the body by the time the tumor is detected. In short, there is a long road ahead for scientists to establish any causation between specific microbes and CRC incidence—but we are making steady progress.

Cancer and Antibiotic-Resistant Infections

Infections are a major and life-threatening danger to all cancer patients given that the cancer and its therapies prevent the immune system from working at full capacity. Several pathogens that cause infections are resistant to many antibiotics, which makes treatment extremely difficult. We have used the same drugs so widely and for so long that the infectious organisms have adapted and are now often resistant to traditional antibiotics. This makes our need for new solutions dire.

Although the research is in its infancy, there is significant optimism that altering the microbiome could help counter these antibiotic-resistant infections. It is well established that a healthy microbiome can block pathogens by outcompeting them for nutrients and sites to colonize. Patients undergoing any kind of treatment can work to maintain a healthy microbiome and encourage this internal environment. This includes promoting healthy, diverse microbiota by eating a diet that includes foods such as kefir and active-culture yogurts, fermented plant-based foods (e.g., tempeh, miso, sauerkraut), fruits, and leafy greens.

A healthy microbiome also improves the gut barrier by decreasing its permeability, which further prevents unwanted microbes or their molecules from entering the body—especially from reaching the bloodstream. Excitingly, patients undergoing stem cell transplants colonized with certain microbes were protected against subsequent infection of vancomycin-resistant enterococcus (VRE). There are over fifty-four thousand infections and five thousand deaths annually from VRE. Enterococci cause a range of infections, including bloodstream, surgical site, and urinary tract infections. There are few or no antibiotic treatment options left, as these bacteria continue to outwit our current drug supply. This is why this discovery of microbe-boosted protection is so exciting. The potential to save lives is immense, and there is significant hope that in the future we will utilize the microbiome to decrease the risk of infections in cancer patients.

Stem Cell Transplants

Deep in the bone marrow live stem cells, which are the precursor cells forming all the cells in our blood. Sometimes, the cancer cells that arise in the bone marrow result in blood and bone marrow cancers (e.g., multiple myeloma and leukemia). To treat these cancers, all of a patient's bone marrow is destroyed through chemotherapy or radiation. Blood-derived stem cells from a related donor, such as a sibling, are then placed into the patient where they localize to the bone marrow and "reboot" the production of normal blood and immune cells. This technique is called Allogeneic Hematopoietic Stem Cell Transplantation (Allo-HCT). It is still fraught with problems such as infections and graft-versus-host disease (GVHD), where the donor's immune cells mistakenly attack the recipient's body. The condition can range from mild to life-threatening. And the older the person, the higher the risk for GVHD.

Several recent reports suggest that the microbiota may influence the outcome of bone marrow transplants before and after the procedure. Pre-transplant microbiome dysbiosis has been linked to higher risk of infections, GVHD, and reduced overall survival. In a study of eighty recipients, low bacterial diversity was also associated with significantly worse outcomes following transplantation. This suggests that a robust microbiome is important to help prevent these complications. In an exciting recent clinical pilot study, fecal transfers were successfully used to treat GVHD following transplantation. Moreover, researchers can now predict GVHD by measuring microbial molecules that affect the immune system, which also correlates with survival and lower rates of remission. These represent major and unexpected steps forward for the field, and a groundbreaking avenue toward more effective cancer treatments.

Increased GVHD mortality is also associated with the broad-spectrum antibiotic use that often follows bone marrow transplantation and would also decrease microbial diversity. Because patients' immune systems are destroyed by the procedure, they are at high risk of infection and need to rely on strong antibiotics to fight it off. Breaking this cycle of antibiotic dependence is crucial, and microbes can provide the much-needed new methods to boost the immune system first and lessen problematic dependence on antibiotics after. In a retrospective study of 541 microbiomes of Allo-HCT transplantation individuals, a particular microbe, *Eubacterium limosum*, was associated with a decreased risk of relapse and progression of the disease. Interestingly, this microbe is also found extensively in centenarians.

There is exciting potential in applying this knowledge to medical practices. We may be able to better predict clinical outcomes based on individual patients' microbiome composition. We could also replenish the microbiome post-transplantation to reduce intestinal inflammation and improve health outcomes.

Cancer Therapy and Microbes

Besides surgical removal, traditional cancer treatments include radiation therapy and chemotherapy, which use toxic chemicals and work by preferentially killing fast-growing cancer cells. Given the toxicity of these treatments, it is not surprising they both significantly diminish microbial diversity.

One promising potential new solution to this problem is using our microbiota to predict the success of chemotherapy. Microbes can affect the bioavailability (degree and rate at which a drug is absorbed) of chemotherapy agents by affecting either drug metabolism or uptake of the drug. In animal studies using chemotherapy, subcutaneous (under the skin) tumors failed to respond to chemotherapy following antibiotic treatment. Cyclophosphamide, a common chemotherapy agent, requires a healthy gut microbiota to achieve efficacy. Studies indicated that the microbiota were needed to potentiate (to activate) the full activity of the immune system. A recurrent theme is that a strong immune system is essential to control tumor growth, and microbes can influence this immune response. We are awaiting studies in humans to confirm these findings.

Most exciting is the potential of the microbiome not just to predict but also to improve immunotherapy outcomes. To explain this, we need to take a couple of steps back. Cancer immunotherapy works by blocking checkpoints—pathways that impede the immune system. It essentially boosts the body's natural defenses to fight cancer by unleashing the immune system. Immunotherapy improves or restores immune system function to stop or slow the growth of cancer cells, and to stop cancer from spreading to other parts of the body. There are several types of therapies, including monoclonal antibodies, nonspecific immunotherapies, oncolytic virus therapy, T cell therapy, and cancer vaccines. Immune therapies are relatively new and are often used after traditional treatments of radiation or chemotherapy have failed. The treatments work in some cases, but not in others.

Two papers published in late 2015 upended the entire immunotherapy field by showing that microbes can affect cancer therapy outcomes, bringing the role of microbes in traditional treatments to the forefront. In the first paper, Dr. Thomas Gajewski led a team of researchers at the University of Chicago. They asked the fairly simple question: Will manipulating microbial composition change the efficacy of an immunotherapy? His team tested this question on an immunotherapy that uses an anti-PDL1 monoclonal antibody as a checkpoint inhibitor. PDL1 constrains the production of specific immune cells (CD8+ T cells) that actively seek out and destroy tumors. Dr. Gajewski's team began by looking at the anti-tumor effect in a strain of lab mice that were bred at two different mouse facilities. These mice purposefully had different gut microbiota. The scientists then implanted melanoma tumors in the mice. They found a difference: Tumors grew less aggressively in mice from one breeder than the other. They also found a more robust T cell response in the mice with slower tumor growth. These experiments suggested that different microbiota affected T cell responses differently, and importantly, affected tumor growth rate. To confirm this result, they let the mice live together, which enabled the mixing of the microbiota, due to general contact and the fact that mice are coprophagic, meaning that they eat each other's feces—the ultimate FMT! After swapping microbes, the two mice strains no longer had detectable tumor growth differences. Similarly, when feces were deliberately transplanted from one mouse strain to another, the anti-tumor and

T cell effects were also transferred. By combining fecal transfer and immunotherapy in more susceptible animals, even greater tumor control was observed. This suggested that the microbiome can play a central role in cancer immunotherapy treatment.

This discovery sparked another question: Are any particular microbes specifically involved in this effect on the immunotherapy? By sequencing the gut microbiota, these researchers found that *Bifidobacterium* species are the ones linked to anti-tumor immune responses. When they added a cocktail of these microbes to the susceptible animals, they were able to transfer the ability to control tumors in susceptible mice to the same extent as a fecal transfer. What really cinched things was that when they fed the *Bifidobacterium* mixture to mutant mice that lacked CD8+ T cells (needed for cancer surveillance), they were unable to control tumors–meaning that both CD8+ T cells and this microbe are needed. Further, if they killed the bacteria before giving it to mice, there was no effect. This suggests that live bacteria are needed for the effect to work.

The second study, led by Dr. Laurence Zitvogel in France, offers further evidence–but with different players. Her team used lab mice with various sarcoma, melanoma, or colorectal tumors to investigate the effect of immunotherapy against a different checkpoint protein, CTLA-4. This immunotherapy is approved for treatment of patients with metastatic melanoma (skin cancer). Dr. Zitvogel's team found that neither germ-free nor antibiotic-treated animals responded to the anti-CTLA-4 therapy. The normal mice (with normal microbiota) responded well. Researchers also found that if they added *Bacteroides fragilis* to germ-free or antibiotic-treated animals, the effectiveness of the immunotherapy was restored; this effect was mediated by T cells. In another analysis, studying the gut microbiome of twenty-five skin cancer patients, researchers found that a fecal transfer into germ-free mice of patients' feces that contained *B. fragilis* resulted in a restoration of the anti-CTLA-4 anti-tumor activity.

Two more papers were published back-to-back in the journal *Science* that validated the concepts seen in animal models in humans. Extending their mice findings, Dr. Zitvogel's group showed that resistance to immune checkpoint inhibitors is due to the microbiome, and that antibiotics blocked the efficacy of PDL1 inhibitors. They also found that they could transfer feces from cancer patients, who did or didn't respond, into mice, and show that same response to checkpoint inhibitors could be transferred with the feces. The team further analyzed the microbiome content of cancer patients and found a beneficial correlation to *Akkermansia muciniphila*. They could even spike non-responder feces with this microbe, and in mice, they would now respond to PDL1 immune therapy. In the other paper by Dr. Jennifer Wargo's team, the gut microbiomes of 112 melanoma cancer patients were analyzed. Researchers found that the microbiome of responders to anti-PDL1 immunotherapy had a much higher diversity, and an enrichment in *Ruminococcaceae* organisms. They also showed that the positive response to checkpoint inhibitors could be transferred into mice simply by a fecal transfer.

Researchers are now using microbiome analysis to identify patients who should respond (or not) to these checkpoint inhibitors based on deep microbial sequencing, and have developed microbial signatures for responders and non-responders. Others have found that a fiber-rich diet both altered the microbiome and significantly enhanced responses to treatment. Unexpectedly, they found that probiotics actually worsened the outcome, as they presumably inhibited colonization of beneficial microbes. These findings have now been extended by using FMTs along with anti-PDL1 treatment in advanced stage malignant melanoma patients that were resistant to anti-PDL1 treatment. Remarkably, they found clinical benefit (i.e., a cure) in six of the fifteen patients for a disease that is normally fatal. Results such as these are completely changing how we diagnose and treat CRC.

Looking Ahead

Collectively, these findings have unleashed a flurry of research and excited speculation for cancer therapy. Many scientific groups are now exploring these concepts, and additional clinical trials are underway. While we need a better understanding of exactly which microbes are involved in cancer and how, many believe that very soon, patients being considered for immunotherapy will undergo a microbiota analysis first. Those lacking particular microbes may need to be given certain microbes to enhance treatment. This represents a huge step forward in the pursuit of more effectively preventing and treating cancer.

KEY TIPS

Boost your defenses: A healthy microbiome can help block pathogens and potentially improve cancer treatment outcomes. Maintain a healthy microbiota by eating a range of fresh, whole, and fermented foods.

Drink in moderation (if at all): Consuming less or no alcohol can decrease your risk of breast cancer (in addition to a multitude of other deadly diseases, including dementia and cardiovascular disease). The recommended amount is no more than two drinks per day for men and one for women.

Control what you can to reduce risk of CRC: Aim to get regular physical activity, avoid smoking and drinking heavily, and maintain a healthy weight. Minimize red meat and processed meats in your diet, and eat plenty of fiber.

Get screened: Colon cancer is a preventable and highly treatable cancer when caught in the early stages. Starting at age forty-five, everyone should have regular colonoscopies to screen for colon cancer. Begin screenings even earlier if there is a history of family risk.

Use antibiotics only when necessary: Given that heavy antibiotic usage is linked to greater risk of cancer and infections, take antibiotics only when necessary and exactly as prescribed: Do not skip doses, and complete the course of treatment even if you start to feel better, otherwise you increase the chances of increased antimicrobial resistance to the antibiotic, requiring additional treatment. Do not share or use leftover medications. Shore up your immune system after a course of antibiotics with probiotic and prebiotic foods.

13

Zzz: Sleep and the Microbiome

We spend about a third of our lives sleeping—that's around twenty-six years for the average person. Sleep is a basic biological need that plays a critical role in our lives, and more recently, has been recognized as a key part of healthy living and aging. It is a necessary time to enable our bodies to rest, repair, and recover from the day. Contrary to popular belief, your brain is actually active during sleep, working to process and consolidate the day's memories and improve cognitive function. Sleep helps to stabilize your mood and reduce stress. Your blood pressure and heart rate fall, muscles repair, and tissues regenerate. The immune system gets a boost, and your body conserves energy, which helps with metabolic balance. Long story short, sleep is essential to every process in the body and related to every aspect of health. And several recent studies link the microbiome to sleep and sleep quality.

How much sleep do you need? It varies with age. Newborn babies sleep a lot (fourteen to seventeen hours a day), school-age children need about nine to eleven hours, and teenagers eight to ten hours. The National Sleep Foundation recommends that the average adult (eighteen to sixty-four years) requires seven to nine hours to feel well rested. It is a myth that older adults (sixty-five and up) need less sleep: Seven to eight hours is still recommended. But there are changes in sleep patterns and quality that are common among older ages, resulting in more fragmented sleep and increased napping. Older adults tend to get tired earlier in the evening, wake up earlier, and have less REM and slow wave sleep (often referred to as deep sleep). Finally, is there too much of a good thing? It turns out that yes, sleeping too much (more than ten hours) may be just as detrimental to our health as chronic sleep deprivation. So, aim for the Goldilocks level with seven to nine hours a night.

Unfortunately, more than a third of Americans (about two thirds of Australians) report getting less than seven hours of sleep a night. About 30 percent of adults have symptoms of insomnia. While once an all-nighter may have been viewed as a badge of honor, we now recognize that sleep deprivation has major impacts. Lack of sleep is linked to increased risk for numerous health conditions including obesity, diabetes, hypertension, heart disease, stroke, anxiety, depression, and dementia. The three pillars of health–nutrition, exercise, and sleep–are tightly connected. If you don't sleep well, you tend not to eat as well (e.g., junk food cravings can increase), and often the last thing you want to do is hit the gym. Furthermore, sleep apnea (a potentially serious sleep disorder in which breathing repeatedly pauses while sleeping), which affects between 9 to 38 percent of the US and Australian populations, is associated with increased Alzheimer's risk. REM sleep behavior disorders (vocally and/or physically acting out your dreams) are a major risk factor for Parkinson's.

MYTH: It doesn't matter what time of day you sleep.

FACT: Timing matters.

Our circadian rhythm (the internal "clock" that guides the secretion of the sleep hormone melatonin) is significantly influenced by natural sunlight. When the sun comes up and we're exposed to sunshine, it stops the floodgates of melatonin and activates the "on" phase of our circadian rhythm. At the end of the day, going into a dark environment enables the secretion of melatonin.

So, how do you ensure a good night's sleep? The internet is full of advice that includes having a consistent sleep schedule, a relaxing pre-bedtime routine (e.g., doing calming activities like reading a book), a comfortable sleep environment (a cool, dark room), no large meals or excessive alcohol just before bedtime, staying active during the day, managing stress, limiting naps, and avoiding screen time just before sleeping. The last one is difficult, as so much of our lives are online (including even reading electronic books), but many studies have shown that the blue light emitted from phones and tablets affects the body's production of melatonin, which is triggered for sleep and regulates sleep-wake cycles. The general recommendation is to avoid screen time for at least an hour before bed.

Sleepy Microbes

When we wrote the first edition of this book, good sleep was just being recognized as central to health and longevity, so there were few established microbial connections with sleep. However, the past few years have seen an explosion in studies linking the microbiome to sleep.

We've known for a while that the microbiome is involved in regulating circadian rhythms (this is discussed in detail on page 99), which are key to sleep. It now appears that microbes have their *own* circadian rhythms that may interact with the body's circadian rhythms and potentially affect sleep. These microbial rhythms are affected by diet (which influences microbiome composition) and when you eat. We also know that microbes produce neurotransmitters such as serotonin and gamma-aminobutyric acid (GABA), which play a role in regulating mood and relaxation, and of course, sleep. And finally, the microbiome has a large impact on the immune system and inflammation, which in turn, impacts sleep quality (think back to how you tossed and turned with your last fever).

The connection between the microbiome and sleep works both ways. For example, you are fasting when asleep, so this affects bacterial growth in the gut as there are no new nutrients during those hours. Poor sleep can affect the microbiome in detrimental ways. Lack of sleep increases stress, thereby increasing cortisol (a steroid hormone produced by the adrenal glands), which can have a major impact on the microbiome through its inflammatory activity. Lack of sleep can also lead to increased cravings for carbs, sugars, and trans fats, which we know alter the microbiome. Animal experiments show that if you significantly disrupt the microbiome, you disrupt sleep rhythms. Mice fed broad-spectrum antibiotics had changes in their sleep patterns, including disrupted REM sleep and changes in the neurotransmitter serotonin, which is associated with regulating sleep-wake cycles. This antibiotic treatment affected over two hundred other metabolites, another reason to avoid antibiotics unless absolutely necessary.

Evidence of the connection between the microbiome and sleep in humans, especially through the gut-brain microbiome axis, is increasing. People who sleep poorly have dysbiotic microbiomes, including a decrease in the beneficial SCFA producers. One of the SCFAs, butyrate, enhances sleep. Sleep also seems to enhance certain populations of beneficial microbes. Let's dive into this a bit more to see what really happens in humans, since this data have recently become available.

Sleep-Deprived Microbes

A general (and not surprising) consensus emerging among microbiologists is that poor sleepers have a dysbiotic microbiome, but this varies from person to person. There is no single microorganism linked to good sleep; like many things microbiome-related, a diverse collection of beneficial microbes are associated with good sleep. The other prevalent consensus is that although we know beneficial microbiomes are associated with better sleep, we don't know whether they are *causing* better sleep. However, more and more studies are showing that by changing the microbiome (e.g., through diet, probiotics, or fecal transfers), one can promote good sleep. So, using the microbiome to enhance sleep shows significant promise.

In a recent study of twenty-eight healthy young adults, ten bacterial taxa were associated with better sleep, as were more diverse microbiomes. Measures of poor sleep were inversely associated with decreased microbial diversity. Another study found similar results, and also that these changes were linked to changes in the inflammatory cytokines IL-1-beta and IL-6. However, the specific species involved appeared to differ between studies (a frequent occurrence in microbiome studies). Both found that abundance in Bacteroides and Firmicutes was positively associated with better sleep patterns; these organisms have been linked to regulating circadian rhythm and food intake (both linked to sleep). One study found a link between the presence of *Enterobacteriaceae* or *Anaerofilum* and night owls (people who tend to prefer being active late at night and into the early morning). This study also showed that an abundance of *Ruminococcus torques* is linked to an increased risk of snoring and tends to be more prevalent in people with obesity, while *Senegalimassilia* may decrease snoring risk and appears in those at a healthy weight. Another study looked at "social jet lag," which involves waking for work at specific hours during the week, then staying up late and sleeping in on the weekend. In a cohort of 934 people, researchers found that just a ninety-minute difference in the timing of the midpoint of sleep (i.e., sleeping ninety minutes later on the weekend) was associated with changes in the gut microbiome. Social jet lag was also associated with lower overall diet quality and higher sugar intake, which also influence microbes.

Sleep deprivation is becoming more and more common across society and is known to dysregulate inflammatory processes and cognition. Given the microbiome's role in these processes, it is not surprising to see that sleep deprivation impacts our microbiomes. In a study of twenty-five participants, each participant was kept awake for forty hours following eight hours of sleep. In addition to expected poorer cognition performances due to sleep deprivation, they also found decreases in diversity in the microbiome. Continued episodes of sleep deprivation also had increased effects on microbial diversity. Similar studies have been performed in mice with corresponding results, including cognitive impairment, increases in inflammatory responses, and decreases in microbial diversity.

Sleep Disorders and Microbes

Recent studies have investigated the impact of sleep disorders on the microbiome. Not surprisingly, people with sleep disorders have altered microbiomes. However, the role of the microbiome in these disorders has not been established. For example, insomnia (which can affect half of older adults) is linked to decreased microbial diversity, reduced SCFA production, and changes in inflammatory responses. In a study of seventy-two older adults (average age of 73.2 years), researchers found that certain species were associated with better (*Lachnoclostridium*) or poorer (*Blautia*) sleep patterns. Other studies show that individuals with short-term sleep restrictions, such as military personnel, first responders, health care providers, and other shift workers, have reduced gut microbial richness.

It is estimated that over a billion people worldwide have obstructive sleep apnea (OSA), which is defined as breathing being interrupted for greater than ten seconds at least five times an hour, resulting in decreased sleep quality. This condition is associated with increased risk of cardiovascular diseases and diabetes, as well as a decreased life expectancy. It is also associated with obesity, and significantly increased snoring. People (and experimental mice) with OSA have a disrupted microbiome, including a reduction in SCFA producers and altered inflammatory responses. Further, changes in the microbiome have been observed among people with narcolepsy through altered microbial diversity. Patients with chronic fatigue syndrome also had a dysbiotic microbiome. Again, with all of these sleep issues, it has not been established that the microbiome is involved in the problem, or whether secondary changes occur as a result of the problem. However, there are certainly strong hints that the microbiome is involved.

SUSTENANCE AND SNORING

Jessica used to dread childhood sleepovers. Try as she might—by sleeping on her side or elevating her head—inevitably the next morning she would get teased for snoring. Loudly. Snoring is a common condition in which air can't flow easily through your nose or mouth. While mild or occasional snoring isn't usually a cause for concern, chronic snoring can increase risk for some health conditions, including stroke and heart attack. If snoring occurs in combination with gasping for air in your sleep and other symptoms like fatigue or irritability, it is recommended to talk with a health care provider.

As snoring gets louder, the chances of sleep apnea increase proportionately. Because of the link between obstructive sleep apnea (OSA) and obesity, a few studies have shown that lifestyle interventions such as healthy diet and exercise can decrease sleep apnea. A recent study of over fourteen thousand people showed that obese individuals following a plant-based diet with plentiful vegetables, fruits, nuts, and whole grains were 19 percent less likely to suffer from snoring associated with OSA than those with fewer plant-based foods in their diet. Moreover, individuals who ate a less healthy plant-based diet full of refined carbohydrates like pasta, bread, sweets, and sugary drinks had a significantly higher incidence of OSA and snoring. Although they didn't examine the microbiome, it is well established that high-fiber plant-based diets significantly shift the microbiome and promote anti-inflammatory microbes. So, microbes might have a role in snoring!

Boost Your Microbiome to Improve Sleep

Given all that we have seen above about the potential role of the microbiome in sleep, it begs the question: If we enhance our microbiome, can we improve our sleep? Fortunately, there are significant data to indicate that yes, better sleep is indeed possible (along with all the other benefits a healthy microbiome brings).

The first obvious way is to improve diet, such as by increasing intake of fiber and fermented foods. In a 2018 study of 2,068 participants, researchers found that following a Mediterranean-style diet was associated with adequate sleep and less insomnia. In a 2019 study of 1,314 individuals, better adherence to the Mediterranean diet was associated with a higher likelihood of overall adequate sleep quality. Higher fiber increases beneficial SCFAs and serotonin, both associated with enhanced sleep. Other dietary changes that can help enhance sleep include decreasing alcohol consumption, avoiding caffeine and other stimulants right before bed and reducing intake in general, eating meals at regular times (which enhances circadian rhythm) and not right before bedtime, and staying hydrated.

Perhaps the strongest proof that the microbiome is associated with improved sleep comes from fecal material transfer (FMT) experiments done on people with irritable bowel syndrome (IBS). It is well established that an altered dysbiotic gut microbiome is associated with IBS (see chapter 2). Sleep disturbances and changes in sleep patterns are also associated with IBS. In human FMT studies where healthy feces were transferred into IBS patients, improvements were seen in sleep (in addition to depression and anxiety). Related studies have put human feces into germ-free animals with similar results. Collectively, this work suggests that the microbiome can have direct effects on sleep.

Shut-Eye and Probiotics

Throughout this book, we have been rather skeptical of prebiotics and probiotics, primarily because of a lack of rigorous scientific studies that truly demonstrate their effectiveness. However, there is growing evidence over the past couple of years that probiotics may enhance sleep. Several studies indicate that *Lactobacillus* species may enhance sleep. *L. brevis* administration is known to increase microbial metabolites associated with sleep enhancement (but hasn't been directly shown to improve sleep). A heat-inactivated (i.e., killed) administration of *L. gasseri* seemed to improve sleep problems. A meta-analysis of six studies involving 343 healthy adults who consumed *L. gasseri* daily showed significant improvement in sleep.

A recent randomized, double-blind, placebo-controlled trial (the gold standard clinical study as neither the participants nor the scientists know which randomly selected group any one individual belongs to) using a multi-strain probiotic consisting of *Limosilactobacillus fermentum* LF16, *Lacticaseibacillus rhamnosus* LR06, *Lactiplantibacillus plantarum* LP01, and *Bifidobacterium longum* 04 (all common commercially available probiotic strains) was tested in seventy healthy individuals. They took the probiotic mixture for six weeks and then, after a further three weeks, were tested for sleep parameters. Researchers concluded that this probiotic mixture improved the ability to fall asleep faster and experience fewer sleep disturbances, resulting in overall improved sleep quality.

A 2024 study showed that a single probiotic strain, *Bifidobacterium longum* 1714, was able to improve sleep. This probiotic has already shown positive effects on stress, anxiety, and depressive symptoms. In the randomized, double-blind, placebo-controlled study involving eighty-nine adults with impaired sleep quality, participants were given a capsule of one billion colony forming units of *B. longum* 1714 that also included corn starch (a prebiotic) and magnesium stearate (a muscle relaxant) daily for eight weeks. The strain significantly improved sleep quality and reduced daytime dysfunction due to sleepiness, as well as improving social functioning and vitality compared to the controls. The authors claim that this is the only probiotic strain that also seems to boost mental wellness among recipients. Although the mechanism(s) by which this probiotic may work were not established, it is an excellent trial indicating that this probiotic may enhance not only sleep, but also overall mental health.

Looking Ahead

At this early stage, it seems that the microbiome has significant impacts on sleep and vice versa. A healthy microbiome may promote healthy sleep, which in turns promotes healthy aging. Given that microbes are intricately involved across our body's many systems, it makes sense that they also influence sleep. Take steps now to enhance your microbiome so you don't lose any sleep while scientific research continues to advance.

KEY TIPS

Aim for a consistent sleep schedule: Try to keep a fairly consistent wakeup time throughout the week. Sleeping in every weekend can confuse your brain—and microbes—and cause the release of melatonin at weird hours. The body functions best when it runs on a rhythm.

Make time for sleep: Aim for seven to nine hours of sleep every night. Many studies have shown that lack of sleep impacts every aspect of one's health, including the microbiome.

Follow the Mediterranean diet: Not only can this help enhance sleep, but it is also associated with many additional beneficial health effects such as decreased risk of brain, metabolic, and cardiovascular diseases.

Try a fiber-rich diet for snoring: If you have obstructive sleep apnea and/or heavy snoring, switching to a largely plant-based diet that includes plenty of fruits, vegetables, nuts, seeds, whole grains, and beans may help improve both.

Consider a sleep-enhancing probiotic: Although research is in its early days, *Bifidobacterium longum* 1714 is the one probiotic shown to enhance sleep in controlled clinical trials, in addition to having beneficial effects for overall mental wellness.

14

Too Clean, or Not Too Clean: Environmental Microbes

There is one number that predicts your health and life expectancy more than any other: your zip code. Environmental health researchers and epidemiologists have long recognized the importance of geography to human well-being. This includes physical aspects of the places where we live, learn, work, and play (the built environment); the people we interact with (the social environment); and local characteristics of the natural environment (such as air and water quality, weather, and proximity of green spaces). Having access to healthy foods, quality health care services, and well-maintained parks; ingesting clean water, food, and air; spending time with people who nurture and support us; and living in safe, clean homes all have the potential to influence our overall lifestyles and health.

When we zoom into these various contexts, we once again discover the partners that are silently conducting the symphony of our world: microbes. Microorganisms are present in all these places–the indoor and outdoor spaces we live in, the food and drink we consume, the people we're with every day or pass by only on occasion–and are therefore a key puzzle piece in explaining why some people are healthier and live longer than others.

Jessica focuses her research on this complex relationship between environments and aging. As an environmental gerontologist, she studies where people live as they age and how that affects their health and well-being. Her work examines how environments can "get under our skin" to shape experiences of aging. When interviewing older adults across the Minneapolis metropolitan area as part of her PhD research,

Jessica could not help but notice drastic differences in people's microbial exposures. Some homes were spotless and sterile with freshly scrubbed counters and floors smelling strongly of bleach. More often, homes featured piles of belongings–from clothing to food containers to paperwork–multiple human and pet inhabitants, and evidence of many years of residence. On occasion, Jessica even observed mold from water damage, rotting food on counters, and stuffy unventilated air. This likely put inhabitants at risk through regular contact with pathogens. With this clear-eyed and more holistic view of the aging process, she began to consider invisible and dynamic interactions between the environment, microbiota, and older people.

Nature Versus Nurture

The role of the environment in microbial composition is a subject of much scientific debate in the field of microbiology. To investigate this topic, Dr. Eran Segal and colleagues from the Weizmann Institute of Science collected blood and stool samples from 1,046 healthy Israeli adults (a 2018 study published in *Nature*). These individuals were aged eighteen to seventy; had not used antibiotics within three months prior to participation; did not have a chronic health condition, and were not pregnant; and were from five distinct ancestral origins: Ashkenazi, North African, Yemenite, Sephardi, and Middle Eastern. The relatively recent immigration of genetically diverse populations to Israel, where they share a common environment, created ideal scientific conditions to compare the degree to which environments and genetics shape the microbiome. Segal's group found that ancestry was not significantly associated with microbiome composition; an individual's genetics actually determined a very small fraction (less than 2 percent) of the differences seen across the microbiomes of people.

MYTH: Longevity is determined by genetic factors.

FACT: The everyday social and physical conditions of life—where you live, who you interact with, what you eat, how often you exercise—can influence health and longevity to a much greater extent (about 75 percent in studies) than genes (about 25 percent).

To test this further, Segal and colleagues then analyzed an existing data set from a 2016 study of microbiome composition in 1,126 pairs of twins from the United Kingdom. They determined that between 1.9 and 8.1 percent of the human microbiome is heritable. So, even though twins share the same genetics, they still develop into markedly distinct individuals. Lifestyle factors such as diet, drugs, and home environment account for the remaining 91.9 to 98.1 percent.

In order to examine the degree of environmental influence on the microbiome, Segal's group also looked at the microbial compositions of twenty-four pairs of related individuals who had never lived together. They found no evidence of similar microbiomes among these pairs. By contrast, when investigating fifty-five related pairs with a history of household sharing, they found significant similarities in their microbiomes. They also performed analyses on thirty-two pairs of genetically unrelated pairs who had shared a household, and again found significant microbial similarities. The results of this seminal research all suggest that past or present household sharing contributes to gut microbiome composition, given that relatives with no past household sharing do not have similar microbiomes. In other words, the places you inhabit, and not your genes, define which microbes inhabit you.

Segal's and others' groundbreaking work demonstrates the value of examining non-genetic determinants of health and disease. When considering these factors, new ways to personalize medical treatments and approaches to vitality and healthy aging emerge. Relative to their genes, people's microbiomes are easy to change. We shall see in this chapter that environmental microbiome interventions and treatments, big and small, long-term and short-term, are poised to help us live longer and healthier lives.

Underexposed and Overkilled

Every time you open the front door, a gust of air carries microbes into your home—as do dogs, visitors, Amazon packages, and your own body, which picked up microbes from your car, the sidewalk, your office, etc. These microbes are critical, as Americans, and Australians, now spend about 90 percent of their time indoors. This goes against human nature. We did not evolve in sterile chambers or closed rooms, but rather in close contact with nature. We slept on cave floors, had limited hygiene rituals, and spent most of our time outside with other people and animals. Even as society progressed, livestock still ambled the streets, roofs and walls leaked, sewers overflowed, and windows opened, letting all those microbes in. Until relatively recently, most families lived on farms and were exposed to abundant microbes through daily chores, frequent romps outside, and breezy open windows.

MYTH: All fungi and bacteria in the home are harmful.

FACT: This common misconception inspires unnecessary fears and often excessive cleaning, sterilization, and use of antimicrobial products. The vast majority of microbes found in the built environment are innocuous, and many are even beneficial to human inhabitants.

Modernization sealed us away. This means that we are generally exposed to significantly less diverse microbes on a daily basis. On top of that, we now inhabit a world with thousands of antimicrobial products, ranging from paint and carpeting to cutting boards (more on this later). So, in addition to being exposed to fewer microbes, we're also regularly attempting to kill the ones we actually do come into contact with. We may be more productive, connected, and technologically advanced compared to our ancestors, but we've also alienated ourselves from many of the essential microbes that evolved with us. This shift to the sterilized indoors has had some unintended consequences. It appears that fundamental changes in lifestyle from farm to urban living have led to decreased contact with certain microbes that are essential to immune system development. One result is that respiratory diseases are on the rise: Three hundred million people worldwide suffer from asthma, and more than 40 percent of the world's high-income country population has allergies. Growing scientific evidence links environmental factors known to provide microbial exposure to the reduced risk of developing asthma. In one example, children who grew up on Bavarian or Amish farms, and in close proximity to livestock, had significantly lower rates of asthma than the general, non-farm population. Several factors have been associated with lower prevalence of some allergies, including contact with animals as a child, exposure to stables under the age of one, breast feeding, vaginal birth, and lack of antibiotics early in life.

Being removed from the microbes we knew from farming days doesn't mean that we are alone in our modern-day indoor environments, however. Rather, our homes, workplaces, and public buildings provide new habitats and comfy residence to numerous microbial communities. The problem is that these resident microbes are generally not as diverse or beneficial in composition as outdoor environments. It is therefore important to get outside at any age. Older adults are too often confined to sterile, climate-controlled indoor environments.

We can also find ways to bring the outside in, such as ventilating with fresh air and surrounding ourselves with live greenery. Indoor houseplants and flowers can positively influence health by introducing beneficial bacteria into the indoor microbiome, in addition to stress reduction, boosted creativity, and extra oxygen production. Just like humans, plants harbor distinct microbiomes. Houseplants can also remarkably improve indoor air quality. Leaves filter air to reduce carbon dioxide levels and release oxygen. Indoor plants can stabilize the ecosystem and even counteract pathogens. For example, English ivy, the evergreen vine we so often see climbing the sides of stately buildings, can help eliminate airborne mold spores (but be careful where you place the pot if you bring one home: the leaves are toxic to humans and animals and the sap can irritate skin).

MOISTURE AND MOLD: YOUR UNWANTED ROOMMATES

Fungal growth in damp or water-damaged buildings is an increasing problem. Most indoor water damage is caused by natural disasters (floods) or humans (disrepair). Water can also penetrate buildings through melting snow, heavy rains, or sewer system overflow; water vapor can be produced through daily activities such as cooking, doing laundry, and showering. Mold—a common type of fungus—will easily grow in any place with a lot of moisture.

Most molds are not harmful to healthy humans. They can, however, cause nasal congestion, throat irritation, coughing or wheezing, eye irritation, and sometimes skin irritation in sensitive people. Long-term exposure can particularly affect older adults; infants and children; individuals with respiratory conditions, asthma, and/or allergies; and immune-compromised people.

These groups are at increased risk for respiratory problems and infections, and the exacerbation of asthma and allergies.

The key to minimize mold inside the home is moisture control. The CDC recommends using air conditioners and dehumidifiers to reduce high humidity levels; fixing leaky roofs, windows, and pipes; conducting a thorough cleaning and drying after flooding; and ventilating bathing, laundry, and cooking areas. Mold growth can be scrubbed away on hard surfaces with commercial products, soap and water, or bleach solutions. Most importantly, fix the root cause of any water/moisture problems so that the mold can't grow back.

We Are Family

With scientific advancements in molecular sequencing, we are increasingly able to analyze the individual bacterial, archaeal (a different type of microbe), and fungal species inhabiting the spaces where we live, work, and play. We've learned that indoor microbiomes originate primarily from human skin, pets, and the outside air (see Figure 1). Human depositions of microorganisms have been observed in the microbiome environments of classrooms, households, and athletic spaces. We as human occupants can deposit skin microorganisms at a rate of one million airborne microbial cells per hour. These microbes can then decay, only to be replaced at a rapid rate on the surfaces frequently in contact with humans. The human microbes most commonly shed come from skin bacteria, including high counts of Actinobacteria and Firmicutes, in addition to skin-associated yeasts such as Malassezia. While we normally live in peaceful coexistence with Malassezia yeasts (they are integral components of the skin microbiota), an overabundance can cause skin conditions such as dandruff and atopic dermatitis (eczema), as we saw in chapter 5.

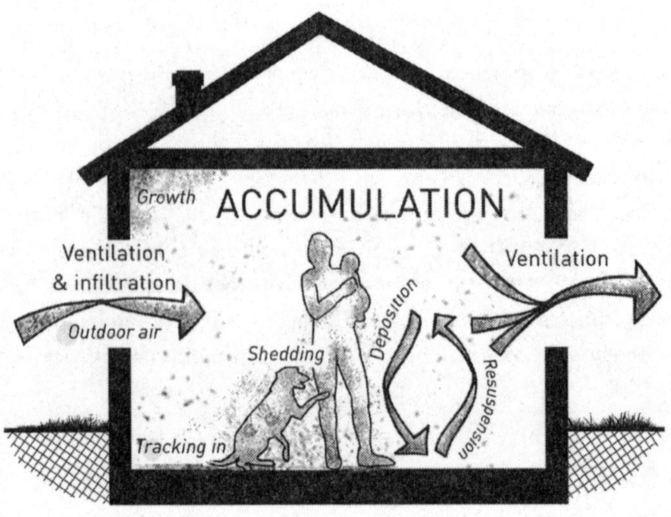

Figure 1: Sources and physical processes that govern assembly of indoor microbial communities. Other potential sources of microbes may include emission from plants, food, and plumbing.

Illustration by Sarah E. Kwan and Jordan Peccia (2016). Buildings, Beneficial Microbes, and Health. *Trends in Microbiology* 24, no. 8. Reprinted with permission.

Scientists in the Home Microbiome Project sequenced bacteria from seven different families, including their pets and shared homes, over four to six weeks. Eighteen participants were trained to collect 1,625 microbial samples from their bodies and from their homes consisting of ten houses, three dogs, and one cat. For three families, samples were taken immediately before and after moving to a new home. Participants swabbed the surfaces of skin, hands, feet, noses, countertops, doorknobs, and many other surfaces that they touched in their homes. Hands were the most microbially similar among family members, while noses remained the most distinct. By contrast, microbial communities differed significantly among homes, and the home microbiome was largely sourced from the humans living inside. Turns out, our bodies release bacteria in almost every encounter we have with our environments—when we scratch our heads, yawn, open the fridge door, or flop onto the couch when we come home at night. Our germ-sharing also happens rapidly. When the three families moved house, it took less than twenty-four hours for the new places to look exactly like their old ones—at least when it came to their microbial roommates. This held true even when the new place was a hotel room that had just been inhabited by other people! Rapid and complete colonization of microbiota in each home was so exact and unique that a swab of any room revealed the family's distinct microbial signature. This was so specific that the researchers were able to successfully predict which family was responsible for a particular sample based solely upon the set of floor microbes they were given.

Social interactions outside our main home also play a major role in facilitating microbe exchanges. Simple acts like shaking hands, passing a friend's phone and scrolling through her photos, and eating off the same dishes all involve swapping microbes. In one study, a volunteer (intentionally) touched a virus-contaminated door handle, then shook hands with a second participant, who then shook hands with a third participant, and so on. The results showed that the virus could be transmitted this way as many as six times. After this person-to-person exchange, the microbes can also be deposited on various surfaces by one person, only to be collected afterward by another. In one study of ten desk surfaces spread across three schools, students deposited microbes from their skin, oral, and gut microbiomes. After desk cleaning, which removed 50 percent of the bacteria, the microbial communities fully reestablished themselves on the surfaces within two to five days.

Both young children and older adults who will be more susceptible to infections should wash their hands regularly with warm, soapy water. Be cognizant of the many people and surfaces you swap microbes with on a daily basis.

CHECK YOUR BACTERIAL BAGGAGE

Lifestyle changes and travel shift our microbiomes in response to the new people, places, and foods we encounter. One of the worst fears of international travel is experiencing traveler's diarrhea (TD) or other enteric (intestinal) infections. In one study, a participant relocated from a major American metropolitan area to the capital of a middle-income nation in Southeast Asia. This individual was exposed to a novel diet and environment while traveling, and experienced two bouts of diarrhea. He also experienced nearly a twofold increase in the Bacteroidetes to Firmicutes ratio, which reversed upon his return to the United States.

The human gut microbiome plays a major role in travelers' health. The density and diversity of one's gut microbiome can prevent and limit pathogenic colonization and growth. This occurs mainly through competitive exclusion. A traveler's unique gut microbiome may predispose them to enteric infection to a greater or lesser extent. For example, Swedish tourists traveling to high-risk destinations for enteric infection were more susceptible to contracting Campylobacter (a cause of diarrhea) if their pre-travel microbiome had a lower diversity. The structure and composition of the gut microbiome can protect against common traveler gut ailments. In another study comparing the gut microbiomes of individuals with TD, researchers found a dysbiotic profile of a high Firmicutes to Bacteroidetes ratio in travelers who developed diarrhea.

There may be ways to manipulate the microbiome to prevent TD. One option is to maintain as normal a diet as possible when abroad. Even short-term changes in eating patterns can have long-term effects on your microbiome—even after returning from travel. However, we recognize that this strategy may notably diminish the quality of one's travels in search of new foods and unique experiences.

Similar to how we get shots to boost our immunity to infectious agents before international travel, we might also consider arming our guts with helpful microbes. Studies have shown that probiotics including the yeast *Saccharomyces boulardii* and bacterium *Lactobacillus rhamnosus* can play a role in the prevention of TD. Prebiotics including a galacto-oligosaccharide mixture (prebiotic fibers that originate from plant sugars) were linked to reduced bouts of diarrhea in travelers, but it was a small study and not a clinically controlled blind trial. Researchers are still investigating whether probiotics and prebiotics can treat acute TD.

Senior Institutional Care

Relocating to a long-term care facility or nursing home has major effects upon the microbiota. If someone moves to a nursing home, it takes about a year for their gut microbes to fully shift to the resident local microbiota. Nursing homes often feature an unhealthy microbial composition that increases inflammation due to lack of microbial diversity. Bacterial infections are also common, given that these facilities provide an ideal environment for the acquisition and spread of infection: Residents share sources of air, food, and health care in often crowded institutional settings, and are already more susceptible to disease. Furthermore, the constant flux of visitors, staff, and residents brings in pathogens from both the hospital and community. Outbreaks of respiratory and gastrointestinal infections are frequent in these settings, and as we know from other chapters, they are caused by microbes and have strong microbial links regarding disease susceptibility.

The bacterium *Streptococcus pneumoniae* (often called the "pneumococcus," which we met in chapter 8) causes many common infections, including pneumonia and ear infections. It is a leading cause of illness and death in the United States, and a significant cause in Australia, each year. We generally use antibiotics to combat bacterial infections like those caused by the pneumococcus. The issue is that because antibiotic usage is so common–and sometimes inappropriately prescribed–in both young and (especially) older populations, care environments often become ideal settings for drug-resistant strains to emerge. The CDC reported that about 30 percent of pneumococcus infections are drug resistant, and these rates are on the rise. Drug-resistant outbreaks can be prevented or minimized with careful use of antibiotics, and pneumococcus pneumonias can be prevented through vaccination. The issue is that vaccines are often underused in nursing homes. Physicians may mistakenly believe that vaccinations are ineffective or harmful in older populations. Only 45 percent of people aged sixty-five and older have been vaccinated against pneumonia in the United States, and less than 40 percent in Australia; and in most nursing homes with outbreaks, fewer than 5 percent of residents have been vaccinated.

A 2017 meta-analysis published in the *American Journal of Infection Control* stated that, on average, 27 percent of nursing home residents are colonized with drug-resistant bacteria. Risk factors included advanced age, comorbid (having two or more) chronic diseases, history of recurrent hospitalization, increased interaction with health care workers, frequent antimicrobial exposure, decreased functional status, advanced dementia, immobility, fecal incontinence, and residency in a long-term care facility. The study's authors emphasize the importance of strong infection prevention programs in nursing homes and long-term care facilities. This is a challenge given frequent understaffing, minimal resources, insufficient training, and inadequate surveillance. The hospital environment also falls under consideration here, given frequent transfers of residents between nursing homes and acute care, which contributes to the influx of pathogens between them.

The Hospital Microbiome Project began in 2013 by collecting microbial samples from surfaces, air, staff, and patients of the University of Chicago's new hospital pavilion. Their goal was to better understand the factors that influence bacterial population development in health care settings. Just as other researchers studied people moving into a new home, this study examines the rate and structure of succession in a hospital microbiome as the hospital starts accepting staff and patients. Environmental variables such as building materials, temperature, humidity, HVAC, and cleaning procedures/schedules play a role. These factors intersect with the patients and staff to affect the complex microbiomes in the hospital. Observing patterns and trends in this sort of data could be critical to the prevention of people becoming sicker in a hospital–the place where they should be recovering–and could also affect the designs of hospitals and medical facilities in the future.

MYTH: Opening the window in a nursing home or hospital room will let in harmful bacteria.

FACT: Health care centers might help thwart the spread of infection by opening the windows. Fresh air lets more microbes in, which can help control previously unchallenged pathogens. In rooms sealed from the outdoors and unventilated by fresh air, harmful bacteria have less competition from other microbes in the environment. A diverse environmental microbiome can act as a protective layer against hospital- and nursing-home-borne infections.

Fido and Her Microbes

One way to bolster the immune system is through exposure to a wider array of the microbial universe, thereby increasing microbial diversity. Remember, more diversity in the biological world is nearly always preferred! One way to do that is to get a pet–especially a dog–to bring more abundant and diverse microbes into the home. In one study, households with pets had more plant and soil bacteria in their homes, which is usually a good thing. Mice fed dust from dog-dwelling homes were more resilient to allergens. And as we've seen, exposure to animals during childhood–including domesticated pets–has been associated with lower prevalence of asthma and allergies. One does not necessarily need to move to a farm, given that dogs can have similar protective effects on their owners as horses (though farms overall likely provide more diverse microbial exposure than city living). Additional benefits of a having a dog include companionship, stress reduction, and an excuse for regular outdoor exercise.

We live with billions of invisible microbial neighbors, and for the most part they are innocuous or even helpful to our health and well-being, including those from pets. On rare occasions, pets can bring detrimental microbes into the home. *Toxoplasma gondii*, for example, is a neurological parasite that can invade all warm-blooded animals, including humans. In immunosuppressed individuals and during pregnancy, its effects can be devastating. Symptoms include aggression, impulsivity, severe mental illness, and even suicide. One can get an infection from *T. gondii* from contact with cat fecal matter. This is why pregnant women are advised to avoid exposure to household cat litter, given that this parasitic infection increases risk of miscarriage, stillbirth, and serious health problems for the baby, including brain and nervous system damage, seizures, and deafness. Dogs can carry it inside on their fur after rolling in cat feces and contaminated soil. If concerned about a furry friend's hygiene, washing your hands after touching them is a good idea (as we well know by now).

MYTH: A dog's mouth is cleaner than a person's mouth.

FACT: A dog's mouth likely contains fewer microbes that are directly harmful to humans. However, that does not mean that the dog's mouth has fewer microbes overall or is "cleaner." Think about how dogs behave–their mouths frequently come into contact with their own and other animals' backsides and feces (unlike humans, they are coprophagic).

In some cases, cat bites (generally to the hand) cause serious bacterial infections, as cats' sharp teeth make relatively deep puncture wounds and can introduce infectious microbes into the body. Bacteria usually invade from the oral microbiota of the biting animal but can even originate from the victim's own skin or physical environment at the time of injury. If bitten, be alert for signs of infection. Seek medical care if you develop swelling, redness, pain, or have difficulty moving your hand.

YOUR CELL PHONE IS TEN TIMES DIRTIER THAN A TOILET SEAT

We are constantly connected to our phones, from reading the news during our morning commute to scrolling through music waiting at the doctor's office, making lists and searching for recipes at the grocery store, and surfing social media in bed. We often don't give it a second thought. Cell phones are the most frequently owned and used electronic devices worldwide and bear the brunt of much negative media for facilitating constant (social) media connectivity, which can impact our mental health and relationships. And now, research shows that cell phones are far dirtier than we might ever expect. They are actually vast reservoirs for bacteria—the more microbes they collect, the more microbes wind up on your hands, face, and everywhere in between.

The text-cramp in your thumb isn't the only way your phone and hand have an unhealthy relationship. Your hands are the biggest culprit when it comes to depositing microbes on the phone's surface. One study showed that Americans check their phones on average 144 times per day (for Australians it's fifty-eight), which provides plenty of opportunities for microbes to move from your fingers and palm to your phone. Research varies on exactly how many and what kinds of bacteria are inhabiting the average cell phone. A 2017 study of twenty-seven secondary school students' cell phones found a median of 17,032 bacterial genes per phone. Most organisms were harmless, including those passed through contact from human skin; potentially pathogenic microbes, however, including *Staphylococcus aureus*, were among the dominant microbes found on these phones. No differences were found based on the phone owner's gender or between phone types (touch screen versus keypad). No antibiotic-resistant microbes were detected.

Researchers at the University of Arizona found that cell phones carry ten times more bacteria than most toilet seats. Ironically, unlike the bathroom, people rarely clean or disinfect their phones, so the bacteria just keep building up. As we use our phones frequently, they remain warm, which creates ideal breeding grounds for bacteria. Fortunately, there are easy ways to minimize contamination. First, do not bring in or use a phone while in the bathroom. When toilets flush, they can spray bacteria into the air, which could contribute to how phones end up covered with fecal bacteria such as *E. coli*. It may be a good idea to generally put the lid down when flushing to prevent fecal matter from spraying onto other bathroom surfaces—like your toothbrush.

There are a few effective ways to clean your phone. A simple soft microfiber cloth will remove many of the surface microbes. For a deeper clean, researchers suggest using a combination of 60 percent water and 40 percent rubbing alcohol. Dip a cloth in this solution before gently wiping it across the phone. Cleaning your phone several times a month is ideal. Or just get used to saying hello to your microbes each time you pick it up!

A Kitchen's Dirty Secrets

Exposure to foodborne microorganisms during food handling in the home is fairly frequent. *Salmonella* is a bacteria that causes foodborne illness, often referred to as food poisoning. The CDC estimates that *Salmonella* causes one million cases of foodborne illness in the US each year (around one hundred and forty thousand cases in Australia). Outbreaks have been linked to contaminated poultry and eggs, as well as cucumbers, pistachios, raw tuna, sprouts, and many other foods. Cattle are sources of *E. coli* 0157, resulting in contamination of hamburger and other meats that have to be recalled. Studies show that improperly cleaning the counter or cutting board used to prep the meat can spread the infection. Another common route of contamination is dipping a BBQ brush back into a bottle of sauce after brushing uncooked meat. We can also indirectly transfer potentially harmful microorganisms via our hands or contact with other surfaces into the nose, mouth, eyes, and open cuts and wounds.

Lab studies show that bacteria and viruses that spread to environmental surfaces from an infected or carrier source can survive in significant numbers for several hours. In some cases, they survive for days, especially on moist surfaces. Organisms can spread rapidly from a contaminated surface via hands, sponges, cleaning cloths, and hand and food contact surfaces around the home. Although raw food is a primary source of unwanted microbes in the kitchen, there is evidence that surfaces such as cutting boards, sinks, dishcloths, and cleaning utensils are major reservoirs for bacteria. Frequently wet and moist sites in particular may act as permanent sources of bacterial populations.

Kitchen sponges are a hotbed of microbes. Researchers in Germany sequenced the microbial DNA of fourteen used kitchen sponges. They found 362 different species of bacteria living within them. Density was incredibly high: About eighty-two billion bacteria were living in just a cubic inch of space. In metric, a single cubic centimeter could be packed with more than forty-five billion bacteria, which corresponds to over five times the number of people inhabiting Earth. Such high bacterial densities found elsewhere are only in feces, the lead scientist told a reporter.

MYTH: Cross-contamination does not occur in the refrigerator as it's too cold in there for microbes to survive.

FACT: Some bacteria can survive, and even thrive, in cool, moist environments like the refrigerator. For example, *Listeria monocytogenes*, a pathogen that contaminates meats and cheeses, loves to grow at 39°F (4°C). Your fridge's crisper compartment may be one of the "germiest" places in the kitchen thanks to its combination of humidity, temperature, and proximity to unwashed produce. Keep fresh fruits and vegetables separate from raw meat, poultry, seafood, and eggs. Clean the fridge on a regular basis with hot water and soap (this includes the walls and undersides of shelves) and clean up any spills immediately. Dry with a clean dish towel and/or let removable parts air-dry outside of the fridge.

Sponges are the perfect environment for bacteria acquired via food, the skin, and other surfaces. They are the ideal incubator for microorganisms: warm, wet, and nutrient-rich. One microbe that particularly excelled among the fourteen sponges studied was *Moraxella osloensis*. This bacterium is extremely common both in nature and on human skin. It is primarily responsible for the smell of dirty laundry, which may be one of the reasons that kitchen sponges can stink so badly. While its risk cannot be assessed from this study alone, it is important to be aware of as you scrub your dishes and counters with that same sponge day after day.

Surprisingly, the popular myth of boiling or microwaving sponges to kill bacteria did not work during the course of the study: Regularly sanitized sponges did not have fewer bacteria than uncleaned ones. In fact, sponges that were regularly sanitized by their owners teemed with a higher percentage of certain bacteria closely related to species that can cause infections in humans. We approach this finding cautiously, however, because the bacteria identified on the sponges are only a weak indicator for pathogenic potential of the identified bacteria. Further, the researchers were not aware of any cases where infections from these particular bacteria were reported from the domestic environments studied.

Given the high bacterial load of sponges, these scientists recommended replacing a kitchen sponge with a new one about once a week. To minimize cross-contamination, give sponges different jobs: one for cleaning the counter, and one for the dishes. Definitely replace if it starts to stink, which is a sign of bacterial inhabitation. To reduce waste, the researchers suggested running it through a washing machine at the hottest setting using detergent and bleach. Then use it elsewhere in the home in less hygiene-sensitive spots like the bathroom. Plenty of companies offer solutions such as bacteria-killing baths for sponges and antimicrobial countertops. However, without enough peer-reviewed scientific studies, it is difficult to evaluate their effectiveness. Plus, antimicrobial products pose risks as we will see later on.

From Cleanliness to . . . Superbugs?

After relocating to the United States, Jessica was alarmed to learn that many Americans keep their shoes on inside the house (generally not a Canadian custom). She cringed at the thought of all the dirt, salt, and grime trailing through the home, especially on her freshly scrubbed floors. Yet, however uncomfortable it may be, while researching for this book, Jessica learned that in general it would better if more people brought the outdoors inside, such as by leaving the windows open on nice days, embracing houseplants, and not stressing as much when tracking in a little dirt. She adjusted some of her everyday habits to find a more holistic approach to "clean."

Many microbiome researchers reason that people are doing themselves a disservice by waging a war on germs at home. Any approach that sterilizes your home gets rid of both the bad and good bacteria with potentially harmful consequences. It leads to a critical question: To what extent do we need to stop protecting people from germs, and instead protect germs from people?

An antimicrobial is designed to kill or inhibit the growth of microorganisms including bacteria (antibacterials), viruses (antivirals), and fungi (antifungals). Until relatively recently, the primary kinds of at-home antimicrobial products were disinfectants, antiseptics, and antibiotics. Disinfectants are products that kill microbes on surfaces like countertops or toilet seats. Antiseptics are products designed for use on skin like for cuts and scrapes. Antibiotics, as we know, are intended to destroy microbes within the body. Now a new class of products is emerging as companies race to put antimicrobial ingredients into all sorts of items.

You can find antimicrobial products in homes, public spaces, workplaces, and schools, ranging from clothes to cutting boards and furniture. The US Environmental Protection Agency (EPA) regulates antimicrobial products as pesticides (disinfectants), while the FDA regulates antimicrobial products as drugs (antiseptics and antibiotics). As pesticides, antimicrobial products are used in everyday objects such as countertops, toys, grocery carts, clothing, utensils, and hospital equipment. As drugs, antimicrobial products are used to treat or prevent diseases on and within people, pets, and other living things. Think of the distinction between these domains as the difference between wipes for the kitchen or bathroom (regulated by the EPA) versus hand-sanitizing wipes (regulated by the FDA). EPA registration is helpful because it ensures that the product actually does what it claims to do, if used properly. Clorox Disinfecting Wipes, for example, require enough wipes to be used so that surfaces remain visibly wet for four whole minutes to disinfect (i.e., kill the bacteria, viruses, and fungi on surfaces or objects), or at least ten seconds to sanitize (i.e., lower the number of microbes). Personal care products like hand soaps, toothpaste, and deodorants are regulated fairly loosely by the FDA. They are more focused on antibiotics and other drugs, which are fastidiously regulated to assure their safety, effectiveness, and security.

The marketing of antimicrobial products preys upon consumer fears, and claim to "kill 99.9 percent of germs." Do these products work? Does overuse of antimicrobial ingredients help breed superbugs? It is a controversial topic in the public health realm today. The US and Australian governments recognize antimicrobial resistance as a growing global threat; at least two million Americans (and twelve thousand Australians) every year are infected with antibiotic-resistant bacteria, and at least twenty-three thousand people die each year as a direct result of these infections. In Australia, it is several hundred to a few thousand.

There is ample scientific evidence to suggest that ubiquitous and careless use of antimicrobials has negative consequences. Many products include the ingredient triclosan, for example, which even in concentrations of 0.2 to 2 percent has antimicrobial activity; it's now less commonly used in Australia. Triclosan kills bacteria but has little to no effect on viruses. This is important because most common household illnesses like colds and the flu are viral, so antibacterial ingredients like triclosan will not prevent them from spreading.

Public health experts fear that overly heavy use of antimicrobials, especially in the uncontrolled home environment, may result in microbes resistant to these chemicals. Triclosan may cause resistance to develop because its mechanism of action is specific, and its use is becoming widespread. In fact, resistance to triclosan has already been observed in laboratory studies. Given this considerable concern about growing resistance and the minimal evidence that they are effective in homes, many experts recommend avoiding household products that contain triclosan. This information is pertinent to independent and assisted-living settings where antimicrobial applications might be overused. These everyday products could do more harm than good for aging residents.

Instead of making our living environments as sterile as possible to support health and longevity, we need to strive for the right kind of hygienic clean. First of all, a very small fraction of the microbes that we encounter in the environment are hazardous. In fact, as we have seen in this chapter, many are beneficial. There is no such thing as a microbe-free home. Disinfectants kill microbes on surfaces temporarily, but they do not provide long-lasting disinfection. In some situations, disinfectants are needed, but on many other occasions they are not. Disinfecting a toilet bowl, for example, is an exercise in futility. While it is important to regularly clean the toilet, given its regular exposure to fecal matter, sterilization is impossible. Another example is spraying a room deodorizer disinfectant. One cannot disinfect air this way. If something smells funny, find the source and clean it up. When might you really need a disinfectant? If the sewer overflows in your basement. Or if highly susceptible individuals with special health problems live in the home. For most other occasions at home, simply cleaning with soap or detergent and clean water should be adequate, as long as it is done frequently and thoroughly. Simple cleaning and handwashing practices generally remain one of the most effective ways to prevent the spread of many types of infections and illnesses.

MICROBES IN SPACE: THE FINAL FRONTIER

According to NASA, a manned trip to Mars will take twenty-one months: nine months of travel in a small spaceship, three months on Mars waiting for the planets to realign, and then another nine months to return. Can we do it?

During space travel, astronauts (and their microbes, both on the skin and inside the body) are exposed to significant amounts of radiation, confined to a small space with microgravity, stressed, and forced to eat diets consisting of packaged foods. A fairly new area of study, astromicrobiology, looks at the impacts of space travel on microbes and is increasingly trying to figure out the impact of long-term space travel on the microbiome.

The constant exposure to radiation and stress on the microbes increase the rate of mutation, including potentially harmful ones that might make an organism more pathogenic or resistant to antimicrobials. They have found that microbes isolated from the International Space Station have increased levels of DNA repair, and other mutations that have allowed them to better adapt to their new home in space. In animal experiments in microgravity systems, researchers have found the ratio of Firmicutes and Bacteroidetes changes, as does the microbiome in general. Another problem is that space travel suppresses the immune system, so astronauts would have increased risk of infections, especially in the confined environment of a spacecraft. Finally, assuming the trip went well, astronauts need to return to living on Earth and reintegrate into society, and they might bring back organisms with increased levels of antimicrobial resistance or other mutations. Work continues to understand the effect of space travel on the microbiome, and we now realize that maintaining a healthy microbiome will be needed for such journeys.

Microbes and Climate Change

When thinking of climate change, melting polar ice sheets and catastrophic weather events often come to mind. However, we need to also consider the microscopic view: that microbes play a major role in climate change. Our response to climate change will depend heavily on the microbiome.

Microbes are central in carbon and nutrient cycling, animal and plant health, agriculture, and the global food web. For example, marine phytoplankton perform over 50 percent of the global photosynthetic carbon fixation, yet they make up less than 1 percent of the global plant biomass. Like humans, ocean microbes will have to adapt to the changing world, including ocean warming and acidification. However, unlike humans, microbes can quickly genetically adapt to these changes.

With global warming, we are seeing increases in the spread of pathogens. For example, as the oceans warm, we are seeing higher incidence of *Vibrio* species (which includes the organism that causes cholera) at higher latitudes in the northern hemisphere. Tropical infectious and vector-borne diseases are also being seen in new areas and for longer seasons due to increased temperatures.

Finally, microbes are essential to agriculture and food safety and are especially important for crop production. Soil microbes drive nutrient turnover and help protect crops from environmental changes such as drought and heat waves. Microbes built this world (they literally made the atmosphere's oxygen that we breathe) and will have a large influence on what happens to the globe as we continue to alter it.

Housekeeping, Microbe-Style

In this chapter, we saw that a tiny fraction of the microbes we are exposed to are as hazardous as we think–and many are actually beneficial. Microbes are constantly all around us, even in interior, supposedly "clean" environments. The indoor microbiome is affected by factors such as air currents and ventilation, surface contact, plants, and human and animal interactions. As we are better able to identify the functions of helpful indoor microbes, we can better plan for building design, operation, and function to maintain the health of people who live and work in these spaces by promoting the right kind of microbe exposure. Instead of nursing homes, hospitals, and care environments that are as "sterile" as possible, we will design environments that are comfortable living spaces for us and our microbial friends. We will work with them to achieve longer and healthier lives.

Current cleaning and hygiene standards in institutional settings, especially hospitals and nursing homes, tend to promote multi-resistant pathogens instead of supporting beneficial microbes. We're beginning to see important steps taken to address mounting concerns regarding the insertion of antimicrobial chemicals into everyday products. This includes the FDA's ban on soaps containing nineteen different antibacterial chemicals (including triclosan and triclocarban). Moving forward, it is essential to rethink our understanding of both sterility and our relationships to surrounding microbes. The next generation of microbial sequencing and microscopic techniques will enable us to better assess indoor microbiomes so that we can develop management strategies for beneficial interactions. Age-friendly environments should foster the health and well-being of all inhabitants–microbes included. For now, removing bad microbes at home requires few interventions.

Ventilate with outdoor air whenever possible, keep surfaces clean, and reduce heavy carpeting and other flooring that traps dust microbes. Indoor houseplants and flowers can positively influence health by introducing beneficial bacteria indoors, in addition to improving air quality. Further increase microbial diversity in the home with pets, regular visits from friends and family, and cleaning with soap and water instead of antimicrobial products. It may even be beneficial to keep your shoes on in the house (just watch where you step!). Do not confine yourself to a climate-controlled, sterilized environment as you age.

KEY TIPS

Expose yourself to diverse microbes: Get outdoors regularly to boost your diversity of microbial exposures. Enhance the biodiversity and air quality of your home by bringing in houseplants and flowers. Open the windows when the weather permits to let in outdoor air and additional plant-associated microbes.

Put the phone down: Microbes are another reason to divorce yourself from your cell phone. Leave it behind on your next trip to the bathroom and ban it from the kitchen table. Clean it regularly to minimize the number of potentially harmful microbes pressed against your face.

Clean the kitchen: To avoid cross-contamination, scrub kitchen surfaces frequently with soap and water. This includes cutting boards, counters, microwaves, and refrigerators. Sponges are a hotbed of microbes and therefore need to be replaced on a regular basis—ideally once a week.

Keep your humidifier clean: If you use a humidifier, make sure to clean it regularly so the parts that come into contact with water cannot develop mold. You don't want mold spores to be potentially released in the mist.

Avoid products with antimicrobial ingredients: Plain old soap will do the job in nearly all instances. Even after handling raw chicken, for example, washing your hands thoroughly with soap and water is completely adequate to remove unwanted bacteria. Same with the surfaces in your home; simply clean with soap or detergent, water, and a rag/towel for everyday purposes. The physical action of scrubbing and then rinsing with water removes substantial numbers of organisms.

Thoroughly vet institutional care centers before moving in: Do your homework beforehand by asking about the institution's cleaning practices, history of infectious outbreaks (such as gastrointestinal and respiratory disease), types of foods served, and scheduled activities. Check out the facility in person and try to speak with current residents and staff about their conditions. Find out what a typical day looks like. How does the food look and taste? What sounds and smells do you pick up on?

15

The New Microbe on the Block: COVID-19

2020. The year everything changed as COVID-19 swept across the globe. We all remember those early days in March: Cities became ghost towns, there was a mad scramble to purchase or make face masks, toilet paper shortages abounded, and grocery store shelves were bare. Parks, schools, and businesses closed; neighbors avoided each other with fearful eyes; and in some cities, a nightly clanging of pots and pans could be heard to recognize and thank first responders and health care workers for their sacrifices. It sent shock waves through the world economy, disrupted shipping and supply chains, and triggered the largest global economic crisis in over a century. Inequalities within and between countries dramatically deepened. A tiny invisible virus brought humankind to its knees while the world as we knew it came to a crashing halt.

How did we get here, from a microbial perspective? Let's backtrack to 2003 when another coronavirus caused the SARS (severe acute respiratory syndrome) outbreak. This virus originated in a meat market in China and spread around the world, infecting about eight thousand people and killing just under eight hundred. SARS impacted Canada particularly severely due to an infected person's travel from Hong Kong to Toronto, where the virus infected many health care workers through very close respiratory contact. Brett co-led a Canadian initiative called SARS Accelerated Vaccine Initiative (SAVI) to develop a SARS vaccine as fast as possible. This effort was a remarkable success, and first-in-the-world prototype vaccines were developed within six months. We originally thought SARS would come back the next flu season (hence the urgent need for a new vaccine), but for some still-unknown reason, SARS just disappeared, aside from a couple of lab-acquired infections. Overall, SARS was a major wake-up call to the world about potential new pandemics.

Fast-forward sixteen years to December 2019 when Brett began hearing worrying reports of a previously unknown respiratory virus originating in China. It bore remarkable similarities to SARS, and when sequenced, was identified as a new coronavirus soon called Severe Acute Respiratory Syndrome Coronavirus 2, or SARS-CoV-2. (Coronaviruses are so named because they have a spiky protein that protrudes from their surface, making the virus look like a crown.) SARS-CoV-2 caused a respiratory infection called COVID-19 ("coronavirus disease of 2019"), with symptoms ranging from minimal or flu-like to severe and life-threatening conditions that were particularly lethal among older populations. As the infections continued to spread, first in China, then throughout Asia and the rest of the world, efforts began to try and control it.

Brett was at a social event at the university on March 11, 2020. All had seemed normal at the gathering (other than continued talk about this potential viral threat). Then, abruptly, the World Health Organization declared COVID-19 a global pandemic, and by the next day, it was the opposite of normal. Everything was suddenly closed, and everyone had to stay home. His university switched to online courses, all lab work halted, and all experimental animals were immediately sacrificed (since researchers and staff couldn't come in to look after them). Jessica's life irrevocably changed a couple of weeks prior to the WHO's declaration. The day after her partner Matt had flown back from a biotech conference, they began hearing reports of numerous conference-goers falling ill. Out of an abundance of caution, Matt asked to work from home (an eyebrow-raising request pre-pandemic), and they pulled their seven-month-old baby out of daycare for the week and quarantined at home to minimize risk of infecting others. Many initially scoffed at this level of precaution, and thankfully, Matt did not contract COVID-19 from the conference. But little did they know that their son would never return to that daycare, or that remote work and quarantining at home would become a global norm. It is now known that Matt's conference was an early superspreader event that set off a chain of around a quarter million estimated cases across the US and Europe.

Now four-plus years later (at the time of writing), it is remarkable how much the world has changed. Although many of us have returned to some normalcy, things are not exactly as they were. Remote work is still highly utilized (we all use "Zoom" as a verb), neighborhoods and cityscapes literally look different (e.g., enlarged outdoor patios and closed pedestrian-only streets in some areas, permanently shuttered storefronts in others), and many of us now react viscerally when someone sneezes or coughs near us without covering their mouth and nose. Approximately eight hundred million people have had COVID-19 and seven million have died, making it the biggest pandemic since the influenza pandemic of 1918 (which killed up to fifty million people). We learned to scale up mask production, epidemiologists and disease control centers tried many tactics to contain the spread, including travel bans and body temperature scans at border crossings, and senior care homes locked down dramatically by blocking visitors and limiting access.

MYTH: I've had COVID-19, so I'm immune.

FACT: It is very possible to become infected with COVID-19 multiple times. Your immune response after having COVID can protect you against reinfection for several months, but this protection decreases over time and is not effective against other constantly evolving strains of the virus. Individuals with weakened immune systems who get an infection may have a limited immune response or none at all. Reinfections are most often mild, but severe illness can still occur.

The pandemic fueled major scientific accomplishments, including rapid sequencing and detection of the virus (even as it changed), and most spectacular of all, the incredibly rapid development of highly effective vaccines (see "COVID-19 Vaccines: A Nobel Prize" on page 269). It also provided many lessons on how the microbiome can impact pandemics, and reinforced the dilemma about healthy microbial exposure versus avoiding microbial infections. As we will see in this chapter, the microbiome influences the severity of a COVID infection, long COVID symptoms, and our body's response to COVID vaccines. From a microbiologist's viewpoint, it put microbiology right back into society's focus (where it should be!), with physician-scientists such as Dr. Anthony Fauci becoming massive public figures with celebrity status.

The Hygiene Hypothesis: Cleaning Up Our World

In the late 1800s, two famous microbiologists, Robert Koch and Louis Pasteur, made the stunning discovery that bacteria cause infectious diseases! Up until then, no one had any idea what caused diseases such as anthrax and tuberculosis, with many theories circulating, such as bad air and swamp gas being the culprits. Louis Pasteur took their discovery one step further: If you killed the bacterium, it couldn't cause disease (hence the name for pasteurization, in which foods such as milk or cider are treated with heat to eliminate pathogens and extend shelf life). Once society realized that bacteria were the cause of diseases and that killing them blocked disease transmission, we went on a major hygiene campaign. Sewers and sanitation were introduced, antibiotics were invented during World War II, and hand sanitizers were invented in the 1960s. Deaths due to infectious diseases plummeted, even causing the US Surgeon General in 1969 to prematurely declare that "it is time to close the book on infectious diseases."

This quest to kill all microbes has had a significant unintended side effect: It has impacted our microbiota. We call this the "hygiene hypothesis": that increased hygiene, including extensive antibiotic use and urban living in sealed buildings, has reduced our exposure to a diversity of beneficial microbes, which in turn has contributed to a remarkable rise in non-communicable diseases such as asthma, obesity, diabetes, Alzheimer's, and many other diseases discussed throughout this book. As we began to realize that we were living "too clean," there was a major campaign to counter excessive hygiene with normal microbial exposures and not use hand sanitizer at every turn. Brett even cowrote a book and made a documentary, *Let Them Eat Dirt*, discussing how to raise your children with their microbes to maximize health and development. The movement to embrace healthy microbial exposure, countering the century-long quest to eradicate microbes, was gaining traction. And then COVID-19 hit.

COVID-19 brought back decades-old hygiene and epidemiology policies previously used to control infectious disease outbreaks: quarantines, border closures, stay-at-home orders, school closures, physical distancing, and heavy antibiotic use. This reversion to early twentieth-century hygiene practices was, in a sense, a natural experiment done on the grandest scale. What happens to the microbiome when you shut down much of the world's microbial exposures and revert back to extreme hygiene practices?

The answer is mixed. Although we used radical hygiene practices, they weren't in effect for that long in the grand scheme of things–a few months to a couple of years. And while many of us fully isolated for a few months, we were in limited contact with others soon after that through our personal "social bubbles." We have now largely discarded wearing daily face masks, and most people don't use hand sanitizer like they did during the height of the pandemic. Studies are just starting to come out about how the microbiome was disrupted, and it's still inconclusive what, if any, effects this had. The microbiomes of those at the bookends of life (infants and the oldest old) were predicted to be the most affected. Older populations, especially those confined to senior care homes, were dramatically cut off from the outside world with presumably significant impacts on their microbiomes. Visitors were not allowed into these homes, staff were masked and gowned, and for approximately two years, they lived in a state of complete lockdown. Brett was unable to see his parents for over a year, and if they had to go out to see a doctor for a routine visit, they were quarantined afterward for three weeks in their tiny room. If COVID-19 did affect a nursing home, the mortality rates were often high, with many devastatingly dying without being able to see their family.

We are now characterizing the impact of COVID-19 on the infant microbiome. Think of a child born during COVID-19. Most were born in a sterile hospital setting (Jessica remembers birthing her second child while wearing a KN95 face mask), and upon returning home, remained largely in isolation from other children (other than siblings) and adults. Most did not go to daycare. These infants stayed pretty much confined to their home, and if living in an urban environment, with limited microbial exposure (one of the many reasons that prompted Jessica, her partner Matt, and their baby to move from an upper-story apartment to a house with a backyard during the pandemic). We expected that limited microbial exposure would increase a child's risk of asthma, allergies, and obesity, all of which are associated with low microbial diversity. However, a recent study suggests it was actually good for infants! By looking at 351 babies born in Ireland in the first three months of the pandemic, researchers found that these infants had different microbiomes than pre-COVID-19 pandemic infants. Pandemic babies had more beneficial microbes such as Bifidobacteria, and as infants, had lower levels of asthma-related diseases and food allergies. Digging into this surprising result, we can come up with some potential reasons why. Isolated at home, these infants were perhaps breastfed more, which passes along maternal microbes in the breast milk and through skin-to-skin contact. Without daycare, they had fewer infections, which in turn, resulted in fewer courses of antibiotics. They may also have had increased intake of home-cooked foods, instead of ultra-processed foods. Presumably all these factors contributed to a healthier microbiome.

For adults, there are no data yet to say that there were significant changes to the microbiome. Most of us returned to a relatively normal life after a period of isolation. Altered diets from less eating out (although take-out food consumption increased) probably contributed to some microbiome changes. Many reverted to more home cooking and baking–Brett even worked his way through an entire bread recipe book, much to his microbes' chagrin! In closing, COVID-19 had a remarkable short-term effect on human behavior, which presumably impacted our microbiomes to some extent, but the long-term implications are not yet fully understood.

Mustering Our Microbial Defenses

To get technical for a moment, the SARS-CoV-2 virus connects to a specific molecule on human cells called a "receptor," which is angiotensin-converting enzyme 2 or ACE-2. This receptor is expressed on lung cells, and so COVID-19 is thought to be transmitted by aerosol particles, entering the body through the lungs by binding to this molecule. However, ACE-2 is also expressed in the gastrointestinal (GI) tract, and the virus may also enter the blood via the GI tract. In addition to respiratory symptoms, the virus can cause intestinal symptoms including diarrhea, abdominal pain, nausea, and vomiting. Several studies have examined the gut microbiome and its correlation to COVID-19. These general themes emerge.

1. People who get more severe COVID-19 tend to have a dysbiotic microbiome, with a reduction in beneficial anti-inflammatory bacteria and an increase in opportunistic pathogens.

2. Disruptions in the gut microbiome can be used to predict the severity of COVID-19 disease.

3. These microbiome disruptions can last months or longer, even after clearing the virus, and impact long COVID risk.

Not everyone is at the same risk for COVID-19, and risk factors include obesity, diabetes, underlying lung problems, and older age. The often dysbiotic microbiomes of individuals with these health conditions may help explain the differences in COVID-19 susceptibility.

Studies looking at the microbiome in COVID-19 patients compared to controls consistently show that those with COVID-19 have a decrease in bacteria associated with dampening inflammation. Because COVID-19 is thought to be an inflammatory disease, dampening the immune response by increasing SCFA production and other mechanisms would decrease disease severity. In addition, some of these beneficial bacteria downregulate the expression of the COVID-19 receptor (ACE-2) on the body's cell surfaces, indicating that a decrease in the receptor may decrease viral load in the body. However, in COVID-19 patients, there is an increase in opportunistic pathogens (microbes that don't usually cause disease in healthy individuals but may become virulent among immunocompromised and unhealthy individuals). These pathogens can contribute to inflammation, potentially worsening COVID-19. These results are consistent over several studies, suggesting that a dysbiotic microbiome is associated with worse COVID-19 symptoms.

Microbiome analysis has been used to predict the severity of COVID-19 symptoms. Researchers found that by tracking forty-eight different bacterial species, they could predict the severity of COVID-19 disease. The more dysbiotic the microbiome, the more severe the symptoms. However, one caveat is that all these studies compared healthy controls to COVID-19 patients. It has not been proven that a preexisting dysbiotic microbiome leads to increased risk of COVID-19 severity. So, what can we take home from all this? Although it sounds like a broken record throughout this book, maintaining a healthy, diverse gut microbiome that is anti-inflammatory may help decrease the likelihood of getting severe COVID-19, in addition to all the other health benefits that come from a healthy microbiome. So, eat your fiber!

BREATHING BUGS

Since we contract COVID-19 by inhaling tiny, aerosolized SARS-CoV-2 particles, researchers have also looked at the composition of the oral and respiratory tract microbiome (including the lungs) with respect to COVID-19. Although the results are not as robust as those seen with the gut microbiome, there are similar emerging trends. A risk factor for COVID-19 infection appears to be a more inflammatory oral microbiome. Oral inflammation might allow the virus easier entry into the body through the mouth. This might help explain why older adults are more susceptible to COVID-19, as they generally have increased oral inflammation (see chapter 6).

Similarly, dysbiotic respiratory tract and lung microbiomes are associated with COVID-19 infections, however, like we saw with the gut microbiome, it is not known if COVID-19 causes the dysbiosis, or whether it was preexisting and increased the infection. While the mechanisms haven't yet been defined, it is proposed that some microbes may inhibit the virus's ability to bind to the body's cells, and inflammation may enhance viral uptake (and removal) in the lungs. Similarly, because lung inflammation is a central feature of COVID-19, microbes that affect inflammation could impact COVID-19 outcome. The bottom line: Try to keep your oral and respiratory tract microbiomes healthy (see chapters 6 and 8 for specific tips on this), because it may help decrease risk and severity of a COVID-19 infection.

Long COVID

One of the scariest aspects when sick with COVID-19 is the prospect of long-term detrimental health impacts–something that doesn't typically come to mind when you have other respiratory infections such as a cold or mild flu. We can likely all think of at least one person who was otherwise healthy and strong pre-COVID infection but now still suffers from long COVID. Professional athletes such as cyclist Chris Froome and hockey player Jonathan Toews have publicly shared their experiences with long COVID and its detrimental impacts on their athletic performances.

Symptoms associated with COVID-19 usually last less than a month, by which time the virus is gone and health returns to normal. However, many people continue to have symptoms that can last months and even years. It is estimated that 75 percent of people have at least one symptom six months after COVID-19, and that seventeen million people in the US (and possibly hundreds of thousands of Australians) have long COVID. These symptoms vary widely between individuals, often including fatigue, headache, post-exertional malaise, hair loss, and cognitive dysfunction (one paper cited 203 possible symptoms involving ten organ systems). There is not one definition yet of long COVID (also known as Post-COVID Conditions, or PCC), but generally it refers to symptoms that continue or develop four or more weeks following infection. Generally, long COVID is associated with more serious COVID-19 cases, especially prevalent among those who were hospitalized. It is also more prevalent in people who were at increased risk and/or unvaccinated. There is no treatment for long COVID, especially since it includes a wide range of symptoms, nor is there a specific test.

As we saw above, microbiome composition is directly related to COVID-19 severity (including influencing our body's inflammatory response). Not surprisingly, both contracting long COVID and its severity are now also strongly linked to the microbiome. In one study, 106 individuals with COVID-19 and sixty-eight controls were sampled over various time periods up to six months. As in COVID-19, they found a strong correlation between microbiome composition and long COVID, including higher levels of *Ruminococcus gnavus* and *Bacteroides vulgatus*, lower levels of *Faecalibacterium prausnitzii*, and a striking loss in anti-inflammatory butyrate-producing bacteria. This indicates that a patient's gut microbiome profile predicts and affects susceptibility to long COVID and symptom severity. A recent study followed patients with COVID and found that they could predict with 86 percent accuracy which patients would go on to experience long COVID based on their microbiome composition—this prediction was better than all other known risk factors! Yet another study showed that dysbiotic microbiomes were also found in long-COVID patients a year after discharge from hospital. Similar results were seen in the oral and lung microbiome of long COVID patients, with decreased anti-inflammatory bacteria. Collectively, these studies suggest that long COVID is closely associated with dysbiotic microbiomes, including a loss of anti-inflammatory microbes, and that this can be used to successfully predict long COVID.

Vaccine Victory

Probably the most remarkable scientific achievement of the COVID-19 pandemic was the extremely rapid development of an effective, novel type of vaccine that markedly decreased the risk of COVID-19. Nearly fourteen billion vaccine doses have been administered worldwide. Researchers have now shown that, like with other vaccines, the microbiome influences one's response to SARS-CoV-2 vaccines.

It is well established that older populations show reduced vaccine responses, which also holds true for the COVID-19 vaccine. This is likely due to immunosenescence (a weakening of the immune system due to aging). In addition, older adults are more likely to have dysbiotic microbiomes, which may also impact the response to the vaccine. However, it is still strongly recommended to get the COVID-19 vaccine in later life, since it protects against serious disease and death.

Several studies are underway to determine if the microbiome could be altered to enhance responses to the vaccine. Some include taking prebiotics and/or probiotics or improving diet, although the results have not yet been published. Currently, the best advice to optimize protection against COVID-19 is to try to keep your microbiome diverse and healthy through everyday activities such as regular exercise and a fiber-rich diet, and to get a COVID-19 vaccine when suggested by your local public health office.

COVID-19 VACCINES: A NOBEL PRIZE

A vaccine currently takes at least ten years to develop (usually longer). This long time period is due to vaccine component optimization (i.e., formulating the best combination of ingredients) and extensive animal and then human experiments on both safety and efficacy. This whole process typically costs billions of dollars. When Brett was involved in fast-tracking a SARS vaccine, they were able to rapidly develop three prototype SARS vaccines in six months, which was unheard of in the traditional vaccine world back in 2003. However, the fast-tracking and development of a SARS-CoV-2 vaccine blew the doors off rapid vaccine development and established a whole new vaccine type and approach with many other potential medical applications.

The most commonly used COVID-19 vaccines use a new technology with messenger RNA (mRNA), which make spike proteins in order to trigger an immune response. Because this new protein is foreign to the body, the immune system reacts to it much like it would respond to an infection. This immune response "trains" the immune system to be on the lookout for more of this molecule, so that when SARS-CoV-2 enters the body, the immune system recognizes the spike protein and mounts an immune response that kills and removes the virus, thereby protecting the individual from COVID-19.

The concept of using mRNA for potential vaccines is not new. In a now-celebratory underdog story, Dr. Katalin Karikó started work on improving mRNA delivery first in her native country of Hungary and then in the USA in the 1980s. There were major problems in getting it to work initially, as it was unstable and triggered unwanted immune responses. There was much pessimism from the scientific community, and Dr. Karikó was unable to get grants to fund her research and even got demoted. However, she remained undeterred and began collaborating with Dr. Drew Weissman in the late 1990s to further develop the technology. Their work formed the foundation of which the current COVID vaccines are based upon, and in 2023, they both won the Nobel Prize in Physiology or Medicine for their discoveries that enabled the development of effective mRNA vaccines against COVID-19.

An added benefit of this vaccine type is that the mRNA can be easily changed just by cloning in another sequence. So as SARS-CoV-2 mutates, the vaccines can be changed as well. This is why we have new vaccines developed in response to new variants as they arise. The vaccine has been incredibly successful, preventing millions of deaths. It has minimal side effects and is considered an incredibly safe vaccine. New uses for the mRNA technology are now being explored, such as cancer vaccines and gene therapy.

Probiotic Protection Against COVID-19

Given the microbiome's involvement in COVID-19, multiple attempts have been made to alter the microbiome to enhance protection against the disease. Several studies hint that a healthy fiber-rich diet decreases both the likelihood of catching COVID-19 and the severity of the disease if you do catch it. This makes sense, as such a diet would both modify your microbiome and its effect on the immune system in a beneficial way. Vitamin D is known to enhance the immune system, and in an older male population, at-risk individuals with a low vitamin D level were thirteen times more likely to die of COVID-19. However, no studies have yet shown that increasing vitamin D protects against COVID-19.

People with COVID-19 have a decrease in beneficial *Lactobacillus* and *Bifidobacterium* (two common probiotics), and *Faecalibacterium prausnitzii*, as well as an increase in opportunistic pathogens. In other studies, probiotics have been shown to have some beneficial effect on other viral respiratory pathogens and to enhance immune responses. Not surprisingly, there have been a plethora of studies looking at the role of probiotics and COVID-19, especially in the early days when there was no vaccine. Most of the studies used strains of *Lactobacillus*, mainly *L. plantarum* and *L. rhamnosus*, and several showed promising results. However, because so many different strains have been tried, with many diverse outcome measures in small numbers of patients, there are currently no clinically recommended probiotic treatments for COVID-19. What is needed are large-scale clinical studies that intensely focus on a promising probiotic. Until then, the use of probiotics in COVID-19 remains uncertain.

On a more optimistic note, a recent randomized, double-blind, placebo-controlled trial from Hong Kong showed significant promise for a synbiotic (a combination of probiotics and prebiotics) for decreasing the severity of long COVID symptoms: 232 adults with long COVID were given a synbiotic (SIM01, ten billion colony forming units) orally twice daily for six months and compared to 231 individuals who took a placebo. SIM01 is a mixture of three probiotic strains (*Bifidobacterium adolescentis*, *Bifidobacterium bifidum*, and *Bifidobacterium longum*) and three prebiotic compounds (galacto-oligosaccharides, xylo-oligosaccharides, and resistant dextrin) that have been shown to promote the growth of these probiotics. Individuals who got the synbiotic had decreased long COVID symptoms, including less fatigue, general unwellness, memory loss, gastrointestinal upset, and difficulty concentrating. It was also well tolerated and safe in the clinical trial. The microbiomes in those who took SIM01 also showed increased diversity and an increase in SCFA producers, making this the first study to show that improving the microbiome is correlated with improving long COVID symptoms. Of course, more work is needed (including larger trials), however, this study provides significant early evidence.

Looking Ahead

With what feels like a constant cycle of new variants and surges in cases, COVID-19 appears poised to stick around long term. In the past twenty-eight days alone (at the time of writing), nearly one hundred and thirty-five thousand new cases and two thousand deaths have been reported to the WHO worldwide. While overall hospitalization numbers are much lower than the early days of the pandemic, COVID-19 continues to present very real health risks and daily life restrictions, especially for higher-risk individuals. Given emerging evidence of extensive links between the microbiome and COVID-19, the hope is that we can use microbial strategies to decrease our risk of infection, severity of disease, and long COVID symptoms. Our need continues to pursue research and novel treatment options for COVID-19.

Collectively, COVID-19 highlighted the ongoing tension between hygiene and healthy microbial exposure. Increasing angst about "mixing microbes" and overall lack of diverse microbial exposures in an over-sanitized world was gaining traction before 2020. Then society did a 180-degree turn when COVID-19 hit and reverted back to strict hygiene. Where does the balance lie? The answer is in between. For the most part, diverse microbial exposure is really important for lifelong health and well-being. However, at times of extreme contagion–such as early in the COVID-19 outbreak when there were no treatments, vaccines, or even tests, and extreme shortages of medical supplies and hospital beds–strict hygiene is essential and lifesaving. Now that we have entered the endemic phase of COVID-19 with abundant testing, personal protective equipment (PPE), and excellent vaccines available, we need to re-embrace our microbes carefully and thoughtfully. So, ditch the hand sanitizer, open the windows, go outside, and engage with your family, friends, and community.

KEY TIPS

Get your COVID vaccines as directed by public health officials: Staying up-to-date with your vaccines is by far the best way to decrease your chances of getting a severe acute infection and long COVID. Because the virus is constantly changing, you will need booster shots to cover the new strains that arise.

Muster your microbial defenses: Eat a fiber-rich diet and avoid over-sanitization and antibiotics when possible. Keeping your microbiota healthy may help decrease your chances of getting COVID-19, minimize the inflammatory response, and potentially alleviate long COVID symptoms.

Boost your microbial exposures: Get back in touch with more diverse microbial exposures through everyday activities such as going outside and opening the window, having pets and indoor plants, socializing, and exercising.

Fortify yourself for the long haul: If you are navigating long COVID, take whatever steps you can to improve your microbiome. This includes eating a fiber-rich diet and potentially taking probiotics. Emerging findings suggest that improving the gut microbiome may help decrease long COVID symptoms.

16

The Fountain of Youth *Is* Full of Microbes: The Key to Health and Longevity

Back in chapter 3 we met Élie Metchnikoff, the father of immunology, who over a hundred years ago, advocated for consumption of lactic cultures (containing beneficial microbes) to preserve health and longevity. He observed that Bulgarians living in the countryside lived longer than richer Europeans, despite suffering from poverty and a harsher climate. Observing that countryside residents consumed fermented milk, Metchnikoff concluded that the lactic acid bacilli that ferment the milk had anti-aging benefits, and therefore we should consume fermented milk for longevity. He published this work in a now-famous book, *The Prolongation of Life*, and won the 1908 Nobel Prize in Physiology or Medicine for groundbreaking work in immunology. Metchnikoff believed that there were "good" and "bad" microbes in the gut. The "bad" ones produced toxins as part of their metabolism that caused damage to the human body—he called it "intestinal autointoxication"—while the "good" ones produced beneficial fermentation products, such as lactic acid, that could counter harmful products and promote health. This was the birth of probiotics and the concept that gut microbes could be manipulated for health benefits and longevity.

Metchnikoff's hypothesis is eerily prescient of what we are just "learning" today—over a century later—about the role of microbes in our short and long-term health. Reinterpreting his thoughts, we now know that the harmful toxins are inflammation-inducing microbes and their products, while the "good" ones are those that produce anti-inflammatories such as SCFAs. The idea that we might be able to manipulate microbes and their products to benefit health and aging remains a truly exciting one, and great strides in scientific and clinical applications are on the horizon. The microbiome is profoundly affecting fields of health and medicine across all areas of study of the human body, providing new diagnostic techniques and therapies for a host of conditions that couldn't have been imagined a few short years ago. However, even our most "advanced" current therapies used in the clinic, such as fecal transfers, are still very crude. They will require extensive research to fully take advantage of the microbiome, and the various molecules that microbes make that have an effect on our bodies. This final chapter will take a critical and in-depth look at existing methods used to manipulate the microbiome such as diet, probiotics, and prebiotics. The applied field of microbiome research is full of much hype and hope, and many false or exaggerated claims that are not yet based on sound science. Here, we try to provide some guidance based on the current scientific knowledge regarding what you can do today to enhance healthy microbes and their benefits for well-being at any age. We also include a section on what to discuss with your physician based on individual health needs and concerns–or in the case that you are a caregiver, on behalf of the care recipient. At the end, we peer into the future to suggest novel concepts that are on the horizon for this rapidly advancing field.

You Are What You Eat

"Eat your vegetables–they are good for you!" Every child has heard this hundreds of times. However, parents should really say, "Eat your vegetables–they are good for your *microbes*, which are good for you." Diet has a major effect, good and bad, on our microbes. By far the easiest way to improve your microbiome's composition is to change your diet. Despite many undocumented claims, the exact details of a "healthy" microbiota and the type of diet needed to achieve it are not fully understood–and as Jessica saw firsthand in her PhD research, "healthy" won't mean the same thing for every person. However, several guiding principles regarding diet and how foods affect and shape microbiota are becoming well established.

Following these principles may be particularly important to older adults given the significant changes that occur in the microbiome later in life.

Besides fat, fiber was a key dietary factor in the study above. As we discussed in chapter 2, it is broken down into SCFAs by gut microbes. One study showed that supplementing a diet with fiber increased microbial diversity up to 25 percent in those who started with low diversity in their microbiota. Resistant starches (a type of fiber) have been shown to affect the microbiota by improving metabolic measures (such as decreasing glucose spikes) and lessening inflammation. Unfortunately, the typical Western diet has very little fiber in it, while our ancestors ate much more. This change not only affects us today, but there is even concern about long-term changes in the composition of the entire species' microbiome. Mouse studies have shown that while consuming a low-fiber diet has a reversible effect on the microbiome in a single generation, after multiple generations, it is impossible to revert back to a high-fiber microbiome without also adding back the missing microbes (see chapter 2). This suggests that if humans continue to consume low-fiber diets over the generations, beneficial fiber-consuming microbes could go extinct. Current recommendations suggest consuming at least 21 to 25 g of fiber per day for women, and 30 to 38 g per day for men. High-fiber foods include raspberries, pears (with skin), whole wheat spaghetti, barley, bran, split peas, lentils, beans, artichokes, and green peas.

Again, an easy place to look for inspiration on this path are the Mediterranean and MIND diets, which are rich in fiber, vegetables, fruits, nuts, and legumes, and lower in dairy fats and red meat. The Mediterranean diet is constantly ranked as the best diet to follow for many reasons, including decreasing obesity, type 2 diabetes risk, and improving overall health. The MIND diet has been associated with health boosts in multiple studies, including decreased risk of Alzheimer's disease by up to 53 percent. Another study looked at 1,296 aging individuals from five European countries. The experimental group was given dietary instructions and vitamin supplements and asked to follow a Mediterranean diet. Compared to controls, those following the diet instructions lost less bone mass and showed reduced inflammation compared to the controls. Included in the high-fiber diet are whole grains, which, according to studies, appear beneficial to humans on a Western diet. In just a six-week period, those who followed a whole-grain diet saw enhanced beneficial microbiota by increasing SCFA producers, decreasing inflammatory bacteria and inflammation, and enhancing weight loss. Similarly, following a plant-based or predominantly plant-based diet has been associated with many health benefits.

In part produced by microbes, fermented foods are also a good way to increase beneficial microbes traveling through your gut (think of Metchnikoff and his fermented milk). There is little doubt that these probiotic foods, such as sauerkraut and kimchi, provide additional nutritional value, but we lack strong clinical research to confirm their potential health benefits beyond nutrition. Few controlled human trials have been carried out with fermented foods other than probiotic yogurts. This handful of small studies showed improvements in weight maintenance and reduction in cardiovascular disease, type 2 diabetes, and metabolic syndrome. Although these foods seem to have beneficial effects, we still cannot say with certainty that they are working throughout the microbiome.

What has complicated studies about diet and microbiota is the difference in microbiomes between individuals. As we saw in chapter 2, individuals respond differently to various food groups. This suggests that personalized diets based on the microbiome could become a mainstay of diets in the future. It will also allow us to establish the effect of different microbes on food groups, and the effects of different foods on the microbes—this information is urgently needed if we are going to truly understand the role of the microbiome in diets and nutrition.

No matter what nutritional or diet program you follow, aim for stability and continuity. We saw the harms of yo-yo diets in chapter 2 and of travel disruptions in chapter 14. If you go on and off diets, there seems to be a microbial memory that sabotages weight loss efforts. Remember, also, what we saw with artificial sweeteners. In a subset of people, they may actually cause dysbiosis and worsen metabolic symptoms by increasing glucose intolerance. And new research strongly recommends that we stay away from ultra-processed foods! While the exact correlations between food groups and microbiota are still lacking, the general concept of increasing fiber to benefit your microbes and decrease inflammation seems to be a salient one.

Recommendation: *Pursue a diet that is rich in fiber, including fruits, nuts, vegetables, whole grains, berries, fish, and moderate amounts of red wine. Avoid red meats and foods rich in animal fat. Largely plant-based diets such as the Mediterranean and MIND diets are generally excellent ones to follow from both a healthy human and microbial point of view.*

Probiotics for Life

There is no topic that generates more discussion in the microbiome world than probiotics. It is a gigantic industry estimated at over thirty billion dollars per year worldwide. While products such as kombucha have risen rapidly in popularity, a bigger question remains: Do they work? A simple question with a complex answer. In this section, we will dig deep into probiotics so that you can have a more informed opinion on this growing trend and how it might help you.

Probiotic is a term that originates from Greek and means "for life." Using probiotics for health has a long history: In 1917, German scientist Alfred Nissle isolated a non-pathogen *E. coli* strain from the feces of a World War I soldier who did not contract an infectious diarrhea (shigellosis) that was rampant at the time. This bacterial strain became known as *E. coli* Nissle 1917, which is now an accepted probiotic. The current definition of a probiotic, according to the WHO and other organizations, is "live microorganisms which when administered in adequate amounts confer a health benefit on the host." Probiotics are live microbes, usually species of *Lactobacillus*, *Bifidobacterium*, some *E. coli* and *Bacillus*, and the yeast *Saccharomyces boulardii*, that, when taken regularly in sufficient doses, are designed to promote health effects. They can be taken separately or added to food. The problem is that there are many probiotics now available but not much clarity or consensus about what each of them is, what they do, and who should take them. When the average consumer walks into a health food store, they are confronted with a bewildering array of probiotic choices–usually one or more walls covered in shelves, each package with its own enticing but unchecked health claims.

Another problem is that despite a large body of literature on probiotics, we still do not really know how they work. They seem to have a variety of effects, including decreasing gut permeability and decreasing inflammation (which are likely interrelated). They do not seem to have a direct long-term effect on the overall structure of the existing microbiota population given that they rapidly disappear from the gut. One study showed that they actually inhibited beneficial microbial colonization post-antibiotics. Recommended doses are so large—one hundred million to ten billion or more live microbes per day—because they are largely isolated from the environment, animals, or other body sites. They aren't meant to live in the gut, so they don't colonize there.

The third issue is that because probiotics are sold in Canada and the US as foods and dietary supplements, they are not regulated by the FDA or Health Canada. (In Australia, they are regulated by FSANZ or the TGA, depending on if they are marketed as foods or with therapeutic claims.) Therefore, their health claims are often not supported by the kinds of extensive and rigorous clinical trials required for FDA-approved drugs. Although there are over fifteen hundred clinical trials involving many different probiotics, they are often not well-designed studies: Many are not randomized, they are difficult to conduct completely blinded (participants often know or can figure out if they are in the control or study group), and can be sponsored by probiotic companies. There are little good clinical data on the ability of probiotics to promote overall health (as opposed to helping heal a specific disease). Still, many people swear that probiotics make them feel better. Probiotics rarely have any side effects and all are considered safe; they are also quite cheap compared to most prescription drugs one could use for similar conditions.

The fourth issue is that most probiotics indicate how many live bacteria are supposed to be in the supplement, but this does not always reflect the actual viable counts. Factors such as refrigeration and other storage techniques can affect viability. The lack of standardization in the field causes large heterogeneity in the quality of different probiotics. There are significant issues with labeling: One study found that a product did not even contain the supposed *Lactobacillus* on the label, and only 80 percent had the viability that the labels claimed. They are still generally safe to take, they just may be less effective than advertised.

So how does one make sense of all the confusing and often conflicting information out there about probiotics? There are groups dedicated to aligning probiotic information and claims with actual science. One such group is the International Scientific Association for Probiotics and Prebiotics (ISAPP). Dr. Mary Ellen Sanders is the founding president of ISAPP and got in at the "ground floor" of probiotics in the United States, entering the field in 1990. "I was at first a big skeptic. In my graduate school days, I thought that the whole probiotic area was just snake oil. To this day, my graduate advisor teases me that ever since I went out on my own to start a consulting business, probiotics have consumed everything that I work on. My skepticism was not unfounded. At first it was much more a field of faith than science." Now, after decades of serious research and advancements in high-quality human trials, Dr. Sanders feels confident saying that probiotics have important effects on health. She believes that probiotics will flourish if the available products are scientifically validated, responsibly produced, and accurately labeled.

As a steward of the field, Dr. Sanders, along with prebiotic expert Professor Glenn Gibson, formed ISAPP back in 2002 to connect multidisciplinary scientists. This involved researchers from microbiology, biochemistry, gastroenterology, and food technology, as well as the wide range of people more directly involved in probiotics and prebiotics.

With the aim of bringing great minds together, ISAPP has also begun to focus on the abundance of information–and misinformation–out there. The organization offers helpful explanations on what to look for in a probiotic and how they might work. Jargon-free infographics, a few videos, and detailed information are easily accessible to the general public on their website (isappscience.org).

In addition, two excellent websites–Clinical Guide to Probiotic Products (usprobioticguide.com) and the Canadian equivalent (probioticchart.ca)–are designed to give a synopsis of the clinical evidence regarding a particular probiotic and specific conditions. They are updated yearly and provide a wealth of accurate information about which probiotics may work for which condition, based on clinical evidence distilled from the numerous papers describing studies of various probiotics. Although the sites are designed for clinicians, they are terrific tools for everyone wanting to understand which probiotics have actual clinical data and, just as important, how strong that data are. If the websites appear confusing at first glance, it is well worth the effort to work through them (keep reading to find out how) and study the guides to determine what probiotics may work, which ones to use, what doses, and the underlying clinical evidence. (ProbioticAdvisor.com aims to help select quality probiotic products in Australia.)

Both websites include a series of tables for adult health, pediatric health, vaginal health, and functional foods with added probiotics. Each table lists many of the commercially available probiotics in either Canada or the US by their brand name, which probiotic strain(s) they contain, the dosage form, the dose, and the number of doses needed per day. In the center is a ranking of the clinical evidence available for a series of diseases. A ranking of I is the highest, meaning there was efficacy seen in at least one well-designed randomized clinical trial. Levels II and III have less clinical evidence available. These rankings are attributed to a list of diseases, with each disease named and abbreviated by one or more letters (e.g., ID = infectious diarrhea; AAD = antibiotic-associated diarrhea).

There are a few examples where we do have convincing clinical evidence of probiotics' efficacy in treating specific conditions. These include antibiotic-associated diarrhea, irritable bowel syndrome (IBS) and associated depression, prevention of C. *difficile*-associated diarrhea, adjunct therapy with *H. pylori* eradication, colic for breastfed infants, vulvovaginal candidiasis, and bacterial vaginosis. The bottom line is that some probiotics can work for some conditions, although many do not show clinical efficacy in spite of extensive marketing and sales. All these uncertainties about probiotics will hopefully change as scientists rapidly investigate specific mechanisms of the human microbiome and effects of probiotics. Armed with this knowledge, Dr. Sanders expressed excitement regarding the continuing evolution of probiotics to meaningfully intervene in health and disease.

Recommendation: *Some probiotics may work well for conditions including antibiotic-associated diarrhea, C. difficile-associated diarrhea, IBS, colic in breastfed infants, and bacterial vaginosis. However, there are many others that lack proven ability. Take the time to consult the websites (usprobioticguide.com and probioticchart.ca) and talk to an expert before incorporating probiotics into a specific health care regimen.*

Probiotics 2.0

Given the major recent advances in our understanding of the microbiome, there is strong enthusiasm for a future of next-gen probiotics—what we are calling probiotics 2.0. These will be microbes isolated for use in a specific body part, such as using gut microbes for gut disorders or vaginal microbes for gynecological infections. They may be a combination of microbes rather than a single microbe; they may be taken in small doses, since they are designed to live specifically in that one body site, and thus won't be rejected as a foreign invader; they may readily colonize that body site; and most importantly, they will have a defined beneficial function.

A subsection of this new generation of probiotics are being developed and approved by the FDA as drugs, known as live biotherapeutic products (LBPs) or live biotherapeutic agents (LBAs). In chapter 3, we discussed a mixture of *Clostridium* species that had a strong effect on regulatory T cells. Brett is involved with Vedanta Biosciences, Inc., a biotechnology company in Cambridge, Massachusetts. They have successful phase II clinical trials using this mix of microbes for recurrent *C. difficile* infections and are working on other applications. Elsewhere, there is significant interest in using *Faecalibacterium prausnitzii* and *Akkermansia* to increase SCFA production in the gut to decrease inflammation. Many companies are also working on the use of novel bacterial strains as probiotics, based on new knowledge gleaned from studies on the microbiome. Another area of intense interest (but without hard data yet) is "psychobiotics"—probiotics that might affect the brain to treat conditions such as depression and anxiety.

Yet another frontier is genetically engineering bacteria. Work underway includes designing probiotics that express anti-inflammatory cytokines (to directly affect inflammation), or useful metabolic pathways such as producing SCFAs including butyrate, which will hopefully have beneficial health effects. The sky is the limit in designing synthetic microbes, although there are massive regulatory approval hurdles to overcome because this involves releasing a live genetically engineered microbe into the environment. For example, *E. coli* Nissle 1917 has been engineered to inhibit the virulence of *Vibrio cholerae* by disrupting how the *Vibrio* senses its environment. It worked well in a mouse cholera model but has not been tested in humans. Although most of the genetic engineering has been done in approved probiotic strains (*E. coli* Nissle 1917, lactobacilli, and *Bacteroides* species), using novel microbiota strains in combination with genetic modifications might enhance delivery of certain compounds such as anti-inflammatories, as they would colonize body sites more efficiently than current probiotics. Like all new technologies, there are concerns with this approach that need to be seriously addressed. For example, *Akkermansia* has been shown to be extremely beneficial in many gut-associated diseases, yet it is also associated with increased risk of disease in several neurological disorders such as Parkinson's, dementia, Alzheimer's, and multiple sclerosis. This suggests that serious safety concerns need to be addressed before accepting this as a widely used probiotic.

The other concern for any new probiotic is that it would be introduced into the environment and could have unforeseen consequences. The advantage of current probiotics is that they do not stick around for long; however, new microbes that colonize well and propagate have the potential to spread into the environment (including other people) with unknown effects. "Kill switches" can be genetically introduced into microbes and have been used in live engineered vaccine strains; they may be necessary to incorporate into new probiotics.

> **Recommendation:** *Stay tuned; exciting new designer probiotics are coming to a store near you! Keep an eye out for LBPs entering the clinic as FDA-approved medicines, giving new therapeutic solutions to significant health problems.*

Prebiotics

Instead of taking probiotics, which supplement an existing microbiome, how about eating certain foods that enhance the growth or activity of your beneficial microbes from the get-go? These are called "*pre*-biotics." The definition of a prebiotic has evolved over the years, but it generally refers to a substance that is selectively fermented (broken down) and results in a specific change in the composition and/or activity of the gastrointestinal microbiota. This, in turn, confers benefits upon the host's health. Thus, the food itself is not broken down by the host (it is non-digestible) but instead the bacteria metabolize it, with beneficial effects on the microbiome as well as the host.

Prebiotics are a subset of fiber (carbohydrates or sugars, often called "resistant starch") that includes inulin, fructo-oligosaccharides, and galacto-oligosaccharides. These microbial foods selectively enrich the beneficial *Lactobacillus* and/or *Bifidobacterium* species (although we now realize that other microbes are also affected by these prebiotics, especially butyrate producers). They are thought to also increase microbial diversity. Prebiotics are naturally found in plant foods and are usually isolated from biological sources.

There are many hypotheses about how prebiotics work. The theory is that by consuming foods that in turn feed these beneficial microbes, the microbes will increase in number and provide benefits such as increased SCFA production. They could also affect how long it takes materials to move through the intestinal tract (known as gut transit time), viscosity (thickness of the gut material), and how microbes interact with other food components.

Like probiotics, the most pressing question is: Do they actually confer a health benefit to the user? Again, the data are not well established and require more studies. For some, they definitely enhance the number of beneficial microbes, but actual proof of providing health benefits is not yet clinically established. Some studies have also shown that inulin and fructo-oligosaccharide enhance calcium absorption and bone density, especially in teenagers, while contrasting results were obtained in adults. There are reports that they may affect vaccine responses, as well as have beneficial effects for infectious diarrhea and IBS. In studying the collective literature on prebiotics, the general consensus is that they may enhance some health effects, but the data are not as strong as for probiotics. Additional confirmatory clinical studies are needed.

In the meantime, Brett regularly sprinkles a tablespoon of inulin on his morning (whole grain) cereal. Although he can't swear to a health benefit, it is a fun experiment as he then gets a real gut-check and can appreciate firsthand the gut microbes' fermentation in action (think: gas!). Prebiotic foods high in plant fiber include raw chicory root, Jerusalem artichoke, garlic, leeks, onion, and asparagus.

Overall, the concept of prebiotics makes sense: Consume substances that select for beneficial microbes and sit back and let them do their job. However, translating this into reality has been more difficult than it seems.

As with probiotics, the more we learn about microbial metabolism in the gut, the better the prebiotics that will be developed, with health benefits through defined mechanisms.

Recommendation: *There are too few appropriate human intervention trials with prebiotics to definitively say that they work in people and have a beneficial effect, although several more clinical studies are underway. At present, eating a balanced diet rich in a variety of different fibers has a likely beneficial effect on the microbiome, and can contribute to improved overall health. There are currently no reasons not to use them as they have few side effects (other than dose-dependent flatulence as a by-product of fermentation).*

Synbiotics

If there are indications that probiotics and prebiotics each might have beneficial effects, what happens if you combine them? These are called "synbiotics." We saw an exciting new example of synbiotics in the COVID chapter: A combined mixture of three probiotics and three prebiotics showed promising results to help improve long COVID symptoms. In theory it's a great idea, but there are no data yet to say that they work better as a team than prebiotics or probiotics alone. In one study, older adults (aged sixty-five to ninety) were given the probiotic *Bifidobacterium longum* and the prebiotic inulin. This treatment did increase Bifidobacteria numbers (as well as other beneficial microbes) and decreased Proteobacteria (pro-inflammatory). They also saw an increase in butyrate production and a decrease in pro-inflammatory cytokines; however, these beneficial effects soon disappeared after the treatment ended. As great as this increase sounds, even in isolation, there are many other studies that did not see any major effects from doses of synbiotics or found that individually a probiotic or prebiotic was more effective than the combination.

Recommendation: *There are not enough good clinical data yet to recommend the use of synbiotics, although both probiotics and prebiotics on their own can be beneficial. We just don't know yet if their effects are synergistic.*

Antibiotics

Antibiotics are one of the biggest medical discoveries of the twentieth century and have saved countless lives. They are the biggest reason we have a longer lifespan than people did a century ago. However, antibiotics are also a source of new problems, including how they affect the microbiome. Over 80 percent of antibiotics in Canada and the US are not used to treat disease but rather in animal husbandry as growth enhancers; in Europe this practice is banned; in Australia, the percentage is almost zero. North America is finally starting to take notice, with huge companies such as McDonald's, Subway, and Kentucky Fried Chicken committing to using antibiotic-free livestock and poultry. Use of antibiotics in animal husbandry, in addition to overprescription by physicians for conditions that are not improved by antibiotics, and abuse of antibiotics by the public, has led to antibiotic-resistant pathogens. These "superbugs" are extremely difficult to treat and cause legitimate concerns about a global return to a pre-antibiotic era. As we saw earlier, in the United States at least two million people are infected annually with antibiotic-resistant bacteria, and at least twenty-three thousand people die from these infections each year. In 2019, it was estimated that 1.27 million people worldwide died due to antimicrobial resistant bacteria, and they contributed to 4.95 million deaths. Individual overuses of antibiotics increase the risk of antimicrobial resistance for us all.

This may have you wondering: Is it safe to use antibiotics at all?

Without hesitation, yes–but only if they are warranted! If you face a life-threatening infection, they can save your life. However, if you have an ear infection that may be viral (in which case antibiotics won't work anyway), physicians will often suggest waiting a day or two before throwing a microbial carpet bomb at your body with a round of antibiotics. As we saw in earlier chapters, antibiotic use is associated with obesity, asthma, allergies, stress, depression, and many more issues. It really comes down to balancing their use and weighing the risks. If you need to take antibiotics, we have discussed various ways of potentially repairing your microbiome afterward, such as taking certain probiotics that work against antibiotic-associated diarrhea, as well as a varied diet that enriches for microbial diversity and beneficial microbes.

Recommendation: *If there is an evidence-based medical recommendation that antibiotics are warranted (such as a serious bacterial infection), take them. But remember that antibiotics can have long-term effects, and don't work against viral infections. If they are not warranted, don't use them. If you do need antibiotics, consider diet and probiotics to try and repair your microbiome after the treatment is finished.*

RePOOPulation: Fecal Transfers

In all our discussion of fecal transfers, also known as fecal microbiota transplants (FMTs), there's a clear bottom line: They can work very well for infections with *C. difficile* and show significant promise for ulcerative colitis (although it can be donor dependent). Additionally, there is real potential being seen for fecal transfer use with stem cell transplantations, preventing multi-drug-resistant infections such as vancomycin-resistant enterococcus (VRE) and multi-drug-resistant *Enterobacteriaceae*, and possibly for use with checkpoint inhibitor immunotherapy in cancer. For most uses, they are currently experimental and being tested for a variety of conditions.

These advances are exciting, but again, we must stress: Do NOT try this at home. If the bowel is perforated during an attempted transfer, the individual could die of sepsis. There are also no studies yet on long-term risks associated with FMTs, including the concern that an undesirable phenotype (characteristic) may be transferred from the donor feces. Remember the example in chapter 2 of the lean person who gained significant weight after receiving an FMT from an obese donor. Although the FMT successfully cured the patient, it may also have shifted the recipient's microbes toward a pattern of obesity.

In the near future, we will be able to use a defined batch of fecal microbes grown in the lab–a process affectionately known as rePOOPulation amongst microbiologists (see chapter 2). This will eliminate the risk of spreading unknown infectious agents found in feces (which is a body fluid). The use of synthetic communities, or live biotherapeutic agents, as discussed previously, is rapidly being developed by various companies to replace donor FMTs in the future.

Recommendation: *If you have had at least two standard antibiotic treatments for recurrent C. difficile infection without persistent cure, ask your doctor about a fecal transfer or an LBP (a mixture of live microbes). The clinical data to support its efficacy are strong and FMTs are clinically approved. If you have ulcerative colitis, you could try to get into a clinical trial where FMTs are being used. For all other indications, clinical evidence of efficacy is still lacking for FMT treatment, so it is not warranted. Do NOT try an FMT at home.*

Talk to Your Doctor

Playing an active role in your health care is one of the best ways to prevent and treat disease, since you know your body best. Open and honest patient-physician communication is essential to conveying the right information at the right time so you can receive the best and most appropriate care. Medicine is not a one-way relationship where the doctor takes the lead with you (the patient) following without questioning. Rather, think of yourselves as partners, and the two of you as part of an even larger team, including other physicians, nurses, pharmacists, therapists, assistants, and health care providers, all necessary to keeping you healthy. Be honest and upfront about your symptoms and opinions, and don't be afraid to ask for other perspectives.

In talking to a doctor about your microbiome, be upfront about what microbe-friendly practices you are following and/or want to try. Remember, physicians are sworn to the Hippocratic Oath, which means first and foremost, do no harm. They need clinical proof that what they recommend will not harm the patient and will have a proven health benefit. For example, if you have experienced multiple bouts of *C. diff* and want to pursue an FMT, ask your health care providers about safety and effectiveness. Be as informed as possible regarding what the clinical data support versus what is promising but "just not there yet."

We spoke to Dr. David Patrick, a practicing infectious disease doctor, professor in the University of British Columbia School of Population and Public Health, and epidemiologist for the BC Center for Disease Control. Dr. Patrick recommended that in considering any new microbial approaches to your health, science is the first place to start: "In the history of the medical profession, we've done a lot based on impulse without the science to back it up. We first need to prove things in experiments [in humans]—meaning rigorous clinical trials—before any widespread application of a treatment can be considered. The risk is that people will jump all over the coolness of microbial advances and leap to conclusions." He clarified that even though studies may show exciting results in mice or initial small human studies, that does not mean they will necessarily translate into successful results for all. For all new treatments, many expensive and long-term clinical trials need to be done before anything is adopted into mainstream medicine. The microbiome is just too new a field for most practices to be fully clinically approved.

Furthermore, shifting your microbiome will not only affect you. It will also affect those around you. As we saw in chapter 14, we share and swap immense numbers of microbes with our roommates—human and non-human. In the worst-case scenario, an ill-informed microbial experiment can harm not only you but those you live with as well. That being said, "do no harm" does not mean "do nothing." Dr. Patrick explained that the first thing a doctor should do is show compassion regarding a patient's symptoms. With broad and ambiguous illnesses such as chronic exhaustion, there may be a need to turn to new treatments whenever the risk is low and if science can reasonably back it up. Here the placebo effect may be able to help. Dr. Patrick explained: "Placebos can actually do a lot to make people feel better. It's not the sugar pill or saline that works, but rather setting expectations. Having the right expectations can meaningfully aid one's recovery."

Regarding antibiotics, Dr. Patrick told us that his standard response to patients is "only take them when they are needed to resolve a serious disease process." Similar to our recommendations, he recognized that there is a proper time and place to use antibiotics. However, he continued, "Fifty to seventy percent of antibiotic use in humans in North America does not fit that bill. It's not necessary. You can dial it back." You may need to be assertive in the conversation with your doctor regarding a course of antibiotics. If you want your microbiome to take care of you, you have to stand up for it!

The best way to be your own health advocate is to stay informed. Dr. Patrick gave the analogy of the rules for a good journalist: "Have your trusted sources. I often point patients toward WebMD and PubMed; Healthdirect is one Australian option. The amount of unfiltered health information out there on the internet is extremely troubling." In the evolving era of fake news, it's increasingly important to distinguish between credible sources of information and misinformed, biased, and even downright wrong sources. If you are unsure about the accuracy of a medical claim, fact-check it against other studies and consult a health professional who may have more data than you can access.

> **Recommendation:** *When it comes to anything about your health, not just the microbiome, be proactive and start the conversation with your doctor so you can work together to keep you well for the duration of your (long) life.*

The Future Is Bright

The past decade has seen a remarkable renaissance in our understanding of the microbes inside and around us, from recognizing that we coevolved with them to the discovery of the fundamental roles they play in both lifelong health and disease. The exploding knowledge suggests many exciting new possibilities for how we can use microbes' countless beneficial capacities in the future for human health.

The field is rapidly moving from "microbe cataloguing" (identifying exactly which microbes are in and around the body) to figuring out the microbial genes and mechanisms that are responsible for particular effects. As we define particular microbial species and their molecules, it opens up opportunities for novel treatments. For example, we are still in the early days of defining which components of diet that particular microbes utilize. While we now recognize that fiber is converted into SCFAs with beneficial effects, this is just the beginning of what could be a regular partnership between nutrition and microbiology. Specific diet components will be linked to specific microbes, and even metabolic pathways and molecules within them, thus allowing diets to be tailored to individuals for specific defined health benefits. Recommended food guidelines may be adjusted to incorporate the microbiome (e.g., perhaps we will distinguish fermented foods as a new food group), and they are even more likely to be personalized for unique microbiomes and needs. This will include designing specific diets for each stage of life, particularly early on when one's microbiome is being established, and later in life to enhance health and longevity.

Genetic engineering has changed the entire biotechnology sector and will be applied to the microbiome field. We are already starting to see common probiotics engineered to enhance their benefits. However, microbes could be engineered to better regulate energy balance, to detoxify harmful products, or synthesize beneficial molecules including vitamins. A recent major advance in molecular biology involved the development of CRISPR-Cas9, a tool that has made the replacement of genes in practically any organism much, much easier. Additionally, mRNA vaccines such as those pioneered for COVID-19 have completely changed the vaccine world. These and other tools will make the engineering of beneficial microbes much more practical. We also sorely need tools to surgically alter microbiome composition, such that it can be shaped into a more beneficial, less dysbiotic community in individuals (especially older adults) when standard treatments for diseases are unsuccessful or impossible. We are already seeing companies performing early clinical trials that replenish dysbiotic microbiomes with a mixture of specific microbes grown in the laboratory. This opens many exciting avenues that could be used to repair poorly functioning microbiomes that don't respond to other methods.

With each generation, the collective microbiome of humans decreases in diversity and becomes more homogeneous as we share cities, food sources, and each other's company. As Dr. Martin Blaser points out in his book *Missing Microbes*, we are at significant risk of losing microbes that are part of our evolution, and from what we know, this could have significant effects on our health (witness the rise of asthma, obesity, and the many diseases in our society correlated with a decrease in microbial diversity). The real problem is what to do about this. There are some groups that are working on biobanking microbes as a sort of "microzoo." As discussed previously, some current members of our microbiome really may be endangered species, which could have significant effects on humans. We are removing a key component of our evolution as a species.

Similar possibilities can be contemplated about our microbes as we age.

We saw in chapter 5 the beneficial effect of skin microbes from younger women on skin health in older women. We know that our microbes shift as we get older, and at least in mice, transplanting microbes from younger animals into older ones can decrease inflammation. One can imagine a future where you might biobank microbes from your youthful skin in a tube in a freezer, which would become part of your retirement package to boost skin appearance and overall health later in life. This personal biobank could also be useful if you were diagnosed with cancer and needed a bone marrow transplant, or if you suddenly got a *C. difficile* infection and needed to boost your microbiome at a critical time. We might also see the application of younger persons' microbes into commercially available products to cultivate the healthful effects of vigorous youthful microbes later in life.

In chapter 7, we saw an example of "drugging the bugs" with respect to inhibiting TMA production by the gut microbiota (produced from choline and carnitine in animal products such as red meat and egg yolks) to decrease cardiovascular disease. As we establish the exact roles of microbes and their enzymes, we may have at our disposal a vast new set of pharmaceuticals in the future. For example, *Eggerthella lenta* is a gut microbe that can block digoxin activity (a heart medication) by breaking down the drug. Researchers have identified the microbial pathway responsible and have now shown that they can inhibit this pathway, which could provide a new tool to enhance digoxin's effects in more people. One advantage of drugging the microbes, but not ourselves, is that specific adverse reactions to the drug shouldn't affect us. The drugs can act directly upon the microbes with limited side effects to our H. sapiens gene products.

This brings us to the effect of the microbiome on personalized medicine. Personalized medicine is based on the premise that different people respond differently to drugs, and that by understanding a person's genetic composition, one should be able to better predict which drugs should work with each individual. The problem with that theory is that humans are 99.9 percent identical genetically (sex chromosomes excepted). Scientists have been able to identify genetic loci that dictate a particular drug's effect for only a small number of drugs. However, each of us has a unique microbiome, with only a fraction of shared microbes between people—even among those living together. It is the microbiome that gives individuals much of their uniqueness. When you swallow a drug, it is usually the microbes in the gut that break it down or modify it into a molecule that may cause adverse drug effects. In the future, microbiome sequencing may be even more helpful to doctors than genetic sequencing, as it could provide guidance about which drugs to use and at what dosage by considering your particular microbiome's composition and potential interactions.

For every bacterium it is estimated that there are about a hundred bacterial viruses called "bacteriophages" or "phages." Studying the "virome" in the human gut is still new (but advancing rapidly, with lots of promising new findings). There are thousands of viral genotypes in the gut (one study estimated more than 140,000). Each phage has a specific bacterial host, which prompts the idea that phages can be used to specifically target a bacterium. This forms the basis of "phage therapy," a technology pioneered in the Soviet Union in the 1950s and 1960s. However, this technology has problems, as bacteria rapidly become resistant to phages, and it has not withstood Western clinical trials. New uses for phages are on the horizon. For example, CRISPR-Cas9 can be packaged into a phage and used to target a specific pathogen, modulate the microbiome, or even used to engineer a bacterium to treat a disease.

Looking further into the future, it may be possible to engineer microbes that increase longevity. *Caenorhabditis elegans* (frequently called *C. elegans*) is a small nematode (worm) that has been studied extensively in many labs. It feeds off bacteria such as *E. coli* that also colonize its gut. When researchers made individual mutations in every non-essential *E. coli* gene (all 3,983 of them) and then fed them to worms, they identified twenty-nine bacterial genes that increased worm longevity. Some of the gene products affected worm pathways already known to increase longevity, including mitochondria ("powerhouse" organelles that produce the energy for most cellular processes) and unfolded protein responses. Although very far from the world of humans, this work hints that there may be ways to alter the microbiome to enhance longevity. However, these types of experiments in humans would take many generations to reproduce given that the average lifespan of *C. elegans* is twelve to eighteen days, and average time between generations is four days!

Knowing the role of the microbiome in human health and disease has opened up many fascinating possibilities to harness this information to develop beneficial products. However, it is still hindered by the lack of mechanistic knowledge about exactly which microbes, which metabolic pathways, and which molecules are responsible for any particular activity. As science relentlessly progresses in these areas, countless opportunities exist to enter a whole new era of pharmacology based on microbes and their products.

In Pursuit of Health and Longevity

So, what can you do now?

First and foremost, recognize that we live in harmony with most of our microbes. They are a normal, essential part of everyday human life. Choose your lifestyle habits based not only on your needs, but also on your microbes'. Protocols of hygiene and health exist on a spectrum–from hand sanitizer and antibiotics to how you move and what you eat–and can all be calibrated to enable your microbes to thrive along with you. Recognize that as you age, you may need to adjust things to maintain a healthy diversity of microbes.

In his popular book *The Blue Zones*, Dan Buettner originally examined five regions of the world where people live much longer than average: Sardinia (Italy), Okinawa (Japan), Loma Linda (California), Nicoya (Costa Rica), and Ikaria (Greece). He observed and compared many aspects of their lives, including social habits, diet, and exercise. In Buettner's nine lessons learned from those with extraordinary longevity, we found that many are underscored by the microbiome. First, one's diet has obvious connections. These long-lived populations frequently ate plant-based foods, fish, nuts, legumes, and little red meat. The Japanese diet rich in fish and rice and the Mediterranean diets were expected, but southern California? In Loma Linda, there are many Seventh-Day Adventists, who are encouraged to follow a well-balanced vegetarian diet. Given all we have seen with diet and microbe interconnections, this certainly makes sense.

The second theme we noticed is exercise. One does not have to be a marathon runner, but countless studies find that staying active promotes health and longevity. Many in the Blue Zones were sheep herders or walked to the village daily for groceries and social contact. In southern California, the weather is conducive to outdoor activities such as jogging, tennis, and walking. Perhaps their longevity is impacted by active lifestyles that encourage beneficial microbes.

The third theme is strong social bonds with family and friends. This might include an eighty-year-old daughter caring for her one-hundred-year-old father, or simply playing a daily game of cards. People in most of these areas of the world live among their extended families and in multi-generational households. The religious community in Loma Linda acts like an extended family with regular social contact. And we know that social contact is a great way to share and swap microbes. Unfortunately, modern Western societies tend to do the complete opposite in caring for older people. We put them in assisted living and nursing homes, feed them a limited diet, and visit only when we can find a spare moment in our busy lives. As you and loved ones age, keep these lessons in mind to maintain a vibrant and healthy lifestyle.

The fourth theme is decreased stress in one's life. This may be the hardest one to pursue in our fast-paced modern society. However, as we have seen in this book, stress causes significant harm to the microbiome that in turn translates into health issues. All of the Blue Zone areas are known for lower-stress lifestyles and attitudes.

Along with these goals, try to get a full night's sleep. Many studies show that sleep is needed to help maintain body and brain health, and recent studies have uncovered the microbiome's role in sleep. Your body *and* microbes need a bit of down time to process the day, repair, and replenish.

While science is still in the shallow end of this vast pool of exploration, the body's many microbiomes represent a promising and exciting new frontier of aging research—a fountain of youth that's far bigger than we ever could have imagined. Keep an eye out for exciting new scientific advances in "microbe therapies" that we saw glimpses of in this book. At thirty-five and sixty-five years old, we (Jessica and Brett) regularly consider and want to proactively address our own age-related concerns—from wrinkles and declining mobility to Alzheimer's disease. We have adopted many of the diet and lifestyle strategies suggested throughout this book, pursuing them with the knowledge that the more we can learn about their engagement with the microbiome, the more we can improve quality of life in our globally aging population. As new discoveries appear every day, we may soon realize that the fountain of youth we've traveled far and wide to find is right under (and inside, and on) our own noses. We hope that you and your microbes may live long–and prosper.

Selected References

1. THE FOUNTAIN OF YOUTH IS FULL OF . . . MICROBES?

Badal, V. D., Vaccariello, E. D., Murray, E. R., et al., "The gut microbiome, aging, and longevity: A systematic review," *Nutrients* 12, no. 12 (2020): 3759, doi:10.3390/nu12123759.

Biagi, E., Candela, M., Franceschi, C., and Brigidi, P., "The aging gut microbiota: new perspectives," *Ageing Research Reviews* 10, no. 4 (2011): 428–29, doi.org/10.3390/nu12123759

Biagi, E., Nylund, L., Candela, M., et al., "Through ageing, and beyond: gut microbiota and inflammatory status in seniors and centenarians," *PLOS One* 5, no. 5 (2010): e10667, doi:10.1371/journal.pone.0010667.

Brüssow, H., "Microbiota and healthy ageing: observational and nutritional intervention studies," *Microbial Biotechnology* 6, no. 4 (2013): 326–34, doi:10.1111/1751-7915.12048.

Claesson, M. J., Jeffery, I. B., Conde, S., et al., "Gut microbiota composition correlates with diet and health in the elderly," *Nature* 488, no. 7410 (2012): 178–84, doi:10.1038/nature11319.

Conway, J., and Duggal, N. A., "Ageing of the gut microbiome: Potential influences on immune senescence and inflammageing," *Ageing Research Reviews* 68 (2021): 101323, doi:10.1016/j.arr.2021.101323.

Ghosh, T. S., Shanahan, F., and O'Toole, P. W., "The gut microbiome as a modulator of healthy ageing," *Nature Reviews Gastroenterology and Hepatology* 19, no. 9 (2022): 565–84, doi:10.1038/s41575-022-00605-x.

Gilbert, J. A., Blaser, M. J., Caporaso, J. G., Jansson, J. K., Lynch, S. V., and Knight, R., "Current understanding of the human microbiome," *Nature Medicine* 24, no. 4 (2018): 392–400, doi:10.1038/nm.4517.

Heintz, C., and Mair, W., "You are what you host: microbiome modulation of the aging process," *Cell* 156, no. 3 (2014): 408–11, doi:10.1016/j.cell.2014.01.025.

Jackson, M. A., Jeffery, I. B., Beaumont, M., et al., "Signatures of early frailty in the gut microbiota," *Genome Medicine* 8, no. 1 (2016): 8, doi:10.1186/s13073-016-0262-7.

Kong, F., Hua, Y., Zeng, B., Ning, R., Li, Y., and Zhao, J., "Gut microbiota signatures of longevity," *Current Biology* 26, no. 18 (2016): R832–33, doi:10.1016/j.cub.2016.08.015.

"Life Expectancy," Our World in Data, accessed January 1, 2025, ourworldindata.org/life-expectancy.

Lynch, D. B., Jeffery, I. B., and O'Toole, P. W., "The role of the microbiota in ageing: current state and perspectives," *Wiley Interdisciplinary Reviews Systems Biology and Medicine* 7, no. 3 (2015): 131–38, doi:10.1002/wsbm.1293.

Rondanelli, M., Giacosa, A., Faliva, M. A., Perna, S., Allieri, F., and Castellazzi, A. M., "Review on microbiota and effectiveness of probiotics use in older," *World Journal of Clinical Cases* 3, no. 2 (2015): 156–62, doi:10.12998/wjcc.v3.i2.156.

Saraswati, S., and Sitaraman, R., "Aging and the human gut microbiota–from correlation to causality," *Frontiers in Microbiology* 5 (2014): 764, doi:10.3389/fmicb.2014.00764.

Schupack, D. A., Mars, R. A. T., Voelker, D. H., Abeykoon, J. P., and Kashyap, P. C., "The promise of the gut microbiome as part of individualized treatment strategies," *Nature Reviews Gastroenterology and Hepatology* 19, no. 1 (2022): 7–25, doi:10.1038/s41575-021-00499-1.

Smits, S. A., Leach, J., Sonnenburg, E. D., et al., "Seasonal cycling in the gut microbiome of the Hadza hunter-gatherers of Tanzania," *Science* 357 no. 6353 (2017): 802–6, doi:10.1126/science.aan4834.

Stern, J., Moazami, S., Qiu, Y., et al., "Evidence for a distinct gut microbiome in kidney stone formers compared to non-stone formers," *Urolithiasis* 44 no. 5 (2016): 399–407, doi:10.1007/s00240-016-0882-9.

Teng, M., Ng, C., Huang, D., et al., "Global incidence and prevalence of nonalcoholic fatty liver disease," *Clinical and Molecular Hepatology* 14, no. 29 (2023): S32–42, doi:10.3350/cmh.2022.0365.

Thevaranjan, N., Puchta, A., Schulz, C., et al., "Age-Associated Microbial Dysbiosis Promotes Intestinal Permeability, Systemic Inflammation, and Macrophage Dysfunction," *Cell Host & Microbe* 21, no. 4 (2017): 455–66.e4, doi:10.1016/j.chom.2017.03.002.

Tiihonen, K., Ouwehand, A. C., and Rautonen, N., "Human intestinal microbiota and healthy ageing," *Ageing Research Reviews* 9, no. 2 (2010): 107–16, doi:10.1016/j.arr.2009.10.004.

Wilmanski, T., Diener, C., Rappaport, N., et al., "Gut microbiome pattern reflects healthy ageing and predicts survival in humans," *Nature Metabolism* 3, no. 2 (2021): 274–86, doi:10.1038/s42255-021-00348-0.

Zapata, H. J., and Quagliarello, V. J., "The microbiota and microbiome in aging: potential implications in health and age-related diseases," *Journal of the American Geriatrics Society* 63, no. 4 (2015): 776–81, doi:10.1111/jgs.13310.

2. MICROBE MECCA: THE GUT MICROBIOME

Ahmad, S., Moorthy, M. V., Lee, I. M., et al., "Mediterranean Diet Adherence and Risk of All-Cause Mortality in Women," *JAMA Network Open* 7, no. 5 (2024): e2414322, doi:10.1001/jamanetworkopen.2024.14322.

Bala, S., Marcos, M., Gattu, A., Catalano, D., and Szabo, G., "Acute binge drinking increases serum endotoxin and bacterial DNA levels in healthy individuals," *PLOS One* 9, no. 5 (2014): e96864, doi:10.1371/journal.pone.0096864.

Baothman, O. A., Zamzami, M. A., Taher, I., Abubaker, J., and Abu-Farha, M., "The role of Gut Microbiota in the development of obesity and diabetes," *Lipids in Health and Disease* 15, no. 108 (2016), doi:10.1186/s12944-016-0278-4.

Ben-Yacov, O., Godneva, A., Rein, M., et al., "Personalized Postprandial Glucose Response–Targeting Diet Versus Mediterranean Diet for Glycemic Control in Prediabetes," *Diabetes Care* 44, no. 9 (2021): 1980–91, doi:10.2337/DC21-0162.

Biagi, E., Franceschi, C., Rampelli, S., et al., "Gut Microbiota and Extreme Longevity," *Current Biology* 26 no. 11 (2016): 1480–85, doi:10.1016/j.cub.2016.04.016.

Bian, G., Gloor, G. B., Gong, A., et al., "The Gut Microbiota of Healthy Aged Chinese Is Similar to That of the Healthy Young," *mSphere* 2, no. 5 (2017): e00327, doi:10.1128/mSphere.00327-17.

Brandt, L. J., "Fecal Microbiota Therapy With a Focus on Clostridium difficile Infection," *Psychosomatic Medicine* 79, no. 8 (2017): 868–73, doi:10.1097/PSY.0000000000000511.

Brichacek, A. L., Florkowski, M., Abiona, E., and Frank, K. M., "Ultra-Processed Foods: A Narrative Review of the Impact on the Human Gut Microbiome and Variations in Classification Methods," *Nutrients* 16, no. 11 (2024): 1738, doi:10.3390/nu16111738.

Brüssow, H., "Microbiota and healthy ageing: observational and nutritional intervention studies," *Microbial Biotechnology* 6, no. 4 (2013): 326–34, doi:10.1111/1751-7915.12048

Chen, L., He, F. J., Dong, Y., et al., "Modest Sodium Reduction Increases Circulating Short-Chain Fatty Acids in Untreated Hypertensives: A Randomized, Double-Blind, Placebo-Controlled Trial," *Hypertension* 76, no. 1 (2020): 73–79, doi:10.1161/HYPERTENSIONAHA.120.14800.

Chu, H., Khosravi, A., Kusumawardhani, I. P., et al., "Gene-microbiota interactions contribute to the pathogenesis of inflammatory bowel disease," *Science* 352, no. 6289 (2016): 1116–20, doi:10.1126/science.aad9948.

Corbin, K. D., Carnero, E. A., Dirks, B., et al., "Host-diet-gut microbiome interactions influence human energy balance: a randomized clinical trial," *Nature Communications* 14, no. 1 (2023): 3161, doi:10.1038/s41467-023-38778-x.

Daas, M. C., and de Roos, N. M., "Intermittent fasting contributes to aligned circadian rhythms through interactions with the gut microbiome," *Beneficial Microbes* 12, no. 2 (2021): 147–61, doi:10.3920/BM2020.0149.

Deehan, E. C., and Walter, J., "The Fiber Gap and the Disappearing Gut Microbiome: Implications for Human Nutrition," *Trends in Endocrinology and Metabolism* 27, no. 5 (2016): 239–42, doi:10.1016/j.tem.2016.03.001.

Forslund, K., Hildebrand, F., Nielsen, T., et al., "Disentangling type 2 diabetes and metformin treatment signatures in the human gut microbiota," *Nature* 528, no. 7581 (2015): 262–66, doi:10.1038/nature15766.

Ghosh, S., Whitley, C. S., Haribabu, B., and Jala, V. R., "Regulation of Intestinal Barrier Function by Microbial Metabolites," *CMGH* 11, no. 5 (2021): 1463–82, doi:10.1016/j.jcmgh.2021.02.007.

Iyer, N., and Vaishnava, S., "Alcohol Lowers Your (Intestinal) Inhibitions," *Cell Host & Microbe* 19, no. 2 (2016): 131–33, doi:10.1016/j.chom.2016.01.014.

Jayasinghe, T. N., Chiavaroli, V., Holland, D. J., Cutfield, W. S., and O'Sullivan, J. M., "The New Era of Treatment for Obesity and Metabolic Disorders: Evidence and Expectations for Gut Microbiome Transplantation," *Frontiers in Cellular and Infection Microbiology* 6, no. 15 (2016), doi:10.3389/fcimb.2016.00015.

Kant, R., Chandra, L., Verma, V., et al., "Gut microbiota interactions with anti-diabetic medications and pathogenesis of type 2 diabetes mellitus," *World Journal of Methodology* 12, no. 4 (2022): 246–57, doi:10.5662/wjm.v12.i4.246.

Kliemann, N., Rauber, F., Levy, R., et al., "Food processing and cancer risk in Europe: results from the prospective EPIC cohort study," *The Lancet* 7, no. 3 (2023): E219–32, doi: 10.1016/S2542-5196(23)00021-9.

Kong, F., Hua, Y., Zeng, B., Ning, R., Li, Y., and Zhao, J., "Gut microbiota signatures of longevity," *Current Biology* 26, no. 18 (2016): R832–33, doi:10.1016/j.cub.2016.08.015.

König, J., Siebenhaar, A., Högenauer, C., et al., "Consensus report: faecal microbiota transfer–clinical applications and procedures," *Alimentary Pharmacology & Therapeutics* 45, no. 2 (2017): 222–39, doi:10.1111/apt.13868.

Leung, C., Rivera, L., Furness, J. B., and Angus, P. W., "The role of the gut microbiota in NAFLD," *Nature Reviews Gastroenterology & Hepatology* 13, no. 7 (2016): 412–25, doi:10.1038/nrgastro.2016.85.

Li, H., Zhang, L., Li, J., et al., "Resistant starch intake facilitates weight loss in humans by reshaping the gut microbiota," *Nature Metabolism* 6, no. 3 (2024): 578–97, doi:10.1038/s42255-024-00988-y.

Liang, L., Su, X. Y., Guan, Y., Wu, B., Zhang, X., and Nian, X., "Correlation between intestinal flora and GLP-1 receptor agonist dulaglutide in type 2 diabetes mellitus treatment–A preliminary longitudinal study," *iScience* 27, no. 5 (2024): 109784, doi:10.1016/j.isci.2024.109784.

Maher, R. L., Hanlon, J., and Hajjar, E. R., "Clinical consequences of polypharmacy in elderly," *Expert Opinion on Drug Safety* 13, no. 1 (2014): 57–65, doi:10.1517/14740338.2013.827660.

Maifeld, A., Bartolomaeus, H., Löber, U., et al., "Fasting alters the gut microbiome reducing blood pressure and body weight in metabolic syndrome patients," *Nature Communications* 12, no. 1 (2021): 1970, doi:10.1038/s41467-021-22097-0.

Mehta, R. S., Lochhead, P., Wang, Y., et al., "Association of midlife antibiotic use with subsequent cognitive function in women," *PLOS One* 17, no. 3 (2022): e0264649, doi:10.1371/journal.pone.0264649.

Mohr, A. E., Jasbi, P., Bowes, D. A., et al., "Exploratory analysis of one versus two-day intermittent fasting protocols on the gut microbiome and plasma metabolome in adults with overweight/obesity," *Frontiers in Nutrition* 9 (2022): 1036080, doi:10.3389/fnut.2022.1036080.

Mohr, A. E., Sweazea, K. L., Bowes, D. A., et al., "Gut microbiome remodeling and metabolomic profile improves in response to protein pacing with intermittent fasting versus continuous caloric restriction," *Nature Communications* 15, no. 1 (2024): 4155, doi:10.1038/s41467-024-48355-5.

Mousavi, S. N., Rayyani, E., Heshmati, J., Tavasolian, R., and Rahimlou, M., "Effects of Ramadan and Non-ramadan Intermittent Fasting on Gut Microbiome," *Frontiers in Nutrition* 9 (2022): 860575, doi:10.3389/fnut.2022.860575.

Paukkonen, I., Törrönen, E. N., Lok, J., Schwab, U., and El-Nezami, H., "The impact of intermittent fasting on gut microbiota: a systematic review of human studies," *Frontiers in Nutrition* 11 (2024): 1342787, doi:10.3389/fnut.2024.1342787.

Pham, V. T., Dold, S., Rehman, A., Bird, J. K., and Steinert, R. E., "Vitamins, the gut microbiome and gastrointestinal health in humans," *Nutrition Research* 95 (2021): 35–53, doi:10.1016/j.nutres.2021.09.001.

Pinto-Sanchez, M., Hall, G., Ghajar, K., et al., "Probiotic Bifidobacterium longum NCC3001 Reduces Depression Scores and Alters Brain Activity: A Pilot Study in Patients With Irritable Bowel Syndrome," *Gastroenterology* 153 no. 2 (2017): 448–59.e448, doi:10.1053/j.gastro.2017.05.003.

Rong, B., Wu, Q., Saeed, M., and Sun, C., "Gut microbiota—a positive contributor in the process of intermittent fasting-mediated obesity control," *Animal Nutrition* 7, no. 4 (2021): 1283–95, doi:10.1016/j.aninu.2021.09.009.

Salame, C., Javaux, G., Sellem, L., et al., "Food additive emulsifiers and the risk of type 2 diabetes: analysis of data from the NutriNet-Santé prospective cohort study," *The Lancet Diabetes and Endocrinology* 12, no. 5 (2024): 339–49, doi:10.1016/S2213-8587(24)00086-X.

Santoro, A., Ostan, R., Candela, M., et al., "Gut microbiota changes in the extreme decades of human life: a focus on centenarians," *Cellular and Molecular Life Sciences* 75, no. 1 (2018): 129–48, doi:10.1007/s00018-017-2674-y.

Shelton, C. D., Sing, E., Mo, J., et al., "An early-life microbiota metabolite protects against obesity by regulating intestinal lipid metabolism," *Cell Host and Microbe* 31, no. 10 (2023): 1604–19.e10, doi:10.1016/j.chom.2023.09.002.

Sonnenburg, E. D., Smits, S. A., Tikhonov, M., Higginbottom, S. K., Wingreen, N. S., and Sonnenburg, J. L., "Diet-induced extinctions in the gut microbiota compound over generations," *Nature* 529, no. 7585 (2016): 212–15, doi:10.1038/nature16504.

Spragge, F., Bakkeren, E., Jahn, M. T., et al., "Microbiome diversity protects against pathogens by nutrient blocking," *Science* 382, no. 6676 (2023): eadj3502, doi:10.1126/science.adj3502.

Su, J., Wang, Y., Zhang, X., et al., "Remodeling of the gut microbiome during Ramadan-associated intermittent fasting," *American Journal of Clinical Nutrition* 113, no. 5 (2021): 1332–42, doi:10.1093/ajcn/nqaa388.

Suez, J., Korem, T., Zeevi, D., et al., "Artificial sweeteners induce glucose intolerance by altering the gut microbiota," *Nature* 514, no. 7521 (2014): 181–86, doi:10.1038/nature13793.

Thaiss, C. A., Itav, S., Rothschild, D., et al., "Persistent microbiome alterations modulate the rate of post-dieting weight regain," *Nature* 540, no. 7634 (2016): 544–51, doi:10.1038/nature20796.

Zeevi, D., Korem, T., Zmora, N., et al., "Personalized Nutrition by Prediction of Glycemic Responses," *Cell* 163, no. 5 (2015): 1079–94, doi:10.1016/j.cell.2015.11.001.

Zeng, Y., Wu, Y., Zhang, Q., and Xiao, X., "Crosstalk between glucagon-like peptide 1 and gut microbiota in metabolic diseases," *mBio* 15, no. 1 (2024): e0203223, doi:10.1128/mbio.02032-23.

Zhang, C., Zhang, M., Wang, S. et al., "Interactions between gut microbiota, host genetics and diet relevant to development of metabolic syndromes in mice," *The ISME Journal* 4, no. 2 (2010): 232–41, doi:10.1038/ismej.2009.112.

3. MICROBE TUG-OF-WAR: THE IMMUNE SYSTEM

Asghari, K. M., Dolatkhah, N., Ayromlou, H., Mirnasiri, F., Dadfar, T., and Hashemian, M., "The effect of probiotic supplementation on the clinical and para-clinical findings of multiple sclerosis: a randomized clinical trial," *Scientific Reports* 13, no. 1 (2023): 17617, doi:10.1038/s41598-023-46047-6.

Atarashi, K., Tanoue, T., Oshima, K., et al., "Treg induction by a rationally selected mixture of Clostridia strains from the human microbiota," *Nature* 500, no. 7461 (2013): 232–36, doi:10.1038/nature12331.

Berer, K., Gerdes, L. A., Cekanaviciute, E., et al., "Gut microbiota from multiple sclerosis patients enables spontaneous autoimmune encephalomyelitis in mice," *PNAS* 114, no. 40 (2017): 10719–24, doi:10.1073/pnas.1711233114.

Bergot, A. S., Giri, R., and Thomas, R., "The microbiome and rheumatoid arthritis," *Best Practice and Research: Clinical Rheumatology* 33, no. 6 (2019): 101497, doi:10.1016/j.berh.2020.101497.

Caballero, S., and Pamer, E. G., "Microbiota-mediated inflammation and antimicrobial defense in the intestine," *Annual Review of Immunology* 33 (2015): 227–56, doi:10.1146/annurev-immunol-032713-120238.

Calder, P. C., Bosco, N., Bourdet-Sicard, R., et al., "Health relevance of the modification of low grade inflammation in ageing (inflammageing) and the role of nutrition," *Ageing Research Reviews* 40 (2017): 95–119, doi:10.1016/j.arr.2017.09.001.

Cekanaviciute, E., Yoo, B. B., Runia, T. F., et al., "Gut bacteria from multiple sclerosis patients modulate human T cells and exacerbate symptoms in mouse models," *PNAS* 114 no. 40 (2017): 10713–18, doi:10.1073/pnas.1711235114.

Cervantes-Barragan, L., Chai, J. N., Tianero, M. D., et al., "Lactobacillus reuteri induces gut intraepithelial CD4+CD8 + T cells," *Science* 357, no. 6353 (2017): 806–10, doi:10.1126/science.aah5825.

Christovich, A., and Luo, X. M., "Gut Microbiota, Leaky Gut, and Autoimmune Diseases," *Frontiers in Immunology* 13 (2022): 946248, doi:10.3389/fimmu.2022.946248.

Conway, J., and Duggal, N. A., "Ageing of the gut microbiome: Potential influences on immune senescence and inflammageing," *Ageing Research Reviews* 68 (2021): 101323, doi:10.1016/j.arr.2021.101323.

Correale, J., Hohlfeld, R., and Baranzini, S. E., "The role of the gut microbiota in multiple sclerosis," *Nature Reviews Neurology* 18, no. 9 (2022): 544–58, doi:10.1038/s41582-022-00697-8.

Furusawa, Y., Obata, Y., Fukuda, S., et al., "Commensal microbe-derived butyrate induces the differentiation of colonic regulatory T cells," *Nature* 504, no. 7480 (2013): 446–50, doi:10.1038/nature12721.

Gill, N., and Finlay, B. B., "The gut microbiota: challenging immunology," *Nature Reviews Immunology* 11, no. 10 (2011): 636–37, doi:10.1038/nri3061.

Honda, K., and Littman, D. R., "The microbiota in adaptive immune homeostasis and disease," *Nature* 535, no. 7610 (2016): 75–84, doi:10.1038/nature18848.

Hong, S. H., "Influence of Microbiota on Vaccine Effectiveness: 'Is the Microbiota the Key to Vaccine-induced Responses?'," *Journal of Microbiology* 61, no. 5 (2023): 483–94, doi:10.1007/s12275-023-00044-6.

Hooper, L. V., Littman, D. R., and Macpherson, A. J., "Interactions between the microbiota and the immune system," *Science* 336, no. 6086 (2012): 1268–73, doi:10.1126/science.1223490.

Ivanov, I. I., Frutos Rde, L., Manel, N., et al., "Specific microbiota direct the differentiation of IL-17-producing T-helper cells in the mucosa of the small intestine," *Cell Host & Microbe* 4, no. 4 (2008): 337–49, doi:10.1016/j.chom.2008.09.009.

Kau, A. L., Ahern, P. P., Griffin, N. W., Goodman, A. L., and Gordon, J. I., "Human nutrition, the gut microbiome and the immune system," *Nature* 474, no. 7351 (2011): 327–36, doi:10.1038/nature10213.

Lambring, C. B., Siraj, S., Patel, K., Sankpal, U. T., Mathew, S., and Basha, R., "Impact of the microbiome on the immune system," *Critical Reviews in Immunology* 39, no. 5 (2019): 313–28, doi:10.1615/CritRevImmunol.2019033233.

Link, V. M., Subramanian, P., Cheung, F., et al., "Differential peripheral immune signatures elicited by vegan versus ketogenic diets in humans," *Nature Medicine* 30, no. 2 (2024): 560–72, doi:10.1038/s41591-023-02761-2.

Lynn, D. J., Benson, S. C., Lynn, M. A., and Pulendran, B., "Modulation of immune responses to vaccination by the microbiota: implications and potential mechanisms," *Nature Reviews Immunology* 22, no. 1 (2022): 33–46, doi:10.1038/s41577-021-00554-7.

Mazmanian, S. K., Liu, C. H., Tzianabos, A. O., and Kasper, D. L., "An immunomodulatory molecule of symbiotic bacteria directs maturation of the host immune system," *Cell* 122, no. 1 (2005): 107–18, doi:10.1016/j.cell.2005.05.007.

Miyauchi, E., Shimokawa, C., Steimle, A., Desai, M. S., and Ohno, H., "The impact of the gut microbiome on extra-intestinal autoimmune diseases," *Nature Reviews Immunology* 23, no. 1 (2023): 9–23, doi:10.1038/s41577-022-00727-y.

Pan, Q., Guo, F., Huang, Y., et al., "Gut Microbiota Dysbiosis in Systemic Lupus Erythematosus: Novel Insights into Mechanisms and Promising Therapeutic Strategies," *Frontiers in Immunology* 12 (2021): 799788, doi:10.3389/fimmu.2021.799788.

Postler, T. S., and Ghosh, S., "Understanding the Holobiont: How Microbial Metabolites Affect Human Health and Shape the Immune System," *Cell Metabolism* 26, no. 1 (2017): 110–30, doi:10.1016/j.cmet.2017.05.008.

Ragonnaud, E., and Biragyn, A., "Gut microbiota as the key controllers of 'healthy' aging of elderly people," *Immunity and Ageing* 18, no. 1 (2021): 2, doi:10.1186/s12979-020-00213-w.

Salazar, N., Arboleya, S., Valdés, L., et al., "The human intestinal microbiome at extreme ages of life. Dietary intervention as a way to counteract alterations," *Frontiers in Genetics* 5, no. 406 (2014), doi:10.3389/fgene.2014.00406.

Santoro, A., Zhao, J., Wu, L., Carru, C., Biagi, E., and Franceschi, C., "Microbiomes other than the gut: inflammaging and age-related diseases," *Seminars in Immunopathology* 42, no. 5 (2020): 589–605, doi:10.1007/s00281-020-00814-z.

Scher, J. U., Sczesnak, A., Longman, R. S., et al., "Expansion of intestinal Prevotella copri correlates with enhanced susceptibility to arthritis," *eLife* 2 (2013): e01202, doi:10.7554/eLife.01202.

Shaheen, W. A., Quraishi, M. N., and Iqbal, T. H., "Gut microbiome and autoimmune disorders," *Clinical and Experimental Immunology* 209, no. 2 (2022): 161–74, doi:10.1093/cei/uxac057.

Thevaranjan, N., Puchta, A., Schulz, C., et al., "Age-Associated Microbial Dysbiosis Promotes Intestinal Permeability, Systemic Inflammation, and Macrophage Dysfunction," *Cell Host & Microbe* 21, no. 4 (2017): 455–66.e4, doi:10.1016/j.chom.2017.03.002.

Tong, S., Zhang, P., Cheng, Q., et al., "The role of gut microbiota in gout: Is gut microbiota a potential target for gout treatment," *Frontiers in Cellular and Infection Microbiology* 12 (2022): 1051682, doi:10.3389/fcimb.2022.1051682.

Wastyk, H. C., Fragiadakis, G. K., Perelman, D., et al., "Gut-microbiota-targeted diets modulate human immune status," *Cell* 184, no. 16 (2021): 4137–53.e14, doi:10.1016/j.cell.2021.06.019.

Xu, Q., Ni, J. J., Han, B. X., et al., "Causal Relationship Between Gut Microbiota and Autoimmune Diseases: A Two-Sample Mendelian Randomization Study," *Frontiers in Immunology* 12 (2022): 746998, doi:10.3389/fimmu.2021.746998.

Zhang, L., Qing, P., Yang, H., et al., "Gut Microbiome and Metabolites in Systemic Lupus Erythematosus: Link, Mechanisms and Intervention," *Frontiers in Immunology* 12 (2021): 686501, doi:10.3389/fimmu.2021.686501.

Zheng, D., Liwinski, T., and Elinav, E., "Interaction between microbiota and immunity in health and disease," *Cell Research* 30, no. 6 (2020): 492–506, doi:10.1038/s41422-020-0332-7.

Zhong, D., Wu, C., Zeng, X., and Wang, Q., "The role of gut microbiota in the pathogenesis of rheumatic diseases," *Clinical Rheumatology* 37, no. 1 (2018): 25–34, doi:10.1007/s10067-017-3821-4.

Zimmermann, P., "The immunological interplay between vaccination and the intestinal microbiota," *npj Vaccines* 8, no. 1 (2023), doi:10.1038/s41541-023-00627-9.

4. MIND YOUR MICROBES: MICROBES AND THE BRAIN

Bojing, L., Fang, F., Pedersen N. L., et al., "Vagotomy and Parkinson disease," *Neurology* 88, no. 21 (2017): 1996–2002, doi:10.1212/WNL.0000000000003961.

Bosch, J., Nieuwdorp, M., Zwinderman, A., et al., "The gut microbiota and depressive symptoms across ethnic groups," *Nature Communications* 13, no. 1 (2022): 7129, doi10.1038/s41467-022-34504-1.

Chakrabarti, A., Geurts, L., Hoyles, L., et al., "The microbiota-gut-brain axis: pathways to better brain health. Perspectives on what we know, what we need to investigate and how to put knowledge into practice," *Cellular and Molecular Life Sciences* 79, no. 2 (2022): 80, doi:10.1007/s00018-021-04060-w.

Czarnik, W., Fularski, P., Gajewska, A., et al., "The Role of Intestinal Microbiota and Diet as Modulating Factors in the Course of Alzheimer's and Parkinson's Diseases," *Nutrients* 16, no. 2 (2024): 308, doi:10.3390/nu16020308.

"Dementia prevention, intervention, and care 2024," *Lancet Commission*, last modified July 31, 2024, thelancet.com/commissions/dementia-prevention-intervention-care.

Dohnalová, L., Lundgren, P., Carty, J. R. E., et al., "A microbiome-dependent gut-brain pathway regulates motivation for exercise," *Nature* 612, no. 7941 (2022): 739–47, doi:10.1038/s41586-022-05525-z.

Foster, J. A., and McVey Neufeld, K. A., "Gut-brain axis: how the microbiome influences anxiety and depression," *Trends in Neurosciences* 36, no. 5 (2013): 305–12, doi:10.1016/j.tins.2013.01.005.

Hsiao, E. Y., McBride, S. W., Hsien, S., et al., "Microbiota modulate behavioral and physiological abnormalities associated with neurodevelopmental disorders," *Cell* 155, no. 7 (2013): 1451–63, doi:10.1016/j.cell.2013.11.024.

Leone, V., Gibbons, S. M., Martinez, K., et al., "Effects of diurnal variation of gut microbes and high-fat feeding on host circadian clock function and metabolism," *Cell Host & Microbe* 17, no. 5 (2015): 681–89, doi:10.1016/j.chom.2015.03.006.

Lurie, I., Yang, Y. X., Haynes, K., Mamtani, R., and Boursi, B., "Antibiotic exposure and the risk for depression, anxiety, or psychosis: a nested case-control study," *The Journal of Clinical Psychiatry* 76, no. 11 (2015): 1522–28, doi:10.4088/JCP.15m09961.

Mayer, E. A., Nance, K., and Chen, S., "The Gut-Brain Axis," *Annual Review of Medicine* 73 (2022): 439–53, doi:10.1146/annurev-med-042320.

Mehta, R. S., Lochhead, P., Wang, Y., et al., "Association of midlife antibiotic use with subsequent cognitive function in women," *PLOS One* 17, no. 3 (2022): e0264649, doi:10.1371/journal.pone.0264649.

Messaoudi, M., Lalonde, R., Violle, N., et al., "Assessment of psychotropic-like properties of a probiotic formulation (Lactobacillus helveticus R0052 and Bifidobacterium longum R0175) in rats and human subjects," *The British Journal of Nutrition* 105 no. 5 (2011): 755–64, doi:10.1017/ S0007114510004319.

Metcalfe-Roach, A., Yu, A. C., Golz, E., et al., "MIND and Mediterranean Diets Associated with Later Onset of Parkinson's Disease," *Movement Disorders* 36, no. 4 (2021): 977–84, doi:10.1002/mds.28464.

Mohajeri, M., La Fata, G., Steinert, R., and Weber, P., "Relationship between the gut microbiome and brain function," *Nutrition Reviews* 76, no. 7 (2018): 481–96, doi:10.1093/nutrit/nuy009.

Morris, M. C., Tangney, C. C., Wang, Y., Sacks, F. M., Bennett, D. A., and Aggarwal, N. T., "MIND diet associated with reduced incidence of Alzheimer's disease," *Alzheimer's & Dementia: the Journal of the Alzheimer's Association* 11, no. 9 (2015): 1007–14, doi:10.1016/j.jalz.2014.11.009.

Naseribafrouei, A., Hestad, K., Avershina, E., et al., "Correlation between the human fecal microbiota and depression," *Neurogastroenterology and Motility* 26, no. 8 (2014): 1155–62, doi:10.1111/nmo.12378.

Needham, B. D., Funabashi, M., Adame, M. D., et al., "A gut-derived metabolite alters brain activity and anxiety behaviour in mice," *Nature* 602, no. 7898 (2022): 647–53, doi:10.1038/s41586-022-04396-8.

Radjabzadeh, D., Bosch, J. A., Uitterlinden, A. G., et al., "Gut microbiome-wide association study of depressive symptoms," *Nature Communications* 13, no. 1 (2022), doi:10.1038/s41467-022-34502-3.

Ritz, N. L., Brocka, M., Butler, M. I., et al., "Social anxiety disorder-associated gut microbiota increases social fear," *PNAS* 121, no. 1 (2024): e2308706120, doi:10.1073/pnas.2308706120.

Sampson, T. R., Debelius, J. W., Thron, T., et al., "Gut Microbiota Regulate Motor Deficits and Neuroinflammation in a Model of Parkinson's Disease," *Cell* 167, no. 6 (2016): 1469–80.e12, doi:10.1016/j.cell.2016.11.018.

Sampson, T. R., and Mazmanian, S. K., "Control of brain development, function, and behavior by the microbiome," *Cell Host & Microbe* 17, no. 5 (2015): 565–76, doi:10.1016/j.chom.2015.04.011.

Simpson, C. A., Schwartz, O. S., and Simmons, J. G., "The human gut microbiota and depression: widely reviewed, yet poorly understood," *Journal of Affective Disorders* 274 (2020): 73–75, doi:10.1016/j.jad.2020.05.115.

Svensson, E., Horváth-Puhó, E., Thomsen, R. W., et al., "Vagotomy and subsequent risk of Parkinson's disease," *Annals of Neurology* 78, no. 4 (2015): 522–29, doi:10.1002/ana.24448.

Thaiss, C. A., Zeevi, D., Levy, M., et al., "Transkingdom control of microbiota diurnal oscillations promotes metabolic homeostasis," *Cell* 159, no. 3 (2014): 514–29, doi:10.1016/j. cell.2014.09.048.

Tooley, K. L., "Effects of the human gut microbiota on cognitive performance, brain structure and function: A narrative review," *Nutrients* 12, no. 10 (2020): 3009, doi:10.3390/nu12103009.

van Soest, A. P., Beers, S., van de Rest, O., and de Groot, L. C., "The Mediterranean-Dietary Approaches to Stop Hypertension Intervention for Neurodegenerative Delay (MIND) Diet for the Aging Brain: A Systematic Review," *Advances in Nutrition* 15, no. 3 (2024): 100184, doi:10.1016/j.advnut.2024.100184.

Vogt, N. M., Kerby, R. L., Dill-McFarland, K. A., et al., "Gut microbiome alterations in Alzheimer's disease," *Scientific Reports* 7, no. 1 (2017): 13537, doi:10.1038/s41598-017-13601-y.

Wang, D., Ho, L., Faith, J., et al., "Role of intestinal microbiota in the generation of polyphenol-derived phenolic acid mediated attenuation of Alzheimer's disease -amyloid oligomerization," *Molecular Nutrition & Food Research* 59, no. 6 (2015): 1025–40, doi:10.1002/mnfr.201400544.

5. YOUR MICROBES ARE GLOWING: THE SKIN MICROBIOME

Bouslimani, A., da Silva, R., Kosciolek, T., et al., "The impact of skin care products on skin chemistry and microbiome dynamics," *BMC Biology* 17, no. 1 (2019): 47, doi:10.1186/s12915-019-0660-6.

Grice, E. A., and Segre, J. A., "The skin microbiome," *Nature Reviews Microbiology* 9, no. 4 (2011): 244–53, doi:10.1038/nrmicro2537.

Gueniche, A. G., and Bastien, P., "Oral supplementation with probiotic Lactobacillus paracasei st11 improves dandruff condition," presented at the ESDR Annual Meeting, 2009.

Ito, Y., & Amagai, M., "Controlling skin microbiome as a new bacteriotherapy for inflammatory skin diseases," *Inflammation and Regeneration* 42, no. 1 (2022): 26, doi:10.1186/s41232-022-00212-y.

Knödlseder, N., Fábrega, M. J., Santos-Moreno, J., et al., "Delivery of a sebum modulator by an engineered skin microbe in mice," *Nature Biotechnology* 42, no. 11 (2024): 1661–66, doi:10.1038/s41587-023-02072-4.

Lax, S., Hampton-Marcell, J. T., Gibbons, S. M., et al., "Forensic analysis of the microbiome of phones and shoes," *Microbiome* 3, no. 21 (2015), doi:10.1186/s40168-015-0082-9.

Lee, D. E., Huh, C. S., Ra, J., et al., "Clinical Evidence of Effects of Lactobacillus plantarum HY7714 on Skin Aging: A Randomized, Double Blind, Placebo-Controlled Study," *Journal of Microbiology and Biotechnology* 25, no. 12 (2015): 2160–68, doi:10.4014/jmb.1509.09021.

Levkovich, T., Poutahidis, T., Smillie, C., et al., "Probiotic bacteria induce a 'glow of health,'" *PLOS One* 8, no. 1 (2013): e53867, doi:10.1371/journal.pone.0053867.

Nakatsuji, T., Chen, T., Narala, S., et al., "Antimicrobials from human skin commensal bacteria protect against Staphylococcus aureus and are deficient in atopic dermatitis," *Science Translational Medicine* 9, no. 378 (2017): eaah4680, doi:10.1126/scitranslmed.aah4680.

Nodake, Y., Matsumoto, S., Miura, R., et al., "Pilot study on novel skin care method by augmentation with Staphylococcus epidermidis, an autologous skin microbe–A blinded randomized clinical trial," *Journal of Dermatological Science* 79, no. 2 (2015): 119–26, doi:10.1016/j.jdermsci.2015.05.001.

Oh, J., Byrd, A. L., Park, M., Kong, H. H., and Segre, J. A., "Temporal Stability of the Human Skin Microbiome," *Cell* 165, no. 4 (2016): 854–66, doi:10.1016/j.cell.2016.04.008.

Rozas, M., de Ruijter, A. H., Fabrega, M. J., et al., "From dysbiosis to healthy skin: Major contributions of Cutibacterium acnes to skin homeostasis," *Microorganisms* 9, no. 3 (2021): 628, doi:10.3390/microorganisms9030628.

Salem, I., Ramser, A., Isham, N., and Ghannoum, M. A., "The gut microbiome as a major regulator of the gut-skin axis," *Frontiers in Microbiology* 9 (2018): 1459, doi:10.3389/fmicb.2018.01459.

Sfriso, R., Egert, M., Gempeler, M., Voegeli, R., and Campiche, R., "Revealing the secret life of skin–with the microbiome you never walk alone," *International Journal of Cosmetic Science* 42, no. 2 (2020): 116–26, doi:10.1111/ics.12594.

Shin, H., Price, K., Albert, L., Dodick, J., Park, L., and Dominguez-Bello, M. G., "Changes in the Eye Microbiota Associated with Contact Lens Wearing," *mBio* 7, no. 2 (2016): e00198, doi:10.1128/mBio.00198-16.

Yu, Y., Dunaway, S., Champer, J., Kim, J., and Alikhan, A., "Changing our microbiome: probiotics in dermatology," *British Journal of Dermatology* 182, no. 1 (2020): 39–46, doi:10.1111/bjd.18088.

6. HEALTHY SMILE, HEALTHY YOU: THE ORAL MICROBIOME

Adams, S., Arnold, D., Murphy, B., et al., "A randomised clinical study to determine the effect of a toothpaste containing enzymes and proteins on plaque oral microbiome ecology," *Scientific Reports* 7 (2017): 43344, doi:10.1038/srep43344.

Baker, J. L., Mark Welch, J. L., Kauffman, K. M., McLean, J. S., and He, X., "The oral microbiome: diversity, biogeography and human health," *Nature Reviews Microbiology* 22, no. 2 (2024): 89–104, doi:10.1038/s41579-023-00963-6.

Curtis, M. A., Zenobia, C., and Darveau, R. P., "The relationship of the oral microbiota to periodontal health and disease," *Cell Host & Microbe* 10, no. 4 (2011): 302–6, doi:10.1016/j.chom.2011.09.008.

Gao, L., Xu, T., Huang, G., Jiang, S., Gu, Y., and Chen, F., "Oral microbiomes: more and more importance in oral cavity and whole body," *Protein and Cell* 9, no. 5 (2018): 488–500, doi:10.1007/s13238-018-0548-1.

Huang, X., Huang, X., Huang, Y., et al., "The oral microbiome in autoimmune diseases: friend or foe?," *Journal of Translational Medicine* 21, no. 1 (2023): 211, doi:10.1186/s12967-023-03995-x.

Li, X., Liu, Y., Yang, X., Li, C., and Song, Z., "The Oral Microbiota: Community Composition, Influencing Factors, Pathogenesis, and Interventions," *Frontiers in Microbiology* 13 (2022): 895537, doi:10.3389/fmicb.2022.895537.

Matayoshi, S., Tojo, F., Suehiro, Y., et al., "Effects of mouthwash on periodontal pathogens and glycemic control in patients with type 2 diabetes mellitus," *Scientific Reports* 14, no. 2777 (2024), doi:10.1038/s41598-024-53213-x.

Shoemark, D. K., and Allen, S. J., "The microbiome and disease: reviewing the links between the oral microbiome, aging, and Alzheimer's disease," *Journal of Alzheimer's Disease* 43, no. 3 (2015): 725–38, doi:10.3233/JAD-141170.

Spatafora, G., Li, Y., He, X., Cowan, A., and Tanner, A. C. R., "The Evolving Microbiome of Dental Caries," *Microorganisms* 12, no. 1 (2024): 121, doi:10.3390/microorganisms12010121.

Thomas, S. C., Xu, F., Pushalkar, S., et al., "Electronic Cigarette Use Promotes a Unique Periodontal Microbiome," *mBio* 13, no. 1 (2022), doi.org/10.1128/mbio.00075-22.

Wade, W. G., "The oral microbiome in health and disease," *Pharmacological Research* 69, no. 1 (2013): 137–43, doi:10.1016/j.phrs.2012.11.006.

Weyrich, L. S., Dobney, K., and Cooper, A., "Ancient DNA analysis of dental calculus," *Journal of Human Evolution* 79 (2015): 119–24, doi:10.1016/j.jhevol.2014.06.018.

Zarco, M. F., Vess, T. J., and Ginsburg, G. S., "The oral microbiome in health and disease and the potential impact on personalized dental medicine," *Oral Diseases* 18, no. 2 (2012): 109–20, doi:10.1111/j.1601-0825.2011.01851.

7. LOVE BUGS: THE HEART AND THE MICROBIOME

Al Hamdani, A., and Targett, S., "Sedentary Lifestyle: An Alarming Epidemic," *Aspetar Sports Medicine Journal* 5, no. 1 (2016).

Al Samarraie, A., Pichette, M., and Rousseau, G., "Role of the Gut Microbiome in the Development of Atherosclerotic Cardiovascular Disease," *International Journal of Molecular Sciences* 24, no. 6 (2023): 5420, doi:10.3390/ijms24065420.

Bala, S., Marcos, M., Gattu, A., Catalano, D., and Szabo, G., "Acute binge drinking increases serum endotoxin and bacterial DNA levels in healthy individuals," *PLOS One* 9, no. 5 (2014): e96864, doi:10.1371/journal.pone.0096864.

Boytar, A. N., Skinner, T. L., Wallen, R. E., Jenkins, D. G., and Dekker Nitert, M., "The Effect of Exercise Prescription on the Human Gut Microbiota and Comparison between Clinical and Apparently Healthy Populations: A Systematic Review," *Nutrients* 15, no. 6 (2023): 1534, doi:10.3390/nu15061534.

Chen, M. L., Yi, L., Zhang, Y., et al., "Resveratrol Attenuates Trimethylamine-N-Oxide (TMAO)-Induced Atherosclerosis by Regulating TMAO Synthesis and Bile Acid Metabolism via Remodeling of the Gut Microbiota," *mBio* 7, no. 2 (2016): e02210-15, doi:10.1128/mBio.02210-15.

Clarke, S. F., Murphy, E. F., O'Sullivan, O., et al., "Exercise and associated dietary extremes impact on gut microbial diversity," *Gut* 63, no. 12 (2014): 1913–20, doi:10.1136/gutjnl-2013-306541.

Clauss, M., Gérard, P., Mosca, A., and Leclerc, M., "Interplay Between Exercise and Gut Microbiome in the Context of Human Health and Performance," *Frontiers in Nutrition* 8 (2021): 637010, doi:10.3389/fnut.2021.637010.

Dohnalová, L., Lundgren, P., Carty, J. R. E., et al., "A microbiome-dependent gut-brain pathway regulates motivation for exercise," *Nature* 612, no. 7941 (2022): 739–47, doi:10.1038/s41586-022-05525-z.

"The Facts on Fats Infographic," American Heart Association, accessed 2024, healthyforgood.heart.org/eat-smart/infographics/the-facts-on-fats.

Gregory, J. C., Buffa, J. A., Org, E., et al., "Transmission of atherosclerosis susceptibility with gut microbial transplantation," *The Journal of Biological Chemistry* 290, no. 9 (2015): 5647–60, doi:10.1074/ jbc.M114.618249.

Koeth, R. A., Wang, Z., Levison, B. S., et al., "Intestinal microbiota metabolism of L-carnitine, a nutrient in red meat, promotes atherosclerosis," *Nature Medicine* 19, no. 5 (2013): 576–85, doi:10.1038/nm.3145.

Li, Y., Fu, R., Li, R., et al., "Causality of gut microbiome and hypertension: A bidirectional mendelian randomization study," *Frontiers in Cardiovascular Medicine* 10 (2023): 1167346, doi:10.3389/fcvm.2023.1167346.

Longoria, C. R., Guers, J. J., and Campbell, S. C., "The Interplay between Cardiovascular Disease, Exercise, and the Gut Microbiome," *Reviews in Cardiovascular Medicine* 23, no. 11 (2022): 365, doi:10.31083/j.rcm2311365.

Masenga, S. K., Hamooya, B., Hangoma, J., et al., "Recent advances in modulation of cardiovascular diseases by the gut microbiota," *Journal of Human Hypertension* 36, no. 11 (2022): 952–59, doi:10.1038/s41371-022-00698-6.

Nesci, A., Carnuccio, C., Ruggieri, V., et al., "Gut Microbiota and Cardiovascular Disease: Evidence on the Metabolic and Inflammatory Background of a Complex Relationship," *International Journal of Molecular Sciences* 24, no. 10 (2023): 9087, doi:10.3390/ijms24109087.

O'Donnell, J. A., Zheng, T., Meric, G., and Marques, F. Z., "The gut microbiome and hypertension," *Nature Reviews Nephrology* 19, no. 3 (2023): 153–67, doi:10.1038/s41581-022-00654-0.

Pavlidou, E., Fasoulas, A., Mantzorou, M., and Giaginis, C., "Clinical Evidence on the Potential Beneficial Effects of Probiotics and Prebiotics in Cardiovascular Disease," *International Journal of Molecular Sciences* 23, no. 24 (2022): 15898, doi:10.3390/ijms232415898.

Prins, F. M., Collij, V., Groot, H. E., et al., "The gut microbiome across the cardiovascular risk spectrum," *European Journal of Preventive Cardiology* 31, no. 8 (2024): 935–44, doi:10.1093/eurjpc/zwad377.

Rahman, M. M., Islam, F., -Or-Rashid, M. H., et al., "The Gut Microbiota (Microbiome) in Cardiovascular Disease and Its Therapeutic Regulation," *Frontiers in Cellular and Infection Microbiology* 12 (2022): 903570, doi:10.3389/fcimb.2022.903570.

Shah, S., Mu, C., Moossavi, S., et al., "Physical activity-induced alterations of the gut microbiota are BMI dependent," *FASEB Journal* 37, no. 4 (2023): e22882, doi:10.1096/fj.202201571R.

Singh, P., Meenatchi, R., Ahmed, Z. H. T., et al., "Implications of the gut microbiome in cardiovascular diseases: Association of gut microbiome with cardiovascular diseases, therapeutic interventions and multi-omics approach for precision medicine," *Medicine in Microecology* 19 (2024): 100096, doi:10.1016/j.medmic.2023.100096.

Song, J. S., Kim, J. O. R., Yoon, S. M., Kwon, M.-J., and Ki, C.-S., "The association between gut microbiome and hypertension varies according to enterotypes: a Korean study," *Frontiers in Microbiomes* 2 (2023), doi:10.3389/frmbi.2023.1072059.

Teicholz, N., *The Big Fat Surprise: Why Butter, Meat and Cheese Belong in a Healthy Diet* (Simon & Schuster, 2014).

Tokarek, J., Budny, E., Saar, M., et al., "Does the Composition of Gut Microbiota Affect Hypertension? Molecular Mechanisms Involved in Increasing Blood Pressure," *International Journal of Molecular Sciences* 24, no. 2 (2023): 1377, doi:10.3390/ijms24021377.

Tonelli, A., Lumngwena, E. N., and Ntusi, N. A. B., "The oral microbiome in the pathophysiology of cardiovascular disease," *Nature Reviews Cardiology* 20, no. 6 (2023): 386–403, doi:10.1038/s41569-022-00825-3.

Wang, Z., Roberts, A. B., Buffa, J. A., et al., "Non-lethal Inhibition of Gut Microbial Trimethylamine Production for the Treatment of Atherosclerosis," *Cell* 163, no. 7 (2015): 1585–95, doi:10.1016/j.cell.2015.11.055.

Yan, D., Sun, Y., Zhou, X., et al., "Regulatory effect of gut microbes on blood pressure," *Animal Models and Experimental Medicine* 5, no. 6 (2022): 513–31, doi:10.1002/ame2.12233

Zhu, W., Gregory, J. C., Org, E., et al., "Gut Microbial Metabolite TMAO Enhances Platelet Hyperreactivity and Thrombosis Risk," *Cell* 165, no. 1 (2016): 111–24, doi:10.1016/j.cell.2016.02.011.

8. TAKE A DEEP BREATH: THE LUNG MICROBIOME

Belizário, J., Garay-Malpartida, M., and Faintuch, J., "Lung microbiome and origins of the respiratory diseases," *Current Research in Immunology* 4 (2023): 100065, doi:10.1016/j.crimmu.2023.100065.

Bowdish, D. M. E., Rossi, L., Loeb, M., et al., "The impact of respiratory infections and probiotic use on the nasal microbiota of frail residents in long-term care homes," *ERJ Open Research* 9, no. 5 (2023): 00212-2023, doi:10.1183/23120541.00212-2023.

Cruz, C. S., Ricci, M. F., and Vieira, A. T., "Gut Microbiota Modulation as a Potential Target for the Treatment of Lung Infections," *Frontiers in Pharmacology* 12 (2021): 724033, doi:10.3389/fphar.2021.724033.

Dickson, R. P., Martinez, F. J., and Huffnagle, G. B., "The role of the microbiome in exacerbations of chronic lung diseases," *Lancet* 384, no. 9944 (2014): 691–702, doi:10.1016/ S0140-6736(14)61136-3.

Faner, R., Sibila, O., Agustí, A., et al., "The microbiome in respiratory medicine: current challenges and future perspectives," *The European Respiratory Journal* 49, no. 4 (2017): 1602086, doi:10.1183/13993003.02086-2016.

Hufnagl, K., Pali-Schöll, I., Roth-Walter, F., and Jensen-Jarolim, E., "Dysbiosis of the gut and lung microbiome has a role in asthma," *Seminars in Immunopathology* 42, no. 1 (2020): 75–93, doi:10.1007/s00281-019-00775-y.

Li, R., Li, J., and Zhou, X., "Lung microbiome: new insights into the pathogenesis of respiratory diseases," *Signal Transduction and Targeted Therapy* 9, no. 1 (2024), doi:10.1038/s41392-023-01722-y.

Li, Z., Li, Y., Sun, Q., et al., "Targeting the Pulmonary Microbiota to Fight against Respiratory Diseases," *Cells* 11, no. 5 (2022): 916, doi:10.3390/cells11050916.

Natalini, J. G., Singh, S., and Segal, L. N., "The dynamic lung microbiome in health and disease," *Nature Reviews Microbiology* 21, no. 4 (2023): 222–35, doi:10.1038/ s41579-022-00821-x.

Pettigrew, M. M., Tanner, W., and Harris, A. D., "The lung microbiome and pneumonia," *Journal of Infectious Diseases* 223 (2021): S241–S245, doi:10.1093/ infdis/jiaa702.

Segal, L. N., and Blaser, M. J., "A brave new world: the lung microbiota in an era of change," *Annals of the American Thoracic Society* 11, Suppl. 1 (2014): S21–27, doi:10.1513/AnnalsATS.201306-189MG.

Shi, C. Y., Yu, C. H., Yu, W. Y., and Ying, H. Z., "Gut-Lung Microbiota in Chronic Pulmonary Diseases: Evolution, Pathogenesis, and Therapeutics," *Canadian Journal of Infectious Diseases and Medical Microbiology* 2021 (2021): 9278441, doi:10.1155/2021/9278441.

Sze, M. A., Dimitriu, P. A., Suzuki, M., et al., "Host Response to the Lung Microbiome in Chronic Obstructive Pulmonary Disease," *American Journal of Respiratory and Critical Care Medicine* 192, no. 4 (2015): 438–45, doi:10.1164/rccm.201502-0223OC.

Wenger, N. M., Qiao, L., Nicola, T., et al., "Clinical trial of a probiotic and herbal supplement for lung health," *Frontiers in Nutrition* 10 (2023): 1168582, doi:10.3389/fnut.2023.1168582.

Whiteside, S. A., McGinniss, J. E., and Collman, R. G., "The lung microbiome: Progress and promise," *Journal of Clinical Investigation* 131, no. 15 (2021): e150473, doi:10.1172/JCI150473.

Yagi, K., Huffnagle, G. B., Lukacs, N. W., and Asai, N., "The lung microbiome during health and disease," *International Journal of Molecular Sciences* 22, no. 19 (2021): 10872, doi:10.3390/ijms221910872.

Yi, X., Gao, J., and Wang, Z., "The human lung microbiome–A hidden link between microbes and human health and diseases," *iMeta* 1, no. 3 (2022): e33, doi:10.1002/imt2.33.

Yuksel, N., Gelmez, B., and Yildiz-Pekoz, A., "Lung Microbiota: Its Relationship to Respiratory System Diseases and Approaches for Lung-Targeted Probiotic Bacteria Delivery," *Molecular Pharmaceutics* 20, no. 7 (2023): 3320–37, doi:10.1021/acs.molpharmaceut.3c00323.

9. BELLY BUGS: THE STOMACH MICROBIOME

Chen, Z., Tang, Z., Li, W., et al., "Weizmannia coagulans BCF-01: a novel gastrogenic probiotic for Helicobacter pylori infection control," *Gut Microbes* 16, no. 1 (2024): 2313770, doi:10.1080/19490976.2024.2313770.

Homan, M., and Orel, R., "Are probiotics useful in Helicobacter pylori eradication?," *World Journal of Gastroenterology* 21, no. 37 (2015): 10644–53, doi:10.3748/wjg.v21.i37.10644.

Jackson, M. A., Goodrich, J. K., Maxan, M. E., et al., "Proton pump inhibitors alter the composition of the gut microbiota," *Gut* 65, no. 5 (2016): 749–56, doi:10.1136/gutjnl-2015-310861.

Kiecka, A., and Szczepanik, M., "Proton pump inhibitor-induced gut dysbiosis and immunomodulation: current knowledge and potential restoration by probiotics," *Pharmacological Reports* 75, no. 4 (2023): 791–804, doi:10.1007/s43440-023-00489-x.

Kienesberger, S., Cox, L. M., Livanos, A., et al., "Gastric Helicobacter pylori Infection Affects Local and Distant Microbial Populations and Host Responses," *Cell Reports* 14, no. 6 (2016): 1395–1407, doi:10.1016/j.celrep.2016.01.017.

Koga, Y., "Microbiota in the stomach and application of probiotics to gastroduodenal diseases," *World Journal of Gastroenterology* 28, no. 47 (2022): 6702–15, doi:10.3748/wjg.v28.i47.6702.

Liu, D., Zhang, R., Chen, S., Sun, B., and Zhang, K., "Analysis of gastric microbiome reveals three distinctive microbial communities associated with the occurrence of gastric cancer," *BMC Microbiology* 22, no. 1 (2022): 184, doi:10.1186/s12866-022-02594-y.

Minoretti, P., Liaño Riera, M., Santiago Sáez, A., Gómez Serrano, M., and García Martín, Á., "Probiotic Supplementation With Saccharomyces boulardii and Enterococcus faecium Improves Gastric Pain and Bloating in Airline Pilots with Chronic Non-atrophic Gastritis: An Open-Label Study," *Cureus* 16, no. 1 (2024): e52502, doi:10.7759/cureus.52502.

Peng, R., Zhang, Z., Qu, Y., and Chen, W., "The impact of Helicobacter pylori eradication with vonoprazan-amoxicillin dual therapy combined with probiotics on oral microbiota: a randomized double-blind placebo-controlled trial," *Frontiers in Microbiology* 14 (2023): 1273709, doi:10.3389/fmicb.2023.1273709.

Wang, Y., Han, W., Wang, N., et al., "The role of microbiota in the development and treatment of gastric cancer," *Frontiers in Oncology* 13 (2023): 1224669, doi:10.3389/fonc.2023.1224669.

Wen, J., Lau, H. C. H., Peppelenbosch, M., and Yu, J., "Gastric microbiota beyond H. Pylori: An emerging critical character in gastric carcinogenesis," *Biomedicines* 9, no. 11 (2021): 1680, doi:10.3390/biomedicines9111680.

Yang, I., Nell, S., and Suerbaum, S., "Survival in hostile territory: the microbiota of the stomach," *FEMS Microbiology Reviews* 37, no. 5 (2013): 736–61, doi:10.1111/1574-6976.12027.

Yang, I., Woltemate, S., Piazuelo, M. B., et al., "Different gastric microbiota compositions in two human populations with high and low gastric cancer risk in Colombia," *Scientific Reports* 6, (2016): 18594, doi:10.1038/srep18594.

Yang, J., Zhou, X., Liu, X., Ling, Z., and Ji, F., "Role of the Gastric Microbiome in Gastric Cancer: From Carcinogenesis to Treatment," *Frontiers in Microbiology* 12 (2021): 641322, doi:10.3389/fmicb.2021.641322.

Zhou, S., Li, C., Liu, L., et al., "Gastric microbiota: an emerging player in gastric cancer," *Frontiers in Microbiology* 14 (2023): 1130001, doi:10.3389/fmicb.2023.1130001.

10. MICROBES DOWN UNDER: THE UROGENITAL TRACT MICROBIOME

Baker, J. M., Al-Nakkash, L., and Herbst-Kralovetz, M. M., "Estrogen-gut microbiome axis: Physiological and clinical implications," *Maturitas* 103 (2017): 45–53, doi:10.1016/j.maturitas.2017.06.025.

Chen, X., Lu, Y., Chen, T., and Li, R., "The Female Vaginal Microbiome in Health and Bacterial Vaginosis," *Frontiers in Cellular and Infection Microbiology* 11 (2021), doi:10.3389/fcimb.2021.631972.

Günther, V., Allahqoli, L., Watrowski, R., et al., "Vaginal Microbiome in Reproductive Medicine," *Diagnostics* 12, no. 8 (2022): 1948, doi:10.3390/diagnostics12081948.

Hall, B., Levy, S., Dufault-Thompson, K., et al., "BilR is a gut microbial enzyme that reduces bilirubin to urobilinogen," *Nature Microbiology* 9, no. 1 (2024): 173–84, doi:10.1038/s41564-023-01549-x.

Koebele, S., and Bimonte-Nelson, H., "Modeling menopause: The utility of rodents in translational behavioral endocrinology research," *Maturitas* 87 (2016): 5–17, doi:10.1016/j.maturitas.2016.01.015.

Lebeer, S., Ahannach, S., Gehrmann, T., et al., "A citizen-science-enabled catalogue of the vaginal microbiome and associated factors," *Nature Microbiology* 8, no. 1 (2023): 2183–95, doi:10.1038/s41564-023-01500-0.

Lehtoranta, L., Ala-Jaakkola, R., Laitila, A., and Maukonen, J. "Healthy Vaginal Microbiota and Influence of Probiotics Across the Female Life Span," *Frontiers in Microbiology* 13 (2022), doi:10.3389/fmicb.2022.819958.

Lev-Sagie, A., Goldman-Wohl, D., Cohen, Y., et al., "Vaginal microbiome transplantation in women with intractable bacterial vaginosis," *Nature Medicine* 25, no. 10 (2019): 1500–4, doi:10.1038/s41591-019-0600-6.

Lewis, F. M. T., Bernstein, K. T., and Aral, S. O., "Vaginal microbiome and its relationship to behavior, sexual health, and sexually transmitted diseases," *Obstetrics and Gynecology* 129, no. 4 (2017): 643–54, doi:10.1097/AOG.0000000000001932.

Lledo, B., Fuentes, A., Lozano, F. M., et al., "Identification of vaginal microbiome associated with IVF pregnancy," *Scientific Reports* 12, no. 1 (2022): 6807, doi:10.1038/s41598-022-10933-2.

Ma, B., Forney, L. J., and Ravel, J., "Vaginal microbiome: rethinking health and disease," *Annual Review of Microbiology* 66 (2012): 371–89, doi:10.1146/annurev-micro-092611-150157.

Ma, Z., "Microbiome Transmission During Sexual Intercourse Appears Stochastic and Supports the Red Queen Hypothesis," *Frontiers in Microbiology* 12 (2022): 789983, doi:10.3389/fmicb.2021.789983.

Martin, D. H., "The microbiota of the vagina and its influence on women's health and disease," *The American Journal of the Medical Sciences* 343, no. 1 (2012): 2–9, doi:10.1097/MAJ.0b013e31823ea228.

Martinelli, S., Nannini, G., Cianchi, F., Staderini, F., Coratti, F., and Amedei, A., "Microbiota Transplant and Gynecological Disorders: The Bridge Between Present and Future Treatments," *Microorganisms* 11, no. 10 (2023): 2407, doi:10.3390/microorganisms11102407.

Mayer, B. T., Srinivasan, S., Fiedler, T. L., Marrazzo, J. M., Fredricks, D. N., and Schiffer, J. T., "Rapid and profound shifts in the vaginal microbiota following antibiotic treatment for bacterial vaginosis," *Journal of Infectious Diseases* 212, no. 5 (2015): 793–802, doi:10.1093/infdis/jiv079.

Muhleisen, A. L., and Herbst-Kralovetz, M. M., "Menopause and the vaginal microbiome," *Maturitas* 91 (2016): 42–50, doi:10.1016/j.maturitas.2016.05.015.

Osadchiy, V., Belarmino, A., Kianian, R., et al., "Semen microbiota are dramatically altered in men with abnormal sperm parameters," *Scientific Reports* 14, no. 1 (2024): 1068, doi:10.1038/s41598-024-51686-4.

Park, M. G., Cho, S., and Oh, M. M., "Menopausal Changes in the Microbiome–A Review Focused on the Genitourinary Microbiome," *Diagnostics* 13, no. 6 (2023): 1193, doi:10.3390/diagnostics13061193.

Plummer, E. L., Vodstrcil, L. A., Fairley, C. K., et al., "Sexual practices have a significant impact on the vaginal microbiota of women who have sex with women," *Scientific Reports* 9, no. 1 (2019): 19749, doi:10.1038/s41598-019-55929-7.

Qi, X., Yun, C., Pang, Y., and Qiao, J., "The impact of the gut microbiota on the reproductive and metabolic endocrine system," *Gut Microbes* 13, no. 1 (2021): 1–21, doi:10.1080/19490976.2021.1894070.

Schröder, W., Sommer, H., Gladstone, B. P., et al., "Gender differences in antibiotic prescribing in the community: a systematic review and meta-analysis," *The Journal of Antimicrobial Chemotherapy* 71, no. 7 (2016): 1800–6, doi:10.1093/jac/dkw054.

Schwenger, E. M., Tejani, A. M., and Loewen, P. S., "Probiotics for preventing urinary tract infections in adults and children," *The Cochrane Database of Systematic Reviews* 12 (2015), doi:10.1002/14651858.CD008772.pub2.

Sharma, M., Chopra, C., Mehta, M., et al., "An insight into vaginal microbiome techniques," *Life* 11, no. 11 (2021): 1229, doi:10.3390/life11111229.

Shen, J., Song, N., Williams, C. J., et al., "Effects of low dose estrogen therapy on the vaginal microbiomes of women with atrophic vaginitis," *Scientific Reports* 6, (2016): 24380, doi:10.1038/srep24380.

Thomas-White, K., Brady, M., Wolfe, A. J., and Mueller, E. R., "The bladder is not sterile: History and current discoveries on the urinary microbiome," *Current Bladder Dysfunction Reports* 11, no. 1 (2016): 18–24, doi:10.1007/s11884-016-0345-8.

Thunander Sundbom, L., Bingefors, K., Hedborg, K., and Isacson, D., "Are men under-treated and women over-treated with antidepressants? Findings from a cross-sectional survey in Sweden," *BJPsych Bulletin* 41 no. 3 (2017): 145–50, doi:10.1192/pb.bp.116.054270.

Tuddenham, S., Ghanem, K. G., Caulfield, L. E., et al., "Associations between dietary micronutrient intake and molecular-Bacterial Vaginosis," *Reproductive Health* 16, no. 1 (2019): 151, doi:10.1186/s12978-019-0814-6.

Tuniyazi, M., and Zhang, N., "Possible Therapeutic Mechanisms and Future Perspectives of Vaginal Microbiota Transplantation," *Microorganisms* 11, no. 6 (2023): 1427, doi:10.3390/microorganisms11061427.

Vitale, S. G., Ferrari, F., Ciebiera, M., et al., "The role of genital tract microbiome in fertility: A systematic review," *International Journal of Molecular Sciences* 23, no. 1 (2022): 180, doi:10.3390/ijms23010180.

Wrønding, T., Vomstein, K., Bosma, E. F., et al., "Antibiotic-free vaginal microbiota transplant with donor engraftment, dysbiosis resolution and live birth after recurrent pregnancy loss: a proof of concept case study," *eClinicalMedicine* 61 (2023): 102070, doi:10.1016/j.eclinm.2023.102070.

Yockey, L. J., Hussain, F. A., Bergerat, A., et al., "Screening and characterization of vaginal fluid donations for vaginal microbiota transplantation," *Scientific Reports* 12, no. 1 (2022): 17948, doi:10.1038/s41598-022-22873-y.

Younes, J. A., Lievens, E., Hummelen, R., van der Westen, R., Reid, G., and Petrova, M. I., "Women and Their Microbes: The Unexpected Friendship," *Trends in Microbiology* 26, no. 1 (2018): 16–32, doi:10.1016/j.tim.2017.07.008.

11. FLEX YOUR MICROBES: THE MUSCULOSKELETAL SYSTEM

Allen, J. M., Mailing, L. J., Niemiro, G. M., et al., "Exercise Alters Gut Microbiota Composition and Function in Lean and Obese Humans," *Medicine and Science in Sports and Exercise* 50, no. 4 (2018): 747–57, doi:10.1249/MSS.0000000000001495.

Bressa, C., Bailen-Andrino, M., Perez-Santiago, J., et al., "Differences in gut microbiota profile between women with active lifestyle and sedentary women," *PLOS One* 12, no. 2 (2017): e0171352, doi:10.1371/journal.pone.0171352.

Castaneda, M., Strong, J. M., Alabi, D. A., and Hernandez, C. J., "The Gut Microbiome and Bone Strength," *Current Osteoporosis Reports* 18, no. 6 (2020): 677–83, doi:10.1007/s11914-020-00627-x.

Choi, N., Choi, B., DiNitto, D., et al., "Fall-related emergency department visits and hospitalizations among community-dwelling older adults: examination of health problems and injury characteristics," *BMC Geriatrics* 19, no. 1 (2019): 303, doi:10.1186/s12877-019-1329-2.

Claesson, M. J., Jeffery, I. B., Conde, S., et al., "Gut microbiota composition correlates with diet and health in the elderly," *Nature* 488, no. 7410 (2012): 178–84, doi:10.1038/nature11319.

Cooney, O. D., Nagareddy, P. R., Murphy, A. J., and Lee, M. K. S., "Healthy Gut, Healthy Bones: Targeting the Gut Microbiome to Promote Bone Health," *Frontiers in Endocrinology* 11 (2021), doi:10.3389/fendo.2020.620466.

Cronin, O., Lanham-New, S. A., Corfe, B. M., et al., "Role of the Microbiome in Regulating Bone Metabolism and Susceptibility to Osteoporosis," *Calcified Tissue International* 110, no. 3 (2022): 273–84, doi:10.1007/s00223-021-00924-2.

Das, M., Cronin, O., Keohane, D., et al., "Gut microbiota alterations associated with reduced bone mineral density in older adults," *Rheumatology* 58, no. 12 (2019): 2295–304, doi:10.1093/rheumatology/kez302.

Duffuler, P., Bhullar, K. S., and Wu, J., "Targeting gut microbiota in osteoporosis: impact of the microbial based functional food ingredients," *Food Science and Human Wellness* 13, no. 1 (2024): 1–15, doi:10.26599/FSHW.2022.9250001.

Jackson, M. A., Jeffery, I. B., Beaumont, M., et al., "Signatures of early frailty in the gut microbiota," *Genome Medicine* 8, no. 1 (2016): 8, doi:10.1186/s13073-016-0262-7.

Kelaiditi, E., Jennings, A., Steves, C. J., et al., "Measurements of skeletal muscle mass and power are positively related to a Mediterranean dietary pattern in women," *Osteoporosis International* 27, no. 11 (2016): 3251–60, doi:10.1007/s00198-016-3665-9.

Liu, C., Cheung, W. H., Li, J., et al., "Understanding the gut microbiota and sarcopenia: a systematic review," *Journal of Cachexia, Sarcopenia and Muscle* 12, no. 6 (2021): 1393–1407, doi:10.1002/jcsm.12784.

Locantore, P., Del Gatto, V., Gelli, S., Paragliola, R. M., and Pontecorvi, A., "The Interplay between Immune System and Microbiota in Osteoporosis," *Mediators of Inflammation* (2020): 3686749, doi:10.1155/2020/3686749.

Mach, N., and Fuster-Botella, D., "Endurance exercise and gut microbiota: A review," *Journal of Sport and Health Science* 6, no. 2 (2017): 179–97, doi:10.1016/j.jshs.2016.05.001.

O'Sullivan, O., Cronin, O., Clarke, S. F., et al., "Exercise and the microbiota," *Gut Microbes* 6, no. 2 (2015): 131-36, doi:10.1080/19490976.2015.1011875.

Rankin, A., O'Donavon, C., Madigan, S. M., O'Sullivan, O., and Cotter, P. D., "'Microbes in sport'–The potential role of the gut microbiota in athlete health and performance," *British Journal of Sports Medicine* 51, no. 9 (2017): 698–99, doi:10.1136/bjsports-2016-097227.

Rettedal, E. A., Ilesanmi-Oyelere, B. L., Roy, N. C., Coad, J., and Kruger, M. C., "The Gut Microbiome Is Altered in Postmenopausal Women With Osteoporosis and Osteopenia," *JBMR Plus* 5, no. 3 (2021): e10452, doi:10.1002/jbm4.10452.

Scheiman, J., Luber, J., Chavkin, T., et al., "Meta-omics analysis of elite athletes identifies a performance-enhancing microbe that functions via lactate metabolism," *Nature Medicine* 25, no. 7 (2019): 1104–9, doi:10.1038/s41591-019-0485-4.

Seely, K. D., Kotelko, C. A., Douglas, H., Bealer, B., and Brooks, A. E., "The human gut microbiota: A key mediator of osteoporosis and osteogenesis," *International Journal of Molecular Sciences* 22, no. 17 (2021), doi:10.3390/ijms22179452.

Shah, S., Mu, C., Moossavi, S., et al., "Physical activity-induced alterations of the gut microbiota are BMI dependent," *FASEB Journal* 37, no. 4 (2023): e22882, doi:10.1096/fj.202201571R.

"Stay Strong: Four Ways to Beat the Frailty Risk," Johns Hopkins Medicine, accessed January 10, 2025, hopkinsmedicine.org/health/wellness-and-prevention/stay-strong-four-ways-to-beat-the-frailty-risk.

Steves, C. J., Bird, S., Williams, F. M., and Spector, T. D., "The Microbiome and Musculoskeletal Conditions of Aging: A Review of Evidence for Impact and Potential Therapeutics," *Journal of Bone and Mineral Research* 31, no. 2 (2016): 261–69, doi:10.1002/jbmr.2765.

Ticinesi, A., Nouvenne, A., Cerundolo, N., et al., "Gut microbiota, muscle mass and function in aging: A focus on physical frailty and sarcopenia," *Nutrients* 11, no. 7 (2019): 1633, doi:10.3390/nu11071633.

Vaishya, R., and Vaish, A., "Falls in Older Adults are Serious," *Indian Journal of Orthopaedics* 54, no. 1 (2020): 69–74, doi:10.1007/s43465-019-00037-x.

Villa, C. R., Ward, W. E., and Comelli, E. M., "Gut microbiota-bone axis," *Critical Reviews in Food Science and Nutrition* 57, no. 8 (2017): 1664–72, doi:10.1080/10408398.2015.1010034.

Wang, J., Wang, Y., Gao, W., et al., "Diversity analysis of gut microbiota in osteoporosis and osteopenia patients," *PeerJ* 5 (2017): e3450, doi:10.7717/peerj.3450.

Wang, Y., Zhang, Y., Lane, N. E., et al., "Population-based metagenomics analysis reveals altered gut microbiome in sarcopenia: data from the Xiangya Sarcopenia Study," *Journal of Cachexia, Sarcopenia and Muscle* 13, no. 5 (2022): 2340–51, doi:10.1002/jcsm.13037.

Weaver, C. M., "Diet, gut microbiome, and bone health," *Current Osteoporosis Reports* 13, no. 2 (2015): 125–30, doi:10.1007/s11914-015-0257-0.

Wu, Y., Xia, Y., Huang, S., et al., "The composition of the gut microbiome in patients with sarcopenia," *Turkish Journal of Biochemistry* 47, no. 3 (2022): 327–34, doi:10.1515/tjb-2021-0197.

Zhang, T., Cheng, J. K. and Hu, Y. M., "Gut microbiota as a promising therapeutic target for age-related sarcopenia," *Ageing Research Reviews* 81 (2022): 101739, doi:10.1016/j.arr.2022.101739.

Zhao, J., Liang, R., Song, Q., Song, S., Yue, J., and Wu, C., "Investigating association between gut microbiota and sarcopenia-related traits: a Mendelian randomization study," *Precision Clinical Medicine* 6, no. 2 (2023), doi:10.1093/pcmedi/pbad010.

12. MICROBES MEET CANCER

Bacchus, C. M., Dunfield, L., Gorber, S. C., et al., "Recommendations on screening for colorectal cancer in primary care," *CMAJ: Canadian Medical Association Journal = Journal de l'Association Medicale Canadienne* 188, no. 5 (2016): 340–48, doi:10.1503/cmaj.151125.

Barot, S. V., Sangwan, N., Nair, K. G., et al., "Distinct intratumoral microbiome of young-onset and average-onset colorectal cancer," *eBioMedicine* 100 (2024): 104980, doi:10.1016/j.ebiom.2024.104980.

Cao, Y., Wu, K., Mehta, R., et al., "Long-term use of antibiotics and risk of colorectal adenoma," *Gut* 67, no. 4 (2018): 672–78, doi:10.1136/gutjnl-2016-313413.

Davar, D., Dzutsev, A. K., McCulloch, J. A., et al., "Fecal microbiota transplant overcomes resistance to anti-PD-1 therapy in melanoma patients," *Science* 371, no. 6529 (2021): 595–602, doi:10.1126/science.abf3363.

Garrett, W. S., "Cancer and the microbiota," *Science* 348, no. 6230 (2015): 80–86, doi:10.1126/science.aaa4972.

Giampazolias, E., Pereira da Costa, M., Lam, K. C., et al., "Vitamin D regulates microbiome-dependent cancer immunity," *Science* 384, no. 6694 (2024): 428–37, doi.org/10.1126/science.adh7954.

Gihawi, A., Ge, Y., Lu, J., et al., "Major data analysis errors invalidate cancer microbiome findings," *mBio* 14, no. 5 (2023): e0160723, doi:10.1128/mbio.01607-23.

Gopalakrishnan, V., Spencer, C. N., Nezi, L., et al., "Gut microbiome modulates response to anti-PD-1 immunotherapy in melanoma patients," *Science* 359 no. 6371 (2018): 97–103, doi:10.1126/science.aan4236.

Gunjur, A., Shao, Y., Rozday, T., et al., "A gut microbial signature for combination immune checkpoint blockade across cancer types," *Nature Medicine* 30, no. 3 (2024): 797–809, doi:10.1038/s41591-024-02823-z.

Hullar, M. A., Burnett-Hartman, A. N., and Lampe, J. W., "Gut microbes, diet, and cancer," *Cancer Treatment and Research* 159 (2014): 377–99, doi:10.1007/978-3-642-38007-5_22.

Huynh, M., Crane, M. J., and Jamieson, A. M., "The lung, the niche, and the microbe: Exploring the lung microbiome in cancer and immunity," *Frontiers in Immunology* 13 (2023), doi:10.3389/fimmu.2022.1094110.

Kostic, A. D., Chun, E., Robertson, L., et al., "Fusobacterium nucleatum potentiates intestinal tumorigenesis and modulates the tumor-immune microenvironment," *Cell Host & Microbe* 14, no. 2 (2013): 207–15, doi:10.1016/j.chom.2013.07.007.

"Key Statistics for Colorectal Cancer," American Cancer Society, accessed January 1, 2025, cancer.org/cancer/types/colon-rectal-cancer/about/key-statistics.html.

Martins, D., Mendes, F., and Schmitt, F., "Microbiome: A Supportive or a Leading Actor in Lung Cancer?," *Pathobiology* 88, no. 2 (2021): 198–207, doi:10.1159/000511556.

Najafi, S., Abedini, F., Azimzadeh Jamalkandi, S., Shariati, P., Ahmadi, A., and Gholami Fesharaki, M., "The composition of lung microbiome in lung cancer: a systematic review and meta-analysis," *BMC Microbiology* 21, no. 1 (2021): 315, doi:10.1186/s12866-021-02375-z.

Orberg, E. T., Meedt, E., Hiergeist, A., et al., "Bacteria and bacteriophage consortia are associated with protective intestinal metabolites in patients receiving stem cell transplantation," *Nature Cancer* 5, no. 1 (2024): 187–208, doi:10.1038/s43018-023-00669-x.

Poore, G. D., Kopylova, E., Zhu, Q., et al., "Microbiome analyses of blood and tissues suggest cancer diagnostic approach," *Nature* 579, no. 7800 (2020): 567–74, doi:10.1038/s41586-020-2095-1.

Routy, B., Le Chatelier, E., Derosa, L., et al., "Gut microbiome influences efficacy of PD-1-based immunotherapy against epithelial tumors," *Science* 359, no. 6371 (2018): 91–97, doi:10.1126/science.aan3706.

Roy, S., and Trinchieri, G., "Microbiota: a key orchestrator of cancer therapy," *Nature Reviews Cancer* 17, no. 5 (2017): 271–85, doi:10.1038/nrc.2017.13.

Sehrawat, N., Yadav, M., Singh, M., Kumar, V., Sharma, V. R., and Sharma, A. K., "Probiotics in microbiome ecological balance providing a therapeutic window against cancer," *Seminars in Cancer Biology* 70 (2021): 24–36, doi:10.1016/j.semcancer.2020.06.009.

Shono, Y., Docampo, M. D., Peled, J. U., et al., "Increased GVHD-related mortality with broad-spectrum antibiotic use after allogeneic hematopoietic stem cell transplantation in human patients and mice," *Science Translational Medicine* 8, no. 339 (2016): 339ra71, doi:10.1126/scitranslmed.aaf2311.

Sivan, A., Corrales, L., Hubert, N., et al., "Commensal Bifidobacterium promotes antitumor immunity and facilitates anti-PD-L1 efficacy," *Science* 350, no. 6264 (2015): 1084–89, doi:10.1126/science.aac4255.

Urbaniak, C., Gloor, G. B., Brackstone, M., Scott, L., Tangney, M., and Reid, G., "The Microbiota of Breast Tissue and Its Association with Breast Cancer," *Applied and Environmental Microbiology* 82, no. 16 (2016): 5039–48, doi:10.1128/AEM.01235-16.

Vétizou, M., Pitt, J. M., Daillère, R., et al., "Anticancer immunotherapy by CTLA-4 blockade relies on the gut microbiota," *Science* 350, no. 6264 (2015): 1079–84, doi:10.1126/science.aad1329.

Weber, D., Jenq, R. R., Peled, J. U., et al., "Microbiota Disruption Induced by Early Use of Broad-Spectrum Antibiotics Is an Independent Risk Factor of Outcome After Allogeneic Stem Cell Transplantation," *Biology of Blood and Marrow Transplantation* 23, no. 5 (2017): 845–52, doi:10.1016/j.bbmt.2017.02.006.

Yang, Y., Xia, Y., Chen, H., et al., "The effect of perioperative probiotics treatment for colorectal cancer: short-term outcomes of a randomized controlled trial," *Oncotarget* 7, no. 7 (2016): 8432–40, doi:10.18632/oncotarget.7045.

Zepeda-Rivera, M., Minot, S. S., Bouzek, H., et al., "A distinct Fusobacterium nucleatum clade dominates the colorectal cancer niche," *Nature* 628, no. 8007 (2024): 424–32, doi:10.1038/s41586-024-07182-w.

Zhu, X., Huang, X., Hu, M., et al., "A specific enterotype derived from gut microbiome of older individuals enables favorable responses to immune checkpoint blockade therapy," *Cell Host & Microbe* 32, no. 4 (2024): 489–505.e5, doi:10.1016/j.chom.2024.03.002.

Zitvogel, L., Daillère, R., Roberti, M. P., Routy, B., and Kroemer, G., "Anticancer effects of the microbiome and its products," *Nature Reviews Microbiology* 15, no. 8 (2017): 465–78, doi:10.1038/nrmicro.2017.44.

13. ZZZ: SLEEP AND THE MICROBIOME

Anderson, J. R., Carroll, I., Azcarate-Peril, M. A., et al., "A preliminary examination of gut microbiota, sleep, and cognitive flexibility in healthy older adults," *Sleep Medicine* 38 (2017): 104–7, doi:10.1016/j.sleep.2017.07.018.

Bikov, A., Szabo, H., Piroska, M., et al., "Gut Microbiome in Patients with Obstructive Sleep Apnoea," *Applied Sciences* 12, no. 4 (2022): 2007, doi:10.3390/app12042007.

Cai, Y., Juszczak, H. M., Cope, E. K., and Goldberg, A. N., "The microbiome in obstructive sleep apnea," *Sleep* 44, no. 8 (2021), doi:10.1093/sleep/zsab061.

Dos Reis Lucena, L., Terra Loyola, V., Leopoldino de Bortolli, C., Levy Andersen, M., Tufik, S., and Hachul, H., "Effects of Supplementation with *Lactobacillus* Probiotics on Insomnia Treatment," *Alternative Therapies in Health and Medicine* 27, no. S1 (2021): 178–84.

dos Santos, A., and Galiè, S., "The Microbiota-Gut-Brain Axis in Metabolic Syndrome and Sleep Disorders: A Systematic Review," *Nutrients* 16, no. 3 (2024): 390, doi:10.3390/nu16030390.

Godos, J., Ferri, R., Caraci, F., et al., "Adherence to the Mediterranean Diet Is Associated with Better Sleep Quality in Italian Adults," *Nutrients* 11, no. 5 (2019): 976, doi: 10.3390/nu11050976.

Grosicki, G. J., Riemann, B. L., Flatt, A. A., Valentino, T., and Lustgarten, M. S., "Self-reported sleep quality is associated with gut microbiome composition in young, healthy individuals: a pilot study," *Sleep Medicine* 73 (2020): 76–81, doi:10.1016/j.sleep.2020.04.013.

Haimov, I., Magzal, F., Tamir, S., et al., "Variation in Gut Microbiota Composition Is Associated with Sleep Quality and Cognitive Performance in Older Adults with Insomnia," *Nature and Science of Sleep* 14 (2022): 1753–67, doi:10.2147/NSS.S377114.

Han, M., Yuan, S., and Zhang, J., "The interplay between sleep and gut microbiota," *Brain Research Bulletin* 180 (2022): 131–46, doi:10.1016/j.brainresbull.2021.12.016.

Holzhausen, E. A., Peppard, P. E., Sethi, A. K., et al., "Associations of gut microbiome richness and diversity with objective and subjective sleep measures in a population sample," *Sleep* 47, no. 3 (2024), doi:10.1093/sleep/zsad300.

Karl, J. P., Whitney, C. C., Wilson, M. A., et al., "Severe, short-term sleep restriction reduces gut microbiota community richness but does not alter intestinal permeability in healthy young men," *Scientific Reports* 13, no. 1 (2023): 213, doi:10.1038/s41598-023-27463-0.

Li, Y., Deng, Q., and Liu, Z., "The relationship between gut microbiota and insomnia: a bi-directional two-sample Mendelian randomization research," *Frontiers in Cellular and Infection Microbiology* 13 (2023), doi:10.3389/fcimb.2023.1296417.

Morwani-Mangnani, J., Giannos, P., Belzer, C., Beekman, M., Eline Slagboom, P., and Prokopidis, K., "Gut microbiome changes due to sleep disruption in older and younger individuals: a case for sarcopenia?," *Sleep* 45, no. 12 (2022), doi:10.1093/sleep/zsac239.

Neroni, B., Evangelisti, M., Radocchia, G., et al., "Relationship between sleep disorders and gut dysbiosis: what affects what?," *Sleep Medicine* 87 (2021): 1–7, doi:10.1016/j.sleep.2021.08.003.

Nie, L., Xiang, Q., Lin, Y., et al., "Correlation between symptoms and cognitive function changes in patients with primary insomnia and pathways in gut microbiota," *Biochemistry and Biophysics Reports* 37 (2024): 101629, doi:10.1016/j.bbrep.2023.101629.

Ogawa, Y., Miyoshi, C., Obana, N., et al., "Gut microbiota depletion by chronic antibiotic treatment alters the sleep/wake architecture and sleep EEG power spectra in mice," *Scientific Reports* 10, no. 1 (2020): 19554, doi:10.1038/s41598-020-76562-9.

Patterson, E., Tan, H. T. T., Groeger, D., et al., "Bifidobacterium longum 1714 improves sleep quality and aspects of well-being in healthy adults: a randomized, double-blind, placebo-controlled clinical trial," *Scientific Reports* 14, no. 1 (2024): 3725, doi:10.1038/s41598-024-53810-w.

Santi, D., Debbi, V., Costantino, F., et al., "Microbiota Composition and Probiotics Supplementations on Sleep Quality–A Systematic Review and Meta-Analysis," *Clocks and Sleep* 5, no. 4 (2023): 770–92, doi:10.3390/clockssleep5040050.

Smith, R. P., Easson, C., Lyle, S. M., et al., "Gut microbiome diversity is associated with sleep physiology in humans," *PLOS One* 14, no. 10 (2019): e0222394, doi:10.1371/journal.pone.0222394.

Sun, J., Fang, D., Wang, Z., and Liu, Y., "Sleep Deprivation and Gut Microbiota Dysbiosis: Current Understandings and Implications," *International Journal of Molecular Sciences* 24, no. 11 (2023): 9603, doi:10.3390/ijms24119603.

Wagner-Skacel, J., Dalkner, N., Moerkl, S., et al., "Sleep and microbiome in psychiatric diseases," *Nutrients* 12, no. 8 (2020): 1–18, doi:10.3390/nu12082198.

Wang, Z., Chen, W. H., Li, S. X., et al., "Gut microbiota modulates the inflammatory response and cognitive impairment induced by sleep deprivation," *Molecular Psychiatry* 26, no. 11 (2021): 6277–92, doi:10.1038/s41380-021-01113-1.

Wu, J., Zhang, B., Zhou, S., et al., "Associations between gut microbiota and sleep: a two-sample, bidirectional Mendelian randomization study," *Frontiers in Microbiology* 14 (2023), doi:10.3389/fmicb.2023.1236847.

Zhang, Q., Yun, Y., An, H., et al., "Gut Microbiome Composition Associated With Major Depressive Disorder and Sleep Quality," *Frontiers in Psychiatry* 12 (2021), doi:10.3389/fpsyt.2021.645045.

14. TOO CLEAN, OR NOT TOO CLEAN: ENVIRONMENTAL MICROBES

Aliyu, S., Smaldone, A., and Larson, E., "Prevalence of multidrug-resistant gram-negative bacteria among nursing home residents: A systematic review and meta-analysis," *American Journal of Infection Control* 45, no. 5 (2017): 512–18, doi:10.1016/j.ajic.2017.01.022.

Andersen, B., Frisvad, J. C., Søndergaard, I., Rasmussen, I. S., and Larsen, L. S., "Associations between fungal species and water-damaged building materials," *Applied and Environmental Microbiology* 77, no. 12 (2011): 4180–88, doi:10.1128/AEM.02513-10.

Berg, G., Mahnert, A., and Moissl-Eichinger, C., "Beneficial effects of plant-associated microbes on indoor microbiomes and human health?," *Frontiers in Microbiology* 5, no. 15 (2014), doi:10.3389/fmicb.2014.00015.

Bloomfield, S. F., Stanwell-Smith, R., Crevel, R. W. R., and Pickup, J., "Too clean, or not too clean: the Hygiene Hypothesis and home hygiene," *Clinical & Experimental Allergy* 36, no. 4 (2006): 402–25, doi:10.1111/j.1365-2222.2006.02463.x.

Bosch, T. C. G., Wigley, M., Colomina, B., et al., "The potential importance of the built-environment microbiome and its impact on human health," *PNAS* 121, no. 20 (2024): e2313971121, doi:10.1073/pnas.2313971121.

Bruno, A., Fumagalli, S., Ghisleni, G., and Labra, M., "The Microbiome of the Built Environment: The Nexus for Urban Regeneration for the Cities of Tomorrow," *Microorganisms* 10, no. 12 (2022): 2311, doi:10.3390/microorganisms10122311.

Cardinale, M., Kaiser, D., Lueders, T., Schnell, S., and Egert, M., "Microbiome analysis and confocal microscopy of used kitchen sponges reveal massive colonization by Acinetobacter, Moraxella and Chryseobacterium species," *Scientific Reports* 7, no. 1 (2017): 5791, doi:10.1038/s41598-017-06055-9.

Cavicchioli, R., Ripple, W. J., Timmis, K. N., et al., "Scientists' warning to humanity: microorganisms and climate change," *Nature Reviews Microbiology* 17, no. 9 (2019): 569–86, doi:10.1038/s41579-019-0222-5.

David, L. A., Materna, A. C., Friedman, J., et al., "Host lifestyle affects human microbiota on daily timescales," *Genome Biology* 15, no. 7 (2014): R89, doi:10.1186/gb-2014-15-7-r89.

Hoisington, A. J., Brenner, L. A., Kinney, K. A., Postolache, T. T., and Lowry, C. A., "The microbiome of the built environment and mental health," *Microbiome* 3, (2015): 60, doi:10.1186/s40168-015-0127-0.

Hoisington, A. J., Stamper, C. E., Bates, K. L., et al., "Human microbiome transfer in the built environment differs based on occupants, objects, and buildings," *Scientific Reports* 13, no. 1 (2023): 6446, doi:10.1038/s41598-023-33719-6.

Jansson, J. K., and Hofmockel, K. S., "Soil microbiomes and climate change," *Nature Reviews Microbiology* 18 (2020): 35–46, doi:10.1038/s41579-019-0265-7.

Kõljalg, S., Mändar, R., Sõber, T., Rööp, T., and Mändar, R., "High level bacterial contamination of secondary school students' mobile phones," *Germs* 7, no. 2 (2017): 73–77, doi:10.18683/germs.2017.1111.

Kwan, S., Shaughnessy, R., Hegarty, B., Haverinen-Shaughnessy, U., and Peccia, J., "The reestablishment of microbial communities after surface cleaning in schools," *Journal of Applied Microbiology* 125, no. 3 (2018): 897–906, doi:10.1111/jam.13898.

Lax, S., Smith, D. P., Hampton-Marcell, J., et al., "Longitudinal analysis of microbial interaction between humans and the indoor environment," *Science* 345, no. 6200 (2014): 1048–52, doi:10.1126/science.1254529.

Meadow, J. F., Altrichter, A. E., and Green, J. L., "Mobile phones carry the personal microbiome of their owners," *PeerJ* 2 (2014): e447, doi:10.7717/peerj.447.

Mortazavi, S. M. J., Said-Salman, I., Mortazavi, A. R., El Khatib, S., and Sihver, L., "How the adaptation of the human microbiome to harsh space environment can determine the chances of success for a space mission to Mars and beyond," *Frontiers in Microbiology* 14 (2023): 1237564, doi:10.3389/fmicb.2023.1237564.

Mughini-Gras, L., Smid, J., Wagenaar, J., et al., "Campylobacteriosis in returning travellers and potential secondary transmission of exotic strains," *Epidemiology and Infection* 142, no. 6 (2014): 1277–88, doi:10.1017/S0950268813002069.

Peccia, J., and Kwan, S. E., "Buildings, Beneficial Microbes, and Health," *Trends in Microbiology* 24, no. 8 (2016): 595–97, doi:10.1016/j.tim.2016.04.007.

Rai, S., Singh, D. K., and Kumar, A., "Microbial, environmental and anthropogenic factors influencing the indoor microbiome of the built environment," *Journal of Basic Microbiology* 61, no. 4 (2021): 267–92, doi:10.1002/jobm.202000575.

Riddle, M. S., and Connor, B. A., "The Traveling Microbiome," *Current Infectious Disease Reports* 18, no. 9 (2016): 29, doi:10.1007/s11908-016-0536-7.

Rothschild, D., Weissbrod, O., Barkan, E., et al., "Environment dominates over host genetics in shaping human gut microbiota," *Nature* 555, no. 7695 (2018): 210–15, doi:10.1038/nature25973.

Young, G. R., Sherry, A., and Smith, D. L., "Built environment microbiomes transition from outdoor to human-associated communities after construction and commissioning," *Scientific Reports* 13, no. 1 (2023): 15854, doi:10.1038/s41598-023-42427-0.

15. THE NEW MICROBE ON THE BLOCK: COVID-19

Alqedari, H., Altabtbaei, K., Espinoza, J. L., et al., "Host-microbiome associations in saliva predict COVID-19 severity," *PNAS Nexus* 3, no. 4 (2024), doi:10.1093/pnasnexus/pgae126.

Álvarez-Santacruz, C., Tyrkalska, S. D., and Candel, S., "The Microbiota in Long COVID," *International Journal of Molecular Sciences* 25, no. 2 (2024): 1330, doi:10.3390/ijms25021330.

Ancona, G., Alagna, L., Alteri, C., et al., "Gut and airway microbiota dysbiosis and their role in COVID-19 and long-COVID," *Frontiers in Immunology* 14 (2023): 1080043, doi:10.3389/fimmu.2023.1080043.

Bernard-Raichon, L., Venzon, M., Klein, J., et al., "Gut microbiome dysbiosis in antibiotic-treated COVID-19 patients is associated with microbial translocation and bacteremia," *Nature Communications* 13, no. 1 (2022): 5926, doi:10.1038/s41467-022-33395-6.

Davis, H. E., Assaf, G. S., McCorkell, L., et al., "Characterizing long COVID in an international cohort: 7 months of symptoms and their impact," *eClinicalMedicine* 38 (2021): 101019, doi:10.1016/j.eclinm.2021.101019.

Finlay, B. B., Amato, K. R., Azad, M., et al., "The hygiene hypothesis, the COVID pandemic, and consequences for the human microbiome," *PNAS* 118, no. 6 (2021): e2010217118, doi:10.1073/pnas.2010217118.

Hong, M., Lan, T., Li, Q., et al., "A comprehensive perspective on the interaction between gut microbiota and COVID-19 vaccines," *Gut Microbes* 15, no. 1 (2023), doi:10.1080/19490976.2023.2233146.

Hu, C., Hu, W., Tang, B., et al., "Plasma and urine proteomics and gut microbiota analysis reveal potential factors affecting COVID-19 vaccination response," *iScience* 27, no. 2 (2024): 108851, doi:10.1016/j.isci.2024.108851.

Ke, S., Weiss, S. T., and Liu, Y. Y., "Dissecting the role of the human microbiome in COVID-19 via metagenome-assembled genomes," *Nature Communications* 13, no. 1 (2022): 5235, doi:10.1038/s41467-022-32991-w.

Korpela, K., Hurley, S., Ford, S., et al., "Association between gut microbiota development and allergy in infants born during pandemic-related social distancing restrictions," *Allergy* 79, no. 7 (2024): 1938–51, doi:10.1111/all.16069.

Lau, R. I., Su, Q., Lau, I. S. F., et al., "A synbiotic preparation (SIM01) for post-acute COVID-19 syndrome in Hong Kong (RECOVERY): a randomised, double-blind, placebo-controlled trial," *The Lancet Infectious Diseases* 24, no. 3 (2024): 256–65, doi:10.1016/S1473-3099(23)00685-0.

Leung, J. S. M., "Interaction between gut microbiota and COVID-19 and its vaccines," *World Journal of Gastroenterology* 28, no. 40 (2022): 5801–6, doi:10.3748/wjg.v28.i40.5801.

Liu, Q., Mak, J. W. Y., Su, Q., et al., "Gut microbiota dynamics in a prospective cohort of patients with post-Acute COVID-19 syndrome," *Gut* 71, no. 3 (2022): 544–52, doi:10.1136/GUTJNL-2021-325989.

Nguyen, L. H., Okin, D., Drew, D. A., et al., "Metagenomic assessment of gut microbial communities and risk of severe COVID-19," *Genome Medicine* 15, no. 1 (2023): 49, doi:10.1186/s13073-023-01202-6.

Reuben, R. C., Beugnon, R., and Jurburg, S. D., "COVID-19 alters human microbiomes: a meta-analysis," *Frontiers in Cellular and Infection Microbiology* 13 (2023), doi:10.3389/fcimb.2023.1211348.

Su, Q., Lau, R. I., Liu, Q., et al., "The gut microbiome associates with phenotypic manifestations of post-acute COVID-19 syndrome," *Cell Host & Microbe* 32, no. 5 (2024): 651–60.e4, doi:10.1016/j.chom.2024.04.005.

Taquet, M., Skorniewska, Z., Hampshire, A., et al., "Acute blood biomarker profiles predict cognitive deficits 6 and 12 months after COVID-19 hospitalization," *Nature Medicine* 29, no. 10 (2023): 2498–508, doi:10.1038/s41591-023-02525-y.

Villapol, S., "Gastrointestinal symptoms associated with COVID-19: impact on the gut microbiome," *Translational Research* 226 (2020): 57–69, doi:10.1016/j.trsl.2020.08.004.

Wang, B., Zhang, L., Wang, Y., et al., "Alterations in microbiota of patients with COVID-19: potential mechanisms and therapeutic interventions," *Signal Transduction and Targeted Therapy* 7, no. 1 (2022): 143, doi:10.1038/s41392-022-00986-0.

Wang, M., Zhang, Y., Li, C., Chang, W., and Zhang, L., "The relationship between gut microbiota and COVID-19 progression: new insights into immunopathogenesis and treatment," *Frontiers in Immunology* 14 (2023): 1180336, doi:10.3389/fimmu.2023.1180336.

Xie, L., Luo, G., Yang, Z., et al., "The clinical outcome of COVID-19 is strongly associated with microbiome dynamics in the upper respiratory tract," *Journal of Infection* 88, no. 3 (2024): 106118, doi:10.1016/j.jinf.2024.01.017.

Xu, L., Yang, C. S., Liu, Y., and Zhang, X., "Effective Regulation of Gut Microbiota with Probiotics and Prebiotics May Prevent or Alleviate COVID-19 Through the Gut-Lung Axis," *Frontiers in Pharmacology* 13 (2022): 895193, doi:10.3389/fphar.2022.895193.

Yamamoto, S., Saito, M., Tamura, A., Prawisuda, D., Mizutani, T., and Yotsuyanagi, H., "The human microbiome and COVID-19: A systematic review," *PLOS One* 16, no. 6 (2021): e0253293, doi:10.1371/journal.pone.0253293.

Yeoh, Y. K., Zuo, T., Lui, G. C. Y., et al., "Gut microbiota composition reflects disease severity and dysfunctional immune responses in patients with COVID-19," *Gut* 70, no. 4 (2021): 698–706, doi:10.1136/gutjnl-2020-323020.

Zhang, D., Zhou, Y., Ma, Y., et al., "Gut Microbiota Dysbiosis Correlates With Long COVID-19 at One-Year After Discharge," *Journal of Korean Medical Science* 38, no. 15 (2023), doi:10.3346/jkms.2023.38.e120.

Zhang, F., Lau, R. I., Liu, Q., Su, Q., Chan, F. K. L., and Ng, S. C., "Gut microbiota in COVID-19: key microbial changes, potential mechanisms and clinical applications," *Nature Reviews Gastroenterology and Hepatology* 20, no. 5 (2023): 323–37, doi:10.1038/s41575-022-00698-4.

16. THE FOUNTAIN OF YOUTH *IS* FULL OF MICROBES: THE KEY TO HEALTH AND LONGEVITY

Argaw-Denboba, A., Schmidt, T. S. B., Di Giacomo, M., et al., "Paternal microbiome perturbations impact offspring fitness," *Nature* 629, no. 8012 (2024): 652–59, doi:10.1038/s41586-024-07336-w.

Bandyopadhyay, A., Saha, A., Ghosh, D., Dam, B., Samanta, A. K., and Dutta, S., "Microbial repairing of concrete & its role in CO2 sequestration: a critical review," *Beni-Suef University Journal of Basic and Applied Sciences* 12, no. 1 (2023): 7, doi:10.1186/s43088-023-00344-1.

Berendsen, A., van de Rest, O., Feskens, E., et al., "Changes in Dietary Intake and Adherence to the NU-AGE Diet Following a One-Year Dietary Intervention among European Older Adults-Results of the NU-AGE Randomized Trial," *Nutrients* 10, no. 12 (2018): 1905, doi:10.3390/nu10121905.

Biagi, E., Candela, M., Turroni, S., Garagnani, P., Franceschi, C., and Brigidi, P., "Ageing and gut microbes: perspectives for health maintenance and longevity," *Pharmacological Research* 69, no. 1 (2013): 11–20, doi:10.1016/j.phrs.2012.10.005.

Blaser, M. J., *Missing Microbes: How the Overuse of Antibiotics is Fueling Our Modern Plagues* (Henry Holt and Company, 2014).

Bornbusch, S. L., Clarke, T. A., Hobilalaina, S., Reseva, H. S., LaFleur, M., and Drea, C. M., "Microbial rewilding in the gut microbiomes of captive ring-tailed lemurs (Lemur catta) in Madagascar," *Scientific Reports* 12, no. 1 (2022): 22388, doi:10.1038/s41598-022-26861-0.

Brandt, L. J., "Fecal Microbiota Therapy with a Focus on Clostridium difficile Infection," *Psychosomatic Medicine* 79, no. 8 (2017): 868–73, doi:10.1097/PSY.0000000000000511.

Brüssow, H., "Microbiota and healthy ageing: observational and nutritional intervention studies," *Microbial Biotechnology* 6, no. 4 (2013): 326–34, doi:10.1111/1751-7915.12048.

Buettner, D., *The Blue Zones: Lessons for Living Longer From the People Who've Lived the Longest* (National Geographic Society, 2010).

Camarillo-Guerrero, L., Almeida, A., Rangel-Pineros, G., et al., "Massive expansion of human gut bacteriophage diversity," *Cell* 184, no. 4 (2021): 1098–109.e9, doi:10.1016/j.cell.2021.01.029.

Cockburn, D. W., and Koropatkin, N. M., "Polysaccharide Degradation by the Intestinal Microbiota and Its Influence on Human Health and Disease," *Journal of Molecular Biology* 428, no. 16 (2016): 3230–52, doi:10.1016/j.jmb.2016.06.021.

Fond, G., Boukouaci, W., Chevalier, G., et al., "The 'psychomicrobiotic': Targeting microbiota in major psychiatric disorders: A systematic review," *Pathologie Biologie* 63, no. 1 (2015): 35–42, doi:10.1016/j.patbio.2014.10.003.

Gibson, G. R., Hutkins, R., Sanders, M. E., et al., "Expert consensus document: The International Scientific Association for Probiotics and Prebiotics (ISAPP) consensus statement on the definition and scope of prebiotics," *Nature Reviews Gastroenterology & Hepatology* 14, no. 8 (2017): 491–502, doi:10.1038/nrgastro.2017.75.

Han, B., Sivaramakrishnan, P., Lin, C. C. J., et al., "Microbial Genetic Composition Tunes Host Longevity," *Cell* 169, no. 7 (2017): 1249–62.e13, doi:10.1016/j.cell.2017.05.036.

Hod, K., and Ringel, Y., "Probiotics in functional bowel disorders," *Best Practice & Research Clinical Gastroenterology* 30, no. 1 (2016): 89–97, doi:10.1016/j.bpg.2016.01.003.

Horvath, A., Leber, B., Schmerboeck, B., et al., "Randomised clinical trial: the effects of a multispecies probiotic vs. placebo on innate immune function, bacterial translocation and gut permeability in patients with cirrhosis," *Alimentary Pharmacology & Therapeutics* 44, no. 9 (2016): 926–35, doi:10.1111/apt.13788.

Hungin, A. P. S., Mitchell, C. R., Whorwell, P., et al., "Systematic review: probiotics in the management of lower gastrointestinal symptoms–an updated evidence-based international consensus," *Alimentary Pharmacology & Therapeutics* 47, no. 8 (2018): 1054–70, doi:10.1111/apt.14539.

König, J., Siebenhaar, A., Högenauer, C., et al., "Consensus report: faecal microbiota transfer–clinical applications and procedures," *Alimentary Pharmacology & Therapeutics* 45, no. 2 (2017): 222–39, doi:10.1111/apt.13868.

Lewis, B. B., and Pamer, E. G., "Microbiota-Based Therapies for Clostridium difficile and Antibiotic-Resistant Enteric Infections," *Annual Review of Microbiology* 71 (2017): 157–78, doi:10.1146/annurev-micro-090816-093549.

Liu, Y., Fachrul, M., Inouye, M., and Méric, G., "Harnessing human microbiomes for disease prediction," *Trends in Microbiology* 32, no. 7 (2024): 707–19, doi:10.1016/j.tim.2023.12.004.

Lurie, I., Yang, Y. X., Haynes, K., Mamtani, R., and Boursi, B., "Antibiotic exposure and the risk for depression, anxiety, or psychosis: a nested case-control study," *The Journal of Clinical Psychiatry* 76, no. 11 (2015): 1522–28, doi:10.4088/JCP.15m09961.

McCarville, J. L., Caminero, A., and Verdu, E. F., "Novel perspectives on therapeutic modulation of the gut microbiota," *Therapeutic Advances in Gastroenterology* 9, no. 4 (2016): 580–93, doi:10.1177/1756283X16637819.

Pinto-Sanchez, M. I., Hall, G. B., Ghajar, K., et al., "Probiotic Bifidobacterium longum NCC3001 Reduces Depression Scores and Alters Brain Activity: A Pilot Study in Patients with Irritable Bowel Syndrome," *Gastroenterology* 153, no. 2 (2017): 448–59.e8, doi:10.1053/j.gastro.2017.05.003.

Rees, T., and Blaser, M., "Waking up from antibiotic sleep," *Perspectives in Public Health* 136, no. 4 (2016): 202–4, doi:10.1177/1757913916643449.

Rondanelli, M., Giacosa, A., Faliva, M. A., Perna, S., Allieri, F., and Castellazzi, A. M., "Review on microbiota and effectiveness of probiotics use in older," *World Journal of Clinical Cases* 3 no. 2 (2015): 156–62, doi:10.12998/wjcc.v3.i2.156.

Rothschild, D., Weissbrod, O., Barkan, E., et al., "Environment dominates over host genetics in shaping human gut microbiota," *Nature* 555, no. 7695 (2018): 210–15, doi:10.1038/nature25973.

Salazar, N., Arboleya, S., Valdés, L., et al., "The human intestinal microbiome at extreme ages of life. Dietary intervention as a way to counteract alterations," *Frontiers in Genetics* 5, no. 406 (2014), doi:10.3389/fgene.2014.00406.

Sanders, M. E., "Probiotics and microbiota composition," *BMC Medicine* 14, no. 1 (2016): 82, doi:10.1186/s12916-016-0629-z.

Schwiertz, A., *Microbiota of the Human Body: Implications in Health and Disease* (Springer, 2016).

Steenbergen, L., Sellaro, R., van Hemert, S., Bosch, J. A., and Colzato, L. S., "A randomized controlled trial to test the effect of multispecies probiotics on cognitive reactivity to sad mood," *Brain, Behavior, and Immunity* 48 (2015): 258–64, doi:10.1016/j.bbi.2015.04.003.

Suez, J., Zmora, N., Zilberman-Schapira, G., et al., "Post-Antibiotic Gut Mucosal Microbiome Reconstitution Is Impaired by Probiotics and Improved by Autologous FMT," *Cell* 174 no. 6 (2018): 1406–23.e16, doi:10.1016/j.cell.2018.08.047.

Vanegas, S. M., Meydani, M., Barnett, J. B., et al., "Substituting whole grains for refined grains in a 6-wk randomized trial has a modest effect on gut microbiota and immune and inflammatory markers of healthy adults," *The American Journal of Clinical Nutrition* 105 no. 3 (2017): 635–50, doi:10.3945/ajcn.116.146928.

Veerus, L., Blaser, M. J., Sadovsky, Y., and Jašarević, E., "Dad's gut microbes matter for pregnancy health and baby's growth," *Nature* 629, no. 8012 (2024): 536–37, doi:10.1038/d41586-024-01191-5 .

Wibowo, M. C., Yang, Z., Borry, M., et al., "Reconstruction of ancient microbial genomes from the human gut," *Nature* 594, no. 7862 (2021): 234–39, doi:10.1038/s41586-021-03532-0.

Zhang, C., Li, S., Yang, L., et al., "Structural modulation of gut microbiota in life-long calorie-restricted mice," *Nature Communications* 4, no. 1, (2013): 2163, doi:10.1038/ncomms3163.

Acknowledgments

This book is testament to the enthusiasm and generosity of a large number of people. We were extremely fortunate to receive input from many talented individuals who shared their perspectives, experiences, and collective knowledge.

We thank all of the scientific and medical experts who provided interviews and edits for each chapter: Marty Blaser, Shoki Dedhar, Eran Elinav, Richard Ellen, Stan Hazen, Greg Hillebrand, Jim Hogg, Dan Littman, Brian MacVicar, Anne Martin-Matthews, Heather McKay, Dave Patrick, Mary Ellen Sanders, and Lynn Stothers. They helped ensure that we weren't misinterpreting the scientific data in all our enthusiasm for this burgeoning area. Their wide array of knowledge—most are not experts in microbiology—was fundamental to the framing and content of chapters, and gave us insight into the many ways that microbiology can become more broadly incorporated throughout health care and the daily pursuits of well-being.

Numerous colleagues, friends, and family members read excerpts, provided comments, and sent us relevant articles along the way. This includes Hazel and Wallace Allen, MC Arrieta, Kylynda Bauer, Monica Bennington, John Bienenstock, Mihai Cirstea, Silke Cresswell, Liam Finlay, Derek Gregory, Natasa Jovic, Malcolm Kendall, Roderick MacDonald, Patti Martin, Shaylih Muehlmann, Janet Rossant, and Hillary Waters. We particularly thank Janis Sarra for reading an early draft of the book and providing many valuable comments.

We thank our outstanding agents, Chris Casuccio and John Pearce. Our editors, Jennifer Kurdyla and Sara Zatopek, provided wonderful comments, edits, and compelling questions throughout the writing process.

We appreciate their crucial role in helping us make this book accessible and useful to people of all walks and ages.

Finally, we thank our spouses, Jane and Matt, who were involved in endless discussions, helped brainstorm and "gut-check" ideas, read drafts, and provided countless articles and additional information. We are forever grateful for their unfailing encouragement, patience, and love.

Index

B

C

F

G

H

I

J

K

L

N

O

P

R

S

T

U

V

W

X

Y

Z

About the Authors

B. Brett Finlay, PhD, is a Professor of Microbiology and Biochemistry in the Michael Smith Laboratories at the University of British Columbia and a world leader in researching how bacterial infections work. He has been studying microbes for over forty years and has published over six hundred scientific articles. A cofounder of the biotech companies Commense, Vedanta, and Microbiome Insights, Brett is an Officer of the Order of Canada, the highest Canadian honor given to civilians. He is a coauthor of *Let Them Eat Dirt: How Microbes Can Make Your Child Healthier*. He lives in Vancouver, BC, with his wife, a pediatrician. They have two adult children, one of whom is his coauthor, Jessica.

Jessica M. Finlay, PhD, is an Assistant Professor in the Department of Geography and Institute of Behavioral Science at the University of Colorado Boulder. She trained in geography and gerontology at the University of Minnesota and completed an NIH-funded postdoctoral research fellowship at the University of Michigan. Dr. Finlay is a health geographer and environmental gerontologist who investigates how built, social, and natural environments affect health and well-being across the life course. When not at her desk, Jessica is chasing around after three small children or adventuring outdoors.